How to Survive ACLS!

About the Author

David P. Doernbach, Ed.D., is a professional medical educator. He has been teaching ACLS since 1978, when he initiated the first course at the University of Arkansas for Medical Sciences. During those first formative years, Dr. Doernbach was instrumental in starting the majority of the hospital-based ACLS courses through Arkansas. Each year he teaches over 1000 students spread over 70 separate courses. He currently teaches in six states.

Dr. Doernbach received his undergraduate degree in Biochemistry from the University of California at Riverside. Both his Master's and Doctor of Education degree were awarded by the University of Arkansas majoring in Adult Education.

He was the coauthor of the first and second editions of *ECG Workout: Exercises in Arrhythmia Interpretation* (published by Lippincott–Raven) and is the producer of the *ACLS Survival Hymns*, which set the ACLS protocols to music. He also produced the *Advanced Cardiac Treatment System* (ACTS), which presents all the medications and ACLS algorithms in a more visually appealing and easier to follow format.

Dr. Doernbach has been an ACLS Affiliate Faculty in three states and continues to serve on the ACLS committee in his home state of Arkansas.

How to Survive ACLS!

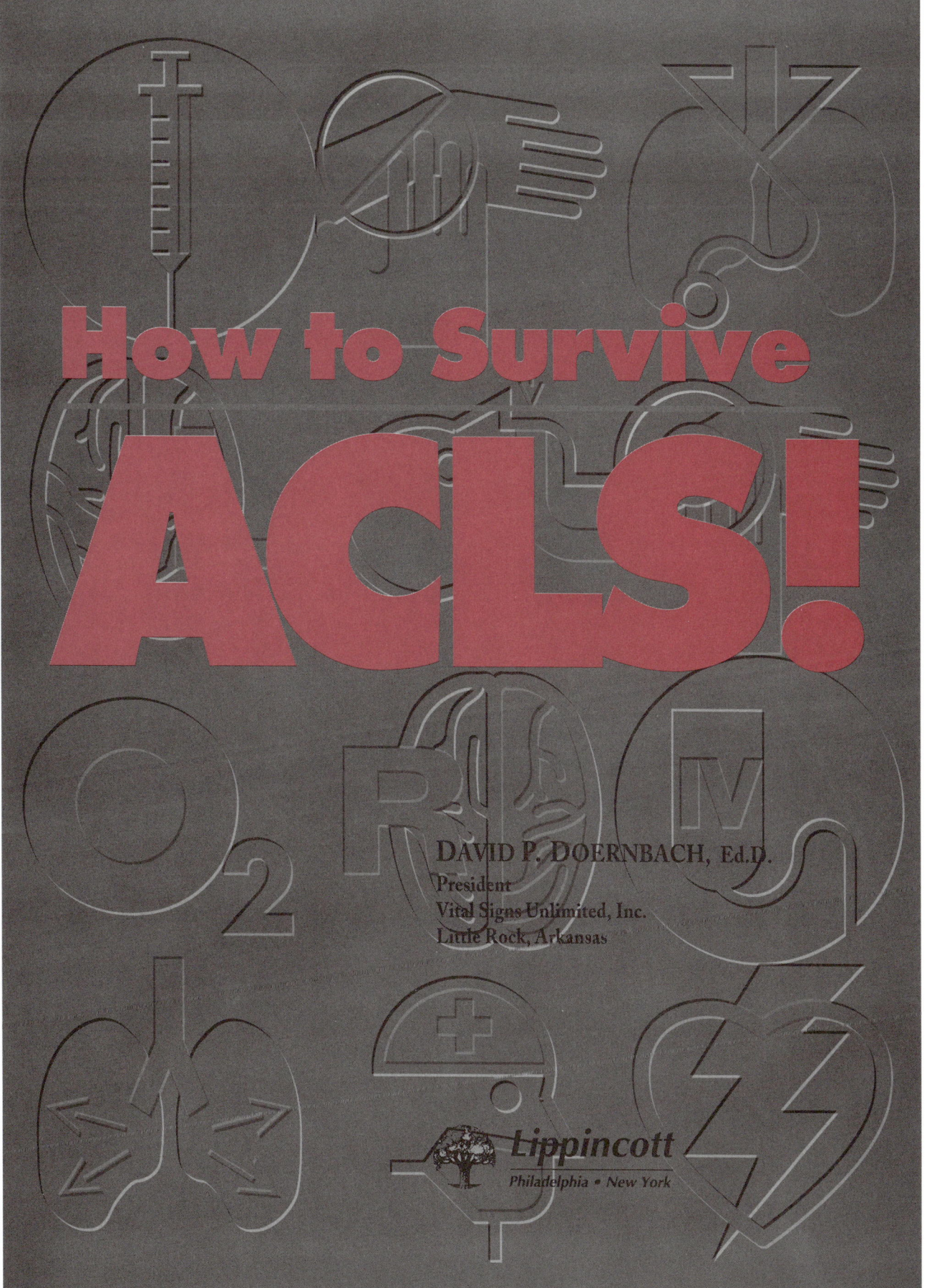

DAVID P. DOERNBACH, Ed.D.
President
Vital Signs Unlimited, Inc.
Little Rock, Arkansas

Lippincott
Philadelphia • New York

Acquisitions Editor: Susan M. Glover, R.N., M.S.N.
Assistant Editor: Bridget Blatteau
Project Editor: Tom Gibbons
Senior Production Manager: Helen Ewan
Production Coordinator: Pat McCloskey
Designer: Doug Smock
Cover Designer: Tom Jackson
Indexer: Victoria Boyle

Copyright © 1998 by Lippincott-Raven Publishers. All rights reserved. This book is protected by copyright. No part of it may be reproduced, stored in a retrieval system, or transmitted, in any form or by any means—electronic, mechanical, photocopy, recording, or otherwise—without the prior written permission of the publisher, except for brief quotations embodied in critical articles and reviews. Printed in the United States of America. For information write Lippincott-Raven Publishers, 227 East Washington Square, Philadelphia, PA 19106.

Library of Congress Cataloging in Publications Data

Doernbach, David P.
    How to survive ACLS! / David P. Doernbach
      p. cm.
    Includes bibliographical references and index.
    ISBN 0-7817-1202-5 (alk. paper)
     1. Cardiac arrest—Treatment. 2. Cardiac resuscitation. 3. Heart Arrest—therapy—case studies. 1. Title.
     [DNLM: 1. Heart Arrest—therapy—examination questions.
2. Resuscitation—examination questions. 3. Life Support Care--examination questions. WG 18.2 D652h 1998]
RC685.C173D64 1998
616.1´23025—dc21
DNLM/DLC
for Library of Congress   97-47792
                                             CIP

    Care has been taken to confirm the accuracy of the information presented and to describe generally accepted practices. However, the authors, editors, and publisher are not responsible for errors or omissions or for any consequences from application of the information in this book and make no warranty, express or implied, with respect to the contents of the publication.
    The authors, editors and publisher have exerted every effort to ensure that drug selection and dosage set forth in this text are in accordance with current recommendations and practice at the time of publication. However, in view of ongoing research, changes in government regulations, and the constant flow of information relating to drug therapy and drug reactions, the reader is urged to check the package insert for each drug for any change in indications and dosage and for added warnings and precautions. This is particularly important when the recommended agent is a new or infrequently employed drug.
    Some drugs and medical devices presented in this publication have Food and Drug Administration (FDA) clearance for limited use in restricted research settings. It is the responsibility of the health care provider to ascertain the FDA status of each drug or device planned for use in their practice.

9 8 7 6 7 6 5 4 3 2 1

• •

I have dedicated this book to the two most important people in my life: my wife Donna and my son Erich.

Donna has been more patient with my writing quirks than I would have been had the situation been reversed. Getting up at all hours of the night and working steadily during weekends usually makes for a shaky relationship. However, her patience, love, and support have allowed me to again write another textbook without fear of losing what I hold most dear—our relationship together. Thank you, Donna!

My son, Erich, occupies a special place in my heart. Most parents hope to instill sufficient moral and ethical values in their children to allow them to live their lives with honor and enjoyment. I consider myself lucky—he survived adolescence and now is a young man of whom I am extremely proud. Erich, I urge you to embrace your love of life as much as Donna and I.

A special dedication to Dr. Gerald Honick, M.D., in memoriam. I wish that you were here to provide your input and guidance, but I am certain that you're still looking out for me.

Contributors

R. Lee Archer, MD
    Associate Professor
    Division of Neurology
    University of Arkansas Center for Medical Sciences
    Little Rock, Arkansas

Eugene S. Smith III, MD
    Assistant Professor of Medicine
    Division of Cardiology
    University of Arkansas Center for Medical Sciences
    Little Rock, Arkansas

Acknowledgments

I wish to acknowledge the individuals who assisted in the creation of this text by supplying hints, tricks, or pertinent knowledge:

Beverly Roam, R.N.
Marilyn Wilson, R.N.
DeAnn Hunt, R.N.
Kristin Hadley, R.N.
J. Derek Gilbreath, EMT-P
Sanford Ward, D.O.
Betty Arnold, R.N.
Don Shelton, R.N.
Thomas E. Harris, M.D.

Jay Holland, M.D.
Ken Gilligan, M.D.
Linda Cartwright, R.N.
Connie Heath, L.P.N.
Catherine McConnell, R.N.
Ray Bollen, M.D.
Linda Seals, R.N.
Hazel Cabrera, RN, BSN
John Dial, M.D.

Some of the art was created by Karen Pipes, R.N., B.S.N., C.C.R.N., and Linda Doernbach. Although Karen is credited with the majority of the illustrations in my interim publication, Linda was my initial artist.

I would also like to acknowledge the addition of torsades de pointes information submitted by Ashok Sachdev, M.D.

The acute coronary syndromes case study is a joint effort with Eugene S. Smith III, M.D. Dr. Smith, a board-certified cardiologist with the University of Arkansas for Medical Sciences, is primarily responsible for the plethora of up-to-date information contained in the lecture. The flow chart, designed to make the treatment protocol more understandable, is reproduced with his permission.

The acute stroke case study is also a joint effort. Dr. R. Lee Archer, a board-certified neurologist with the University of Arkansas for Medical Sciences, made an otherwise cumbersome topic easier to understand. I can't thank him enough for his insight.

I wish to thank the following individuals who assisted in the textbook's review.

Jay Holland, M.D.
Jamin Snarr
Rodney Walker, NREMT-P
Andrea Smith, M.D.

Jeng-Shing Wang, M.D.
Kaye Grimes, M.D.
Michael Layton, NREMT-P
David De Jong, M.D.
William Furlow, M.D.

A special mention to Barbara Gund for the thankless job of the initial edit of the manuscript. I wish that she had survived her bout with cancer to see this work go to publication.

Contents

Unit One
Fundamental Concepts of ACLS — 1

1. *The ACLS Course and This Text* — 3
2. *Respiratory Intervention Case Study* — 9
   - **Case Study 1:** Respiratory Arrest With a Pulse — 9
3. *Lethal Arrhythmia Case Studies* — 29
   - **Case Studies 2 and 3:** Ventricular Fibrillation and Pulseless Ventricular Tachycardia — 30
   - **Case Study 4:** Pulseless Electrical Activity — 50
   - **Case Study 5:** Asystole — 61
4. *Acute Coronary Syndromes Case Study* — 71
   - **Case Study 6:** Coronary Syndromes — 71
5. *Rate-Driven Case Studies* — 93
   - **Case Study 7:** Bradycardias — 98
   - **Case Study 8:** Unstable Tachycardias — 111
   - **Case Study 9:** Stable Tachycardias — 125
6. *Acute Stroke: Acute Ischemic Stroke and Hemorrhagic Stroke* — 147

Comprehensive Posttest — 175

Unit Two
Learning Adjuncts — 215

7 *Megacode Survival Tips* 217

8 *ACLS Drug Therapy* 225

9 *Memorization Techniques* 243

Answers 293

Glossary 339

Index 341

Flash Cards

Unit One
Fundamental Concepts of ACLS

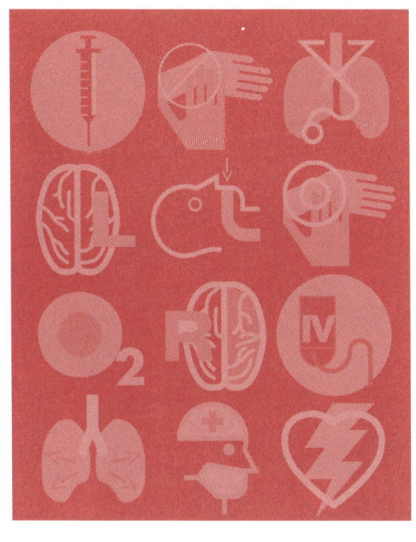

1 The ACLS Course and This Text

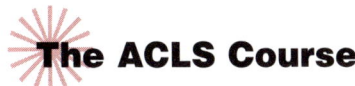 The ACLS Course

Cardiac emergencies are usually controlled chaos. Knowledge gained in an ACLS course will assist you when called on to perform emergency cardiac interventions. Your knowledge and skills in electrocardiogram (ECG) rhythm interpretation, defibrillation, intravenous entry, patient assessment, and medication deployment will be increased significantly by ACLS training. Even though not all members of the team are allowed to perform all of the skills, ACLS training decreases each team member's anxiety during the resuscitation sequence. Each member of the team knows exactly what is needed in advance and thus can better assist the team leader. With ACLS training, team members do not dread an emergency but rather look forward to assisting a stricken patient with their newly acquired skills. They respond in a logical, professional manner according to the standards of the American Heart Association (AHA).

Like all health care professionals who contemplate taking an ACLS course, you are probably anxious. Your anxiety is probably intensified by listening to coworkers discuss a particularly frustrating ACLS experience; recalling your last ACLS course experience; leafing through the *Advanced Cardiac Life Support* textbook by the AHA and noting the enormous amount of information to be read, understood, and memorized; or feeling inadequate in ECG interpretation.

The ACLS course has changed markedly since its inception in 1975. The educational structure is more flexible, with student learning and participation given higher priorities than heavy-handed evaluation. The format of the course has changed from using memorization to focusing on encouraging student learning. Instead of requiring rote memorization of the protocols, the course is now designed to teach students how and why each therapy serves to increase a patient's chance of success. Therefore, regardless of what you have heard from your coworkers or what you may have experienced in the past, the new teaching system is more enjoyable.

> The man who knows "how" will always have a job. The man who knows "why" will always be his boss.

ACLS Enrollment Requirements: Who Can Take the Course?

This course is designed for all health professionals whose daily occupation or volunteer activities demand proficiency in the knowledge and skills of ACLS, including physicians, oral surgeons, registered nurses, licensed practical nurses, licensed vocational nurses, respiratory professionals, and paramedics. Prospective students should be authorized by state law to perform some or all of the functions. The AHA sets the burden of application selection on the course director, an ACLS instructor certified by the AHA to manage an ACLS course. The course director is the only person who can allow you to participate in or audit the course. Entry is usually limited by practical considerations, however, because it is *assumed* that each applicant has a *minimal* knowledge of basic arrhythmia interpretation.

ACLS certification does not mean that you are licensed or certified to perform any of the skills that you learn. It only means that you have successfully completed the course in accordance with the standards of the AHA. An ACLS card is only a *verification* that you have successfully attained the course objectives.

ELECTROCARDIOGRAPHIC SKILLS

Previously, ACLS required an intimate knowledge of ECG interpretation; however, this is no longer the case. There are no specific prerequisites regarding ECG skills. Essentially, all that is important is whether a rhythm has a pulse and whether that pulse is too fast or too slow. The ECG arrhythmia test, which in the past was an integral part of the course, has been deleted by most AHA affiliates. As long as you can recognize asystole, any bradycardia (specific block recognition is not necessary), ventricular tachycardia, ventricular fibrillation, and narrow complex tachycardia, you are prepared for the course.

In an effort to make the experience easier, each case study has an ECG interpretation section of rhythms common to the problem encountered. If you are a novice in this field, the information will be invaluable. Remember, each case study's ECG section has only a quick discussion, not an in-depth look at rhythm interpretation.

CURRENT CARDIOPULMONARY RESUSCITATION CERTIFICATION

Traditionally, a Basic Life Support (BLS) station was tested separately; however, the latest guidelines specify that BLS skills should be evaluated during case studies 2 and 3 (ventricular fibrillation and pulseless ventricular tachycardia.) Nevertheless, to enroll in an ACLS course, each participant must be verified in BLS by the AHA. Most state affiliates accept Red Cross verification; however, you should check with your course director. Bring your BLS verification card with you to the course because the course director will ask to see it. If you have a physical handicap (e.g., pregnancy, back injury, carpal tunnel syndrome), the course director may suggest alternatives, such as taking only the written examination and verbalizing the psychomotor skills.

The Enrollment Packet

Depending on the course, a packet of information will be sent to you after enrollment. This packet usually contains at least the following:

- A welcome letter
- A copy of the ACLS protocols (these may not be included because they are usually only enlarged reproductions found in the *Advanced Cardiac Life Support* textbook)
- The current *Advanced Cardiac Life Support* textbook, published by the American Heart Association
- A pretest

At first glance, this packet of information looks intimidating; however, *How to Survive ACLS* should make the information more understandable. It is therefore ideal to read *this* book before beginning the *Advanced Cardiac Life Support* textbook, which may be difficult to read.

How the ACLS Course Is Organized

A generic ACLS course comprises a series of case studies. The format of the course can vary; however, all courses cover at least case studies 1 through 10. Specific intensive care nursing or specialized physician courses may contain additional case studies, such as hypothermia, but generic ACLS courses cover only case studies 1 through 10.

> ACLS Instruction is the process of moving from cocksure ignorance to thoughtful uncertainty.

DISCUSSION GROUPS

Each case study is covered in a discussion group format. The faculty for each group encourage interaction with and between the participants. Although it is not obvious during the discussion, the faculty are evaluating student answers and skills on *critical actions evaluation checklists*. Psychomotor skills, such as cardiopulmonary resuscitation, defibrillation, intravenous lines, and intubation are covered, practiced, and evaluated in each case study as they appear. For example, defibrillation skills are demonstrated during case studies 2 and 3, which are concerned with ventricular fibrillation, whereas case study 1 primarily evaluates airway maintenance skills.

Pediatrics is not normally covered in a generic ACLS course. The AHA has two courses that deal with children: the Neonatal Resuscitation Program (NRP) and Pediatric Advanced Life Support (PALS). Contact your local AHA affiliate for more information.

EVALUATION

After completion of the group discussions, the evaluation portion begins. This portion is made up of two segments: the ACLS multiple choice evaluation and the megacode. The ACLS evaluation is made up of 50 multiple choice questions supplied by the national office of the AHA. These cover pertinent points of all 10 case studies. The megacode is essentially a mock cardiac arrest. The environment for megacode evaluation has become more relaxed, promoting a learning situation rather than an antagonistic one.

Reverification

Both the original course and the reverification program cover all 10 case studies and therefore are structurally similar. The reverification program, however, assumes that the participants are more knowledgeable. Reverification course participants are expected to demonstrate proficiency in the skills and algorithms, to remain updated on new information, and to complete the course within a minimal time frame. The reverification course time frame does not allow for remedial training. If you are thinking of enrolling in a reverification course, you must be able to (1) provide current verification in both ACLS and cardiopulmonary resuscitation, and (2) demonstrate proficiency in all of the current ACLS protocols and psychomotor skills immediately on arrival. If are not confident in these two areas, sign up for the full provider course. The full provider course has a combined lecture and discussion group format, extends over a longer period, and is taught in a more relaxed atmosphere.

About This Text

The ACLS course is designed as a series of case studies rather than as a more traditional lecture encounter. Although the number of case studies differs according to the level of the participant's medical expertise, a generic ACLS course includes case studies 1 through 10. This text covers 10 case studies and integrates case study 11, on hypotension, shock, and acute pulmonary edema, into the case study on unstable tachycardia. Note that case study 11 is not a required case study. Each of the required 10 case studies represents one or two ACLS protocols.

Unit I of this book mimics the ACLS course by providing case studies, lectures, case study interim evaluations, and a comprehensive posttest. Unit II provides tips for getting through the mock cardiac arrest testing station (the megacode), an in-depth discussion of each of the ACLS drugs, and memorization techniques to help students remember the myriad of drug dosages and intricate ACLS protocols. The appendices to this book include a glossary, an index, and tear-away flash cards that highlight each main drug and ACLS protocol. (See Box 1-1 for an overview of how this text is organized.)

> **Box 1-1.** *How This Text Is Organized*
>
> **This textbook is broken down into two sections:**
>
> Unit I: Fundamental Concepts of ACLS
> Chapter 1: The ACLS Course and This Text
> Chapter 2: Respiratory Intervention Case Study
> Chapter 3: Lethal Arryhthmia Case Studies
> Chapter 4: Acute Coronary Syndromes Case Study
> Chapter 5: Rate-Driven Case Studies
> Chapter 6: Acute Stroke
> Comprehensive Post-test
>
> Unit II: Learning Adjuncts
> Chapter 7: Megacode Techniques
> Chapter 8: ACLS Drug Therapies
> Chapter 9: Memorization Techniques

How To Use This Text Effectively

The following list summarizes the most effective way to use this text:

1. Read this text from cover to cover.
2. Take the case study interim evaluation that appears after each case study.
3. Take the comprehensive posttest.
4. Complete the puzzles found throughout the book.

These steps should be accomplished before the first day of the course and before reading the *Advanced Cardiac Life Support* textbook. You are at an advantage if you arrive on the first day already feeling comfortable with the information and prepared to discuss it (especially if you are enrolled in a 1- or 2-day course). If you received this book on the first day of the course, make certain that you read case study 2 on ventricular fibrillation and pulseless ventricular tachycardia. This will be of the most benefit given your limited time frame for reading and study.

After reading all of this book, you may feel the need for more in-depth information. In this case, read the first chapter in the *Advanced Cardiac Life Support* textbook: "Essentials of ACLS." This chapter summarizes all of the ACLS protocols; the remainder of the textbook is designed to discuss each protocol more thoroughly. Also, refer to the *Advanced Cardiac Life Support* textbook if necessary for clarification when reading *How to Survive ACLS*.

ACLS information is normally conveyed by reading the *Advanced Cardiac Life Support* textbook and listening closely to the faculty during the course. Although they are excellent clinicians, however, most ACLS faculty are not professionals in the field of adult education. Their lectures or discussions may vary in depth, continuity, structure, and entertainment value. In addition, the course offers an abundance of information in a short amount of time. The course director is expected to adjust the pace according to the knowledge base of the participants. Some courses may be completed in a day, while others can be administered on a collegiate basis over a period of a semester.

The *Advanced Cardiac Life Support* textbook is filled with wonderful bits of knowledge; however, only a portion is considered core information (i.e., that necessary to pass a generic course). Each participant wants to get the most out of an ACLS course with the least amount of hassle. So, *How to Survive ACLS* summarizes the core information in a concise yet comprehensive fashion, keeping the amount of extraneous information to a minimum.

> Remember that not all ACLS Faculty have all their faculties.

How the Case Studies Are Organized

SECTION 1: EVALUATION CRITERIA

During each case study, the faculty evaluate each participant using criteria published in the ACLS instructor textbook. Copies of the evaluation checklist are included at the beginning of each case study. These help to reduce your stress by informing you about what the faculty expect you to know. Refer to it frequently as you read each lecture, *but do not memorize it*—that would be a waste of time. The criteria form is only included to: (1) show you what the AHA believes is important during in each case study; (2) describe what the faculty are trying to cover in the station; and (3) provide a summary of the case study after you have read the lecture.

SECTION 2: ACLS ALGORITHM

Complete algorithms are provided to help target what is covered during each case study. These are black-and-white reprints of the full-color algorithms provided in the *Advanced Cardiac Treatment System* (ACTS) published by VSU, Inc. To learn the protocols and drug dosages displayed in these algorithms more easily, refer to Chapter 9, Memorization Techniques. The algorithms printed in this textbook differ slightly in presentation from those in the *Advanced Cardiac Life Support* textbook but contain the same information. Call 1-800-844-ACLS for further information about ACTS.

SECTION 3: IDENTIFYING FEATURES

Many students are asked to take the course but lack a background in basic ECG interpretation skills. Therefore, a quick, basic explanation of pertinent ECGs is provided for each case study.

SECTION 4: PRIMARY AND SECONDARY ASSESSMENTS

Primary and secondary assessment information is provided for each case study. Primary assessment covers: Airway, Breathing, Circulation, and Defibrillation. Secondary assessment covers: Advanced Airway, Beware Blinders, Choice Circulation, and Drugs and Diagnosis.

The first two case studies on (1) respiratory arrest with a pulse, and (2) ventricular fibrillation and pulseless ventricular tachycardia present a comprehensive discussion of each component of the primary and secondary assessments. Rather than print the same assessment information at the beginning of the remaining case studies, however, a graphic representation of each assessment segment is presented during each case study that follows. In any case in which assessment differs from a generic approach, the differing diagnostic data are presented in an abbreviated format.

SECTION 5: LECTURE MATERIAL

Information from the *Advanced Cardiac Life Support* textbook has been scrutinized, and the basic information has been rewritten so that it is easier to read and understand and included in section 5 of each case study. This lecture section is not a substitute for class attendance or for reading the *Advanced Cardiac Life Support* textbook. Because this book is easier to read and comprehend and contains all of the essential information, however, it may suffice if time is limited.

Caution: Many of the drugs in the assessment sections are repeated in different case studies, so do not automatically assume that the information is the same if the first two or three sentences sound familiar. Read the section again because it may contain new facts necessary to understand how the drug relates to a particular cardiovascular problem. Even if the information is the same, remember that *repetition reinforces memory*.

SECTION 6: CASE STUDY INTERIM EVALUATION

Case study interim evaluations are provided so that you can determine whether you retained the information in the case study. There is only one correct answer to each question. A case study interim evaluation answer sheet is provided at the end of the case study. A case study interim evaluation answer key with appropriate rationales is also provided at the end of each case study.

SECTION 7: CROSSWORD PUZZLE

People process information differently, so in the spirit of fun and education, a crossword puzzle is provided after each case study. This makes the educational experience less tedious and more fun. An answer key is provided at the end of the case study.

Comprehensive Posttest

A comprehensive posttest is included in this text. This posttest includes multiple choice questions, associated answers, and the rationale for each. These questions are in addition to the questions that follow each case study. Roughly two thirds of the comprehensive posttest questions ask for specific information gleaned from the 10 case studies. The remaining one third evaluate your ability to recognize an ECG, analyze the history, and then choose the appropriate protocol to employ. There is only one correct answer to each question.

It is important to read and study each of the questions before the final ACLS examination. The comprehensive posttest in this book is similar in format to the Advanced Cardiac Life Support Multiple Choice Evaluation. They are not the same questions, but they are representative of the subject matter on the final examination.

Classification of Therapeutic Interventions in Cardiopulmonary Resuscitation and Electrocardiography

Throughout this book and the *Advanced Cardiac Life Support* textbook are references to a classification structure. This is the AHA's way of assigning priorities to various therapeutic options. For example, defibrillation is a class I therapeutic option, whereas lidocaine and bretylium are considered class IIa options in the ventricular fibrillation protocol. Pay attention to how each therapy is classified.

Class I: A therapeutic option that is usually indicated, always acceptable, and considered useful and effective.
Class II: A therapeutic option that is acceptable, is of uncertain efficacy, and may be controversial.
  Class IIa: A therapeutic option for which the weight of evidence is in favor of its usefulness and efficacy.
  Class IIb: A therapeutic option that is not well established by evidence but that may be helpful and probably is not harmful.
Class III: A therapeutic option that is inappropriate and is without scientific supporting data.

2 Respiratory Intervention Case Study

Case Study 1
Respiratory Arrest With a Pulse

Although ACLS is considered to target improving cardiac function primarily, the health care provider must never forget to consider a patient's airway and respiratory status. This case study demonstrates intervention when only respiratory function is impaired. In addition, the case study provides a blueprint to follow when presented with a patient in any emergency, cardiac or trauma.

Section 1: Critical Actions for Student Evaluation

The ACLS Instructor checklist for case study 1, respiratory arrest with a pulse, was reprinted with permission of the American Heart Association (AHA) and is shown in Table 2-1. This form was designed to guide the faculty when evaluating participants during this particular station. Refer to it frequently as you read the lecture that follows. *Do not memorize it.* The form is only included to: (1) show you what the AHA considers important during this particular case study; (2) describe what the faculty are trying to cover in the station; and (3) provide a summary of the case study after you have read the lecture.

Table 2-1.
Evaluation Checklist—Case 1: Respiratory Arrest With a Pulse

Critical Action	Completed	Not Completed	Comments
Universal algorithm steps			
Primary ABCD survey			
Assesses responsiveness			
Calls for help			
Calls for defibrillator			
Determines breathing			
Determines pulse			
Opens airway			
Initial rescue breathing			
Reassesses adequacy of ventilations			
Right main-stem intubation			
Pneumothorax			
Inadequate airway			
Intubates patient			
Assesses tube placement			
Establishes intravenous line			
Evaluates for cause of problem			
Arranges for further ventilatory support			

(Reproduced with permission. *Instructor's manual for advanced cardiac life support,* 1997 © Copyright American Heart Association, pp. 6–8.)

Section 2: ACLS Universal Algorithm

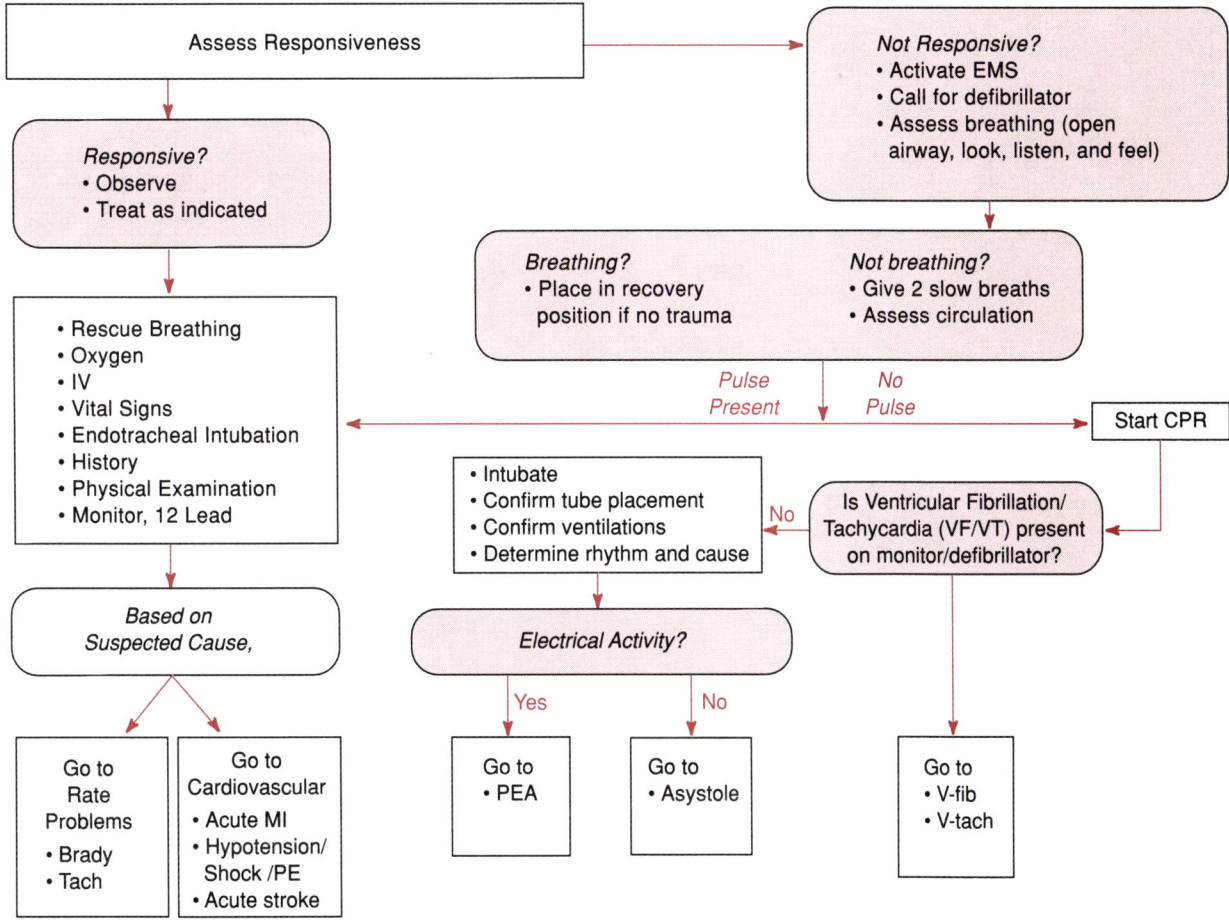

(Reproduced with permission. *Advanced cardiac life support.* Copyright 1997, American Heart Association.)

Section 3: Identifying Features

No one specific electrocardiogram (ECG) can be equated with respiratory arrest. Depending on when you encounter it, the patient's cardiac rhythm may present as a compensatory tachycardia or a decompensating bradycardia. The rhythm is only a symptom of the problem—treat the patient, not the monitor. A patient will initially attempt to compensate for hypoxia by increasing the heart rate (i.e., tachycardia); however, as this compensatory mechanism begins to fail, the heart slows, with a resulting decompensating bradycardia.

Sinus Tachycardia

The ECG strip in Figure 2-1 is identified as sinus tachycardia with a ventricular rate of 130. Because the patient is hypoxic in this case study, the heart is attempting to compensate for the poor oxygenation by increasing the rate. Treatment is not targeted at treating the rhythm; treat the cause, which is apnea.

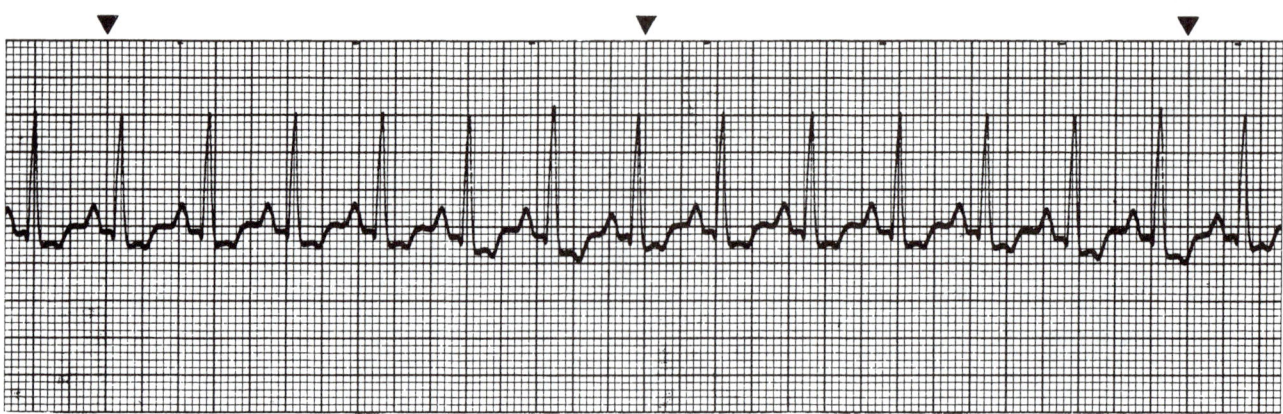

Figure 2-1. Sinus tachycardia.

Identifying features of sinus tachycardia are the presence of P waves with accompanying QRS complexes. The PR intervals are all consistent and last less than 0.20 seconds. The atrial and ventricular rates are equal, and in this instance are greater than 100.

This rhythm could be mistaken for supraventricular tachycardia (SVT); however, it differs in two important ways: (1) the rate is usually less than 170 in sinus tachycardia and greater than 170 in SVT, and (2) P waves are recognizable in sinus tachycardia but not obvious in SVT.

Sinus Bradycardia

The ECG strip in Figure 2-2 is identified as a sinus bradycardia with a ventricular rate of approximately 50. Because the patient is hypoxic in this case study, the heart rate has fallen to 50, reflecting decompensation. Treatment is not targeted at treating the rhythm; treat the cause, which is apnea.

Identifying features of sinus bradycardia are the presence of P waves with accompanying QRS complexes. The PR intervals are all consistent and less than 0.20 seconds. The atrial and ventricular rates are equal and in this instance are less than 60.

Section 4: Assessment

Neither the primary nor secondary assessment should preclude the clinician from initiating treatment in a specific order. The included mnemonics are only intended to help the clinician recall and keep in a prioritized sequence the components of assessment during a potentially chaotic situation. Each clinician is

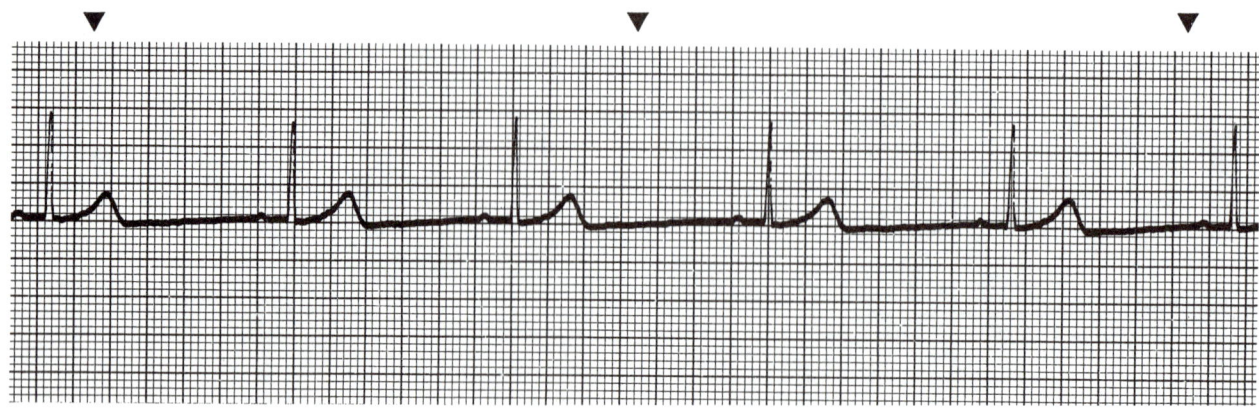

Figure 2-2. Sinus bradycardia.

encouraged to give or receive any orders and—only while carrying them out—repeat the mnemonics to make certain that nothing was forgotten. The mnemonic steps are only there to provide structure. Remember, stress inhibits memory, as is blatantly obvious during the evaluation segment.

Primary Assessment

> When you are up to your rear in alligators, it is hard to remember that your original intention was to drain the swamp.

Any assessment should begin with the primary survey noted in the AHA's universal algorithm: the ABCDs—Airway, Breathing, Circulation, and whether or not Defibrillation should be performed. All thoughts about differential diagnoses and possible causes leading to the arrest (part of the secondary survey) should be put on hold until the primary survey and any specific life-saving modalities have been instituted. Always progress in order—ABCD; do not jump to chest compressions when the airway has not been examined. Think of the primary survey as encompassing only those life-saving procedures that are necessary to keep the patient alive until the more definitive secondary survey is instituted. The entire procedure, with the possible exception of defibrillation, should not take more than a few seconds. Putting the patient on 8 liters of passive-flow oxygen and initiating an intravenous line are not primary survey life-saving tasks; however, aggressive suctioning to secure the airway does qualify as primary.

The patient in this case study is unconscious; thus, after determining unresponsiveness, activate Emergency Medical Services (EMS), call for a defibrillator, or both.

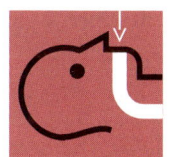

AIRWAY

Immediately inspect the airway. If the airway is open, move on to check breathing; however, if there is an obvious obstruction (e.g., chin to chest, blood or vomitus, massive upper airway trauma), correct the problem *before* checking breathing by a finger sweep or suctioning.

Pharyngeal Suctioning. Remember that few patients vomit only fluid; large food particles are the norm. Do not reach for the suction catheter first. Keeping the spine in alignment, turn the patient and sweep out the large food particles before introducing a rigid pharyngeal suction catheter (e.g., Yankauer; Fig. 2-3). The pressure generated by the device should be higher than -120 mmHg; however, be aware that you are rapidly sucking out the patient's air. It does not make any difference if the patient is apneic if

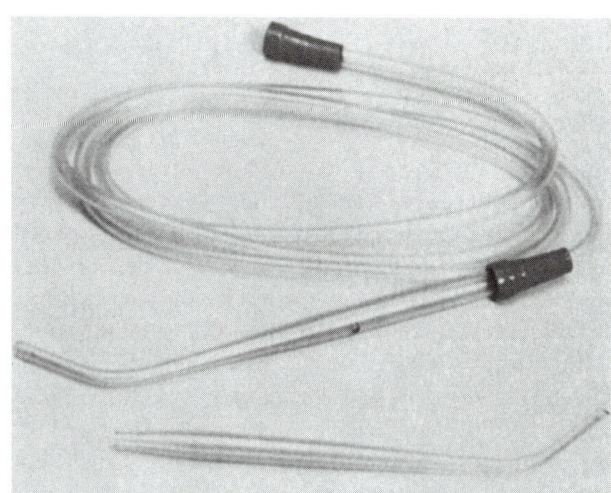

Figure 2-3. (*Top*) Tonsil tip suction catheter with vent control attached to suction tubing. (*Bottom*) Tonsil tip without vent control. (Courtesy of Parr Emergency Sales, Inc., Galloway, OH.)

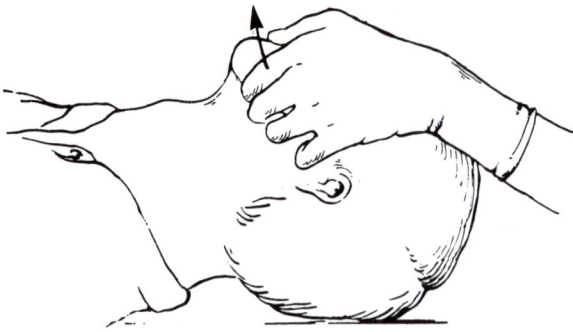

Figure 2-4. The jaw-thrust technique. The hands are placed on either side of the head. The fingers grasp behind the angle of the jaw, bringing it upward, as shown by the arrow. (Jones, S.A., et al. [1992]. *Advanced emergency care*. Philadelphia: Lippincott-Raven.)

the airway is occluded. Remember, if trauma is suspected, open the airway with a jaw-thrust maneuver (Fig. 2-4) rather than the spine-compromising head-tilt and chin-lift technique (Fig. 2-5).

Only after deciding that the airway appears open should you "look, listen, and feel" for breathing attempts. If the patient is adequately ventilating, move to assessing circulation. If, as in this case study, the patient is apneic, or the rate, volume, or effectiveness of the breathing attempts is unacceptable, *and only if immediately available*, place an oropharyngeal airway (OPA) or a nasopharyngeal airway (NPA). If neither of these is *immediately* available, just use the appropriate chin or jaw positioning until you enter the advanced airway portion of the secondary survey.

Oropharyngeal Airways. When properly placed and assisted with a slight head extension, OPAs keep the tongue from blocking the oropharynx. Because an OPA usually precipitates a gag reflex, it should only be employed in unconscious patients. An OPA is a temporary adjunct until a more definitive airway can be employed. It is commonly used to secure an endotracheal (ET) tube so that the patient does not bite down on the tube if he inadvertently regains consciousness. OPAs come in sizes varying from neonate to a large adult. There is no specific empiric measure to determine which size of OPA to introduce. Rule of thumb dictates a direct one-to-one relation between the length of the OPA and the distance from the angle of the jaw to the corner of the mouth.

The OPA is inserted in one of two ways: (1) by the upside-down technique or (2) by the jaw elevation maneuver. The upside-down technique introduces an inverted OPA with the tip sliding across the hard palate of the oral cavity. When the tip reaches the soft palate, the clinician turns it 180 degrees, and the OPA slides down into place. The jaw elevation maneuver slides the OPA directly into the oropharynx, with the tip pointed toward the esophagus, while the clinician elevates the tongue and jaw with a tongue blade (Fig. 2-6).

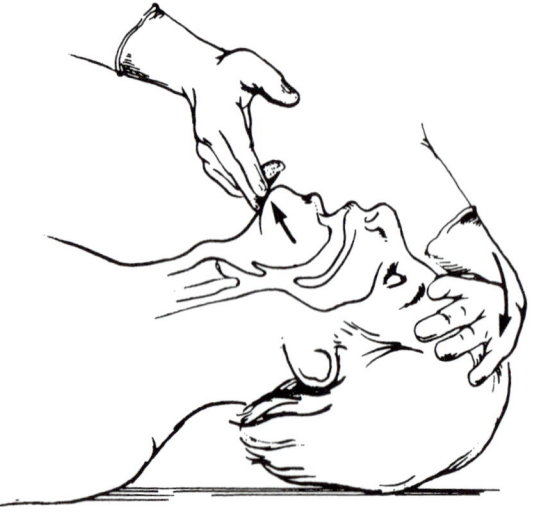

Figure 2-5. The head-tilt and chin-lift technique. The head is tilted backward with one hand (*downward arrow*), while the fingers of the other hand lift the chin forward (*upward arrow*). (Jones, S.A., et al. [1992]. *Advanced emergency care*. Philadelphia: Lippincott-Raven.)

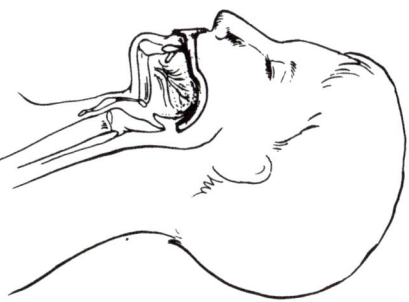

Figure 2-6. Oropharyngeal airway in place. (Jones, S.A., et al. [1992]. *Advanced emergency care*. Philadelphia: Lippincott-Raven.)

Nasopharyngeal Airways. Just like OPAs, NPAs, when properly placed, keep the tongue from blocking the oropharynx. Unlike OPAs, however, NPAs can be used in conscious or unconscious patients; they are commonly employed when repeated nasopharyngeal suctioning is necessary.

Insertion should be preceded by examining for the presence of a deviated septum because insertion through the narrowed side is contraindicated. A prelubricated NPA should be introduced along the floor of the nasal cavity. If resistance is encountered, gently rotate the tube while applying slight pressure (Fig. 2-7).

Important: Always listen to breath sounds to verify proper placement of an OPA or an NPA. It is easy to push the tongue into the oropharynx while introducing an OPA or to twist an NPA, resulting in an obstruction.

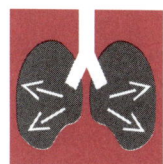

BREATHING

After verifying an open airway, attempt to ventilate with a pocket face mask, barrier device, bag-valve-mask (BVM) device, or demand valve. These devices eliminate direct contact with the patient and result in adequate lung ventilation; however, with the exception of the barrier device, all provide supplemental oxygen.

Mouth-to-Mask Ventilation. The steps for mouth-to-mask ventilation are as follows:

1. Connect the oxygen line to the high-flow oxygen regulator.
2. Open the airway with either the head-tilt and chin-lift or jaw-thrust technique.
3. Insert an OPA or NPA, if immediately available.
4. Secure the mask, establishing a seal between the mask and face.
5. Ventilate through a one-way valve.

Also refer to Figure 2-8.

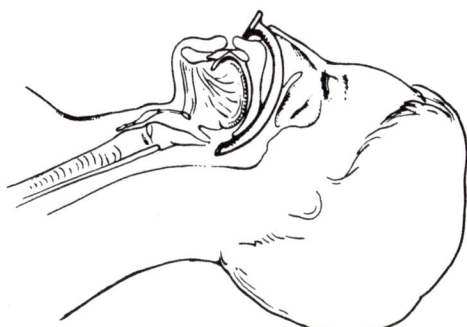

Figure 2-7. Nasopharyngeal airway in place. (Jones, S.A., et al. [1992]. *Advanced emergency care*. Philadelphia: Lippincott-Raven.)

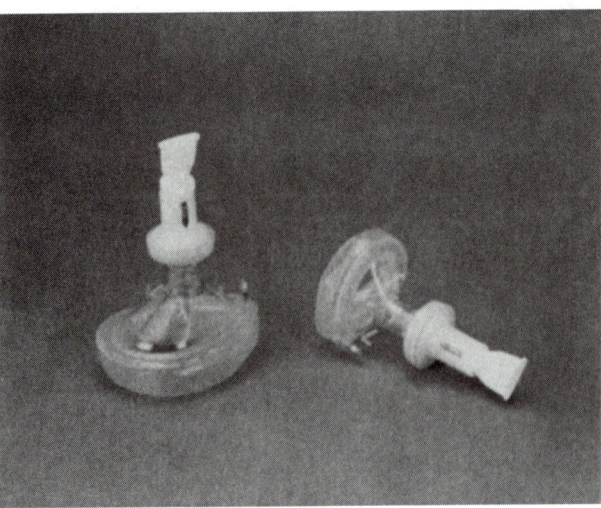

Figure 2-8. Adult (*left*) and pediatric (*right*) pocket face masks. (Courtesy of Parr Emergency Sales, Inc., Galloway, OH.)

Helpful Hints
for Mouth-to-Mask Ventilation

▼ Check and position all equipment before starting the procedure.

▼ It is more efficient to hold the mask under the metacarpal of each thumb than with the phalanges as usually demonstrated. The use of this technique allows the rescuer to add a jaw-thrust maneuver, with the fingers of both hands securing the patient's airway.

▼ If this case study station is equipped with a mannequin for demonstration purposes, it may be necessary to accentuate the head-tilt technique until the airway opens. Be aggressive; it may be necessary to hyperextend the neck significantly until an airway is achieved.

Give two ventilations spread out over 2 to 4 seconds. This accomplishes two goals: it (1) gives adequate time for the patient to exhale, and (2) discourages forceful breaths that might exceed the esophageal opening pressure, resulting in gastric distention. If other professional health care providers are available, direct pressure on the cricoid cartilage during ventilation (Sellick's maneuver) blocks the esophagus, inhibiting air movement into the stomach. This procedure greatly decreases the chance of aspiration. Readjust the airway if the patient still does not ventilate. Replace the mouth-to-mask device with a BVM as soon as possible.

Bag-Valve-Mask Device. By itself, the BVM only delivers room air. To administer 100% oxygen, it is necessary to affix an oxygen supply tube, administer 12 to 15 liters of oxygen, and ensure that the reservoir is attached. Without the reservoir, the concentration of oxygen administered seldom reaches more than 50%.

The approximate volume of a BVM is 1300 mL—a great deal less than the potential volume of a person's lungs. Thus, BVM devices deliver *less* tidal volume than you can deliver with your own lungs through a mouth-to-mask device. It is surprisingly easy to ventilate too forcefully, pushing excess air into the stomach, so consider employing Sellick's maneuver when the patient is not intubated.

Although the BVM allows the operator to feel a sense of chest compliance while supplying high concentrations of oxygen, it is difficult for one person to apply effectively. Proper care must be exercised to

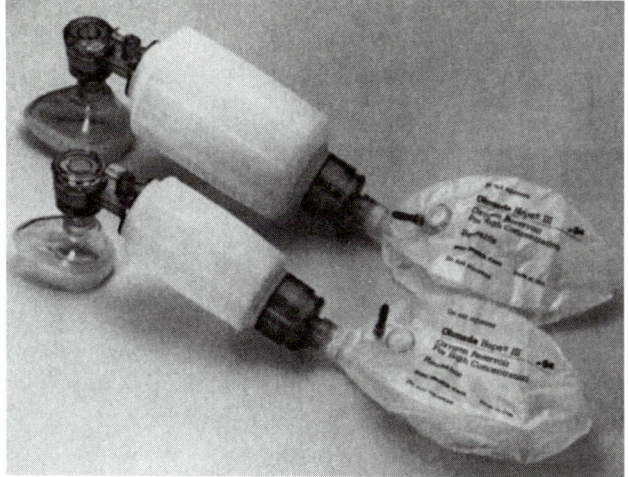

Figure 2-9. Adult (*top*) and pediatric (*bottom*) bag-valve-mask devices with oxygen reservoirs. (Courtesy of Parr Emergency Sales, Inc., Galloway, OH.)

make a proper mask seal. Clinicians are encouraged to use both hands to make the mask seal, while allowing a second professional to squeeze the bag. The BVM is designed to assist or supply all needed ventilations (Fig. 2-9).

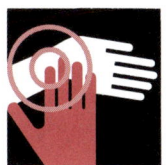

CIRCULATION

After airway and breathing have been secured, check for a carotid pulse. A slow, rapid, or irregular pulse may be difficult to detect; therefore, check it for at least 5 to 10 seconds. If a pulse is present, evaluate its perfusion. If the pulse is absent, begin basic cardiopulmonary resuscitation (CPR). Because this case study is concerned with a living patient in respiratory arrest, just evaluate the perfusion.

DEFIBRILLATION

The last portion of the primary survey, D, stands for defibrillation applicability. Because this patient has a pulse and does not require electrical intervention, move on to the secondary survey, again appropriately again called the ABCDs.

Secondary Survey

To differentiate between the two sets of ABCDs, the secondary set is referred to as AA, BB, CC, and DD. These letters stand for the similar terms as in the primary survey, but at a more *advanced* level.

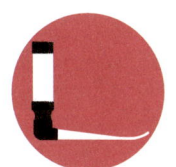

ADVANCED AIRWAY

AA stands for a more *a*dvanced *a*irway—an ET tube. Although intubation is strongly encouraged at this point, use common sense. As long as the airway is secured by other methods (e.g., an OPA and a BVM in conjunction with cricoid pressure) and acceptable ventilations are being delivered, do not hastily attempt to intubate until you are sufficiently prepared. Initiate an intravenous line in the meantime. Only when adequately prepared should you attempt intubation.

Endotracheal Intubation. An ET tube is the best airway of choice for anyone who, for whatever reason, cannot maintain his or her own airway. It is not, however, the initial airway of choice; other methods of positive pressure should be employed to hyperventilate and hyperoxygenate before intubating.

Although they may be placed in conscious patients (e.g., those with inhalation burns, anaphylaxis, or maxillofacial trauma), ET tubes are usually employed in the deeply unconscious patient whose ability to maintain his or her own airway is absent or impaired. *Intubation does not remove the possibility of aspiration, it just reduces the risk.* Intubation allows another route for the administration of certain drugs, including atropine, lidocaine, and epinephrine; the dose is 2 to 2.5 times the intravenous dosage.

Complications of intubation can be recalled using the memory aid DOPE: *d*isplacement, *o*bstruction, *p*neumothorax, and *e*sophagus. The tube may be mistakenly introduced into the esophagus or correctly entered into the trachea but pushed too deep, resulting in intubation of the right main-stem bronchus. If the former occurs, remove the tube immediately, quickly reoxygenate, and reattempt intubation. If the latter occurs, there is no need to extubate; just pull back 1 to 2 cm, and listen again. Common problems that may occur when you only hear breath sounds on the left side of the thorax are mucous plug, pneumothorax, and pneumonectomy.

When attempting to suction endotracheally, remember to both preoxygenate and postoxygenate, to put the patient on a monitor, and to apply suction for no more than 10 seconds while simultaneously withdrawing the catheter.

A brief summary of ET intubation is as follows:

1. Ensure that the patient has been preoxygenated, and check equipment (i.e., appropriate blade [straight or curved], light, ET tube cuff).
2. Holding the laryngoscope in your left hand (regardless of your dominant hand), insert the blade into the right side of the patient's mouth, and sweep the patient's tongue to the left (Fig. 2-10).
3. The tip of the straight blade should pick up the epiglottis, while the curved blade should be inserted in the space between the base of the tongue and the epiglottis, known as the *vallecula*.
4. Pick up the jaw with the laryngoscope angling away from you without prying on the patient's teeth.
5. Visualize the epiglottis and vocal cords.
6. Insert the ET tube through the vocal cords; stop advancing after the cuff passes through the cords.
7. Inflate the cuff with 5 to 10 mL of air, listening for air slipping past the cuff.
8. Check placement by listening over the epigastrium first; then verify bilateral chest excursion at the apex and the base of each lung.

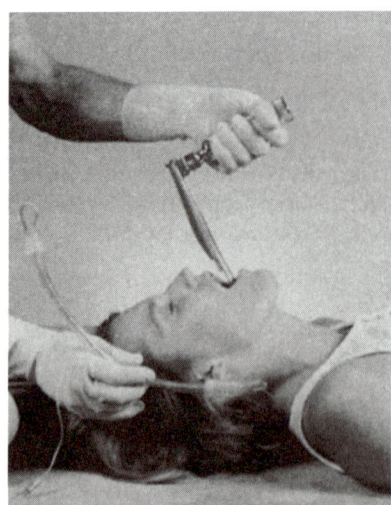

Figure 2-10. Laryngoscope insertion. (Jones, S.A., et al. [1992]. *Advanced emergency care*. Philadelphia: Lippincott-Raven.)

Helpful Hints
for the Intubation Skill Station

- ▼ Inform the faculty member that you would make certain that the patient was adequately preoxygenated (i.e., 2 to 5 minutes) before the procedure.
- ▼ Inflate and deflate the tube cuff before insertion to ensure its integrity.
- ▼ Make certain that the mannequin head is in the "sniffing" position. It is much easier and requires less strength to intubate the mannequin when a pad is placed underneath the head to facilitate positioning.
- ▼ Lubricate the tip and length of tube with silicone spray before insertion.
- ▼ Be sure to state to the faculty member that you would continue serial checks of the lungs to ensure airway integrity.
- ▼ Keep the actual time of intubation (from ceasing ventilations until restarting them) to 30 seconds or less. This can be approximated by holding your breath. If you can no longer comfortably hold your breath during intubation, neither can your patient.
- ▼ The silicone used for lubrication sometimes causes the endotracheal tubes to lose their rigidity. Although the use of stylets is controversial among anesthesiologists, their use in mannequins is helpful because they make the endotracheal tube more form-fitting.
- ▼ The pharynx of the mannequin is manufactured to resemble a human throat; however, it never acts like it. The laryngoscope is introduced into the right side of the mouth, sweeping the tongue to the midline. Depending on the make of mannequin, the tongue may not sweep easily. If this is the case, although it shows poor technique, introduce the blade directly in the midline. Sometimes this works better.
- ▼ Always hold the laryngoscope handle at the base where the blade attaches. This hand position makes it difficult to pry back on the teeth, which could cause dental damage.
- ▼ Some mannequins work better with straight blades than with curved blades. If you encounter difficulty, don't hesitate to try the other blade type.
- ▼ If the batteries in the laryngoscope are low, it is difficult to visualize the laryngeal anatomy. Never hesitate to request that new batteries be inserted if necessary.
- ▼ When lifting the patient's jaw with the blade, point the handle into the top corner of the room across from you. This technique eliminates the possibility of using the teeth as a fulcrum. Remember, lift the jaw structure away from you.
- ▼ Do not worry if, when you elevate the mannequin's jaw, the head lifts off the table. This technique is acceptable as long as the blade does not contact the teeth and the neck is reasonably supported.
- ▼ Sometimes, the only laryngeal structures observable in a patient with a thick neck are the arytenoids. As with a real patient, it is perfectly acceptable for an assistant to apply cricoid pressure to bring the cords into view.
- ▼ Beware of pushing the tube too far through the cords. Watch the cuff go past the cords, and then stop. Do not keep pushing because you will intubate the right main-stem bronchus. If this happens, correction can be achieved by pulling the tube back 1 to 2 cm and listening again.

Remember, do not proceed to circulation until you can secure the airway and provide adequate ventilation. Keep trying to find the cause of the problem, and do not proceed until it is corrected.

Hyperventilate the patient while preparing the equipment and suction if necessary. Make certain that your attempt does not exceed 30 seconds from ventilation to ventilation. If you are not successful, quickly hyperventilate again before making another attempt. After tube placement, listen over the abdomen first to verify that the tube was not placed in the esophagus. Then verify adequate lung sounds by auscultating both lungs during ventilation with a BVM. Make certain that the lung fields are being inflated equally and that both the rate and depth are appropriate. Before moving on, make certain that an OPA is inserted next to the tube to protect it and that the entire apparatus is secured in place. Ensure 100% input with a BVM with an oxygen reservoir coupled with a flow of oxygen of at least 12 to 15 L/minute. Make it a policy to reevaluate airway and breathing on a consistent basis throughout the code. If the patient does not need positive-pressure ventilation, but only needs to be oxygenated, use a passive-flow device (e.g., nasal cannula or adult face mask).

Important: The patient in this case study requires positive-pressure ventilation, but the following passive-flow devices *must* be covered during this case study (Fig. 2-11).

Nasal Cannula. This device is designed for adequately ventilating patients who would profit from increased oxygen concentrations of 24% to 44% at flow rates of 1 to 6 liters/minute. It is designed for simply augmenting the concentrations of oxygen, not hyperoxygenating them.

Oxygen Face Mask. This device is designed for adequately ventilating patients who would profit from increased oxygen concentrations of 40% to 60% at flow rates of 8 to 10 liters/minute. *Important:* Flow rates for this mask must be in excess of 5 liters/minute to wash out exhaled carbon dioxide that accumulates in the mask.

Oxygen Face Mask With Oxygen Reservoir. This device is designed for adequately ventilating patients that would profit from increased oxygen concentrations of 60% (6 liters/minute) to 100% (10 liters/minute), depending on flow rates. This is the device of choice for aggressively increasing an actively ventilated patient's PaO_2.

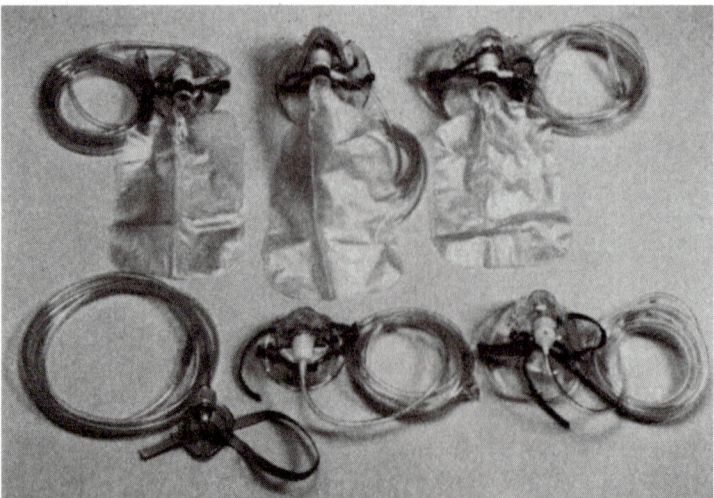

Figure 2-11. Types of oxygen masks (*top*, left to right): Pediatric partial rebreathing, adult nonrebreathing, adult partial rebreathing; (*bottom*, left to right): infant simple mask, pediatric simple mask, adult simple mask. (Courtesy of Parr Emergency Sales, Inc., Galloway, OH.)

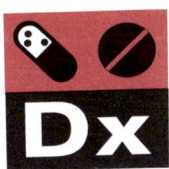

DRUGS AND DIAGNOSIS

The last letters in our secondary survey, DD, provide the mental association to *drugs* as applicable to *diagnosis*. Maybe the patient has some underlying problem that can be treated if the rescuer takes the time to consider the medical, surgical, or traumatic conditions that could have precipitated the respiratory arrest. The patient should be continually evaluated, a history explored, a cardiac monitor hooked up, and a 12-lead ECG obtained.

Section 5: Lecture

The objective of this case study is to familiarize the student with an in-depth study of the *assessment* phase of patient care. Because the patient continues to be apneic, a ventilator is required, which extends past the scope of this case study. The patient should be transferred to a respiratory intensive care unit or a hospital with ventilator capabilities as quickly as possible. Again, serial evaluations are absolutely necessary before and during transport.

Section 6: Respiratory Interim Evaluation

Mark the correct answer.

1. The following is true concerning a BVM (e.g., an Ambu bag) (see ACLS text pp. 2-8 to 2-9): _____
   _____ (a) It should not be used during CPR.
   _____ (b) It is often hampered by a poor seal around the nose and mouth.
   _____ (c) It does not allow the victim to breathe on his or her own.
   _____ (d) It is incapable of providing oxygen concentrations other than 100%.

2. When selecting a BVM, the following are desirable features: (see ACLS text pp. 2-8 to 2-9): (1) a self-expanding bag; (2) a oxygen-supply inlet capable of providing a maximum of 8 liters/minute; (3) a transparent mask; (4) a nonrebreathing valve. _____
   _____ (a) 1, 3, and 4
   _____ (b) 1, 2, and 3
   _____ (c) 1, 2, and 4
   _____ (d) All of the above

3. Improper placement of an OPA may result in tearing of the vocal cords (see ACLS text pp. 2-1 to 2-2). _____
   _____ (a) True
   _____ (b) False

4. Which of the following are part of the primary survey (see ACLS text pp. 1-4 to 1-11): (1) suctioning the airway; (2) starting the IV; (3) placing the patient on 100% O_2; (4) pushing drugs? _____
   _____ (a) All of the above
   _____ (b) 1, 2, and 3
   _____ (c) 1
   _____ (d) 2 and 3

5. A main problem of an NPA is that it is so pliable and soft that it could easily twist during placement, resulting in blockage (see ACLS text pp. 2-2 to 2-3). _____
   _____ (a) True
   _____ (b) False

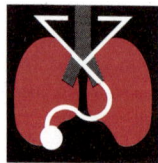

BEWARE BLINDERS

After the advanced airway has been instituted and adequate ventilation verified, consider BB for *b*eware *b*linders. This segment is not a repeat of AA, during which breath sounds were verified, it is a combination:

- Quick thorax examination
- Pertinent patient history

BB reminds the health care professional to assess the thorax specifically for any adventitious sounds, such as rales, rhonchi, and wheezing. Checking for those sounds while assessing for muffled heart tones, subcutaneous emphysema, jugular venous distention, and tracheal deviation is necessary because these are commonly neglected in the chaos of initiating basic life support. Their presence may highlight causes not yet considered. For example, if the BB assessment revealed bilateral rales and rhonchi, large amounts of intravenous fluids might be contraindicated. Additionally, if signs of jugular distention were noted, a more in-depth assessment for a tension pneumothorax or cardiac tamponade would be in order.

If the history reveals that the patient is a diabetic, therapy may include dextrose or insulin. Likewise, if the patient has a preexisting acidosis from an aspirin overdose, sodium bicarbonate would be administered near the beginning of the protocol rather than at the end. Additional treatment for a digitalis overdose might include an antagonist, such as digoxin immune fab (Digibind).

Do not treat BB as just verifying lung sounds; use it to remember that adequate breathing is not just the presence of equal, bilateral lung excursion. It constitutes a specific assessment for other medical or traumatic pathology that might highlight additional problems or might point to a cause of the presenting emergent condition.

CHOICE CIRCULATION

> We get so concerned with urgent, we never have time to deal with the important!

Only after beware blinders has been completed should the next segment in the secondary survey, CC for *c*hoice *c*irculation, be considered. Choice circulation means to obtain a set of vital signs, initiate an intravenous line, and consider appropriate medications.

Start a peripheral intravenous line, which does not interrupt CPR should arrest occur, using lactated Ringer's, normal saline, or D-5-W solution. The AHA encourages the use of normal saline or lactated Ringer's because both solutions:

- Are isotonic and thus expand the intravascular container better than dextrose solutions
- Are less expensive than dextrose solutions
- Have longer shelf-lives than dextrose solutions
- Are compatible with most drugs
- Do not cause pulmonary edema in cardiac patients, as was originally thought

Although D-5-W is being discouraged during code situations because high glucose levels may be linked to poor neurologic outcomes, the patient in this case study is not in arrest, so feel free to start D-5-W if you wish.

Although the letters CC help direct the rescuer's thoughts toward the traditional question of what drugs to use in this protocol, the patient would be ill treated if such a narrow course of action were instituted without diligent thought about the reason for the patient's situation. Considering the causes of a medical condition is common practice; however, during a respiratory emergency, time is so critical that precipitating events of the respiratory arrest may not receive the appropriate scrutiny.

6. During basic life support, if the patient has not been intubated, external pressure is recommended on the cricoid cartilage when using a BVM (see ACLS text pp. 2-8 to 2-9). _____
   _____ (a) True
   _____ (b) False

7. Which of the following correctly states the advantages of ET intubation (see ACLS text pp. 2-3 to 2-6): (1) assists in airway protection from aspiration; (2) provides an alternative route for administration of certain drugs; (3) diminishes the probability of gastric distention; (4) eliminates the need for 100% oxygen source? _____
   _____ (a) 3 and 4
   _____ (b) 1 and 3
   _____ (c) 1, 2, and 4
   _____ (d) 1, 2 and 3

8. ET intubation (see ACLS text pp. 2-3 to 2-6): (1) should be used as the initial means of providing an open airway for an arrested victim; (2) allows adjunctive ventilatory equipment to be used more effectively with less effort on the part of the rescuer; (3) reduces the risk of aspiration of gastric contents; (4) when improperly performed may result in only one lung being inflated. _____
   _____ (a) 1, 2, and 3
   _____ (b) 2, 3, and 4
   _____ (c) 1 and 4
   _____ (d) All of the above

9. Attempts at tracheal intubation may result in (see ACLS text pp. 2-3 to 2-6): (1) laryngeal trauma; (2) esophageal intubation; (3) duodenal perforation; (4) a hiatal hernia. _____
   _____ (a) 1 and 3
   _____ (b) 2 and 3
   _____ (c) 2 and 4
   _____ (d) 1 and 2

10. ET suction (see ACLS text pp. 2-15 to 2-16): (1) should be limited to 25 seconds; (2) should be preceded by increased ventilation with supplemental oxygen; (3) can result in hypoxia; (4) should be performed without applying suction while inserting the catheter. _____
    _____ (a) 1, 3, and 4
    _____ (b) 2, 3, and 4
    _____ (c) 1 and 2
    _____ (d) All of the above

11. In comparing an adult curved with a straight laryngoscope blade, which of the following are true (see ACLS text pp. 2-3 to 2-6): (1) a curved blade should always be initially employed in all patients; (2) the curved blade is designed to be inserted between the vocal cords; (3) the tip of the straight blade is used to lift the epiglottis; (4) the curved blade is designed to fit in the vallecula? _____
    _____ (a) 1 and 4
    _____ (b) 2 and 4
    _____ (c) 2 and 3
    _____ (d) 3 and 4

12. Which of the following statements best describes the optimal position for ET intubation (see ACLS text pp. 2-3 to 2-6)? _____
    _____ (a) Patient supine, neck flexed, head extended
    _____ (b) Patient supine, head flexed forward

_____ (c) Patient prone, head elevated with maximum hyperextension of the neck
_____ (d) Patient left lateral recumbent with head flexed forward

13. You have intubated a cardiac arrest patient. You cannot hear breath sounds on either side of the chest. The most likely possibility is that you have (see ACLS text pp. 2-3 to 2-6): _____
    _____ (a) Intubated the left main-stem bronchus
    _____ (b) Intubated the esophagus
    _____ (c) Pushed the tube firmly against the carina
    _____ (d) Intubated the trachea

14. During the primary survey, you note that the patient is breathing agonally at a rate of 6 breaths/minute. Because the patient is breathing, you can safely assume that the patient has a pulse (see ACLS text pp. 1-4 to 1-11). _____
    _____ (a) True
    _____ (b) False

15. After intubation, which of the following is not a reason for hearing breath sounds only on the left (see ACLS text pp. 2-3 to 2-6)? _____
    _____ (a) Esophageal intubation
    _____ (b) Right-sided tension pneumothorax
    _____ (c) Removal of the right lung
    _____ (d) Mucous plug on right

16. Which of the following would be the passive-flow oxygen delivery device necessary when seeking to deliver high concentrations of oxygen (see ACLS text pp. 2-7 to 2-8)? _____
    _____ (a) Nasal cannula
    _____ (b) Oxygen face mask
    _____ (c) Venti mask
    _____ (d) Oxygen face mask with reservoir

17. Suctioning to clear the airway and obtaining an oxygen tank to get the patient on 100% oxygen are both appropriate during the primary survey (see ACLS text pp. 1-4 to 1-11). _____
    _____ (a) True
    _____ (b) False

18. Which of the following are part of the BB, or beware blinders, section of the secondary survey (see ACLS text pp. 1-4 to 1-11): (1) verifying lung fields directly after intubation; (2) checking for chest symmetry; (3) taking a quick history; (4) noting that the patient is an alcoholic? _____
    _____ (a) 1
    _____ (b) 1 and 2
    _____ (c) 2, 3, and 4
    _____ (d) All of the above

19. The most suitable initial vein for cannulation while CPR is still in progress is the (see ACLS text pp. 1-10 and 6-1): _____
    _____ (a) Femoral vein
    _____ (b) External jugular vein
    _____ (c) Peripheral arm vein
    _____ (d) Subclavian vein

20. Below the inguinal ligament, where is the femoral vein relative to the femoral artery (see ACLS text p. 6-4)? _____
    _____ (a) Lateral
    _____ (b) Medial
    _____ (c) Anterior
    _____ (d) Posterior

21. Which of the following intravenous solutions are considered acceptable in a cardiac arrest (see ACLS text pp. 1-10): (1) lactated Ringer's; (2) normal saline; (3) D-5-W; (4) 5% dextrose in half-normal saline? _____
    _____ (a) 3
    _____ (b) 1 and 2
    _____ (c) 3 and 4
    _____ (d) 1, 2, and 4

26 Unit 1 *Fundamental Concepts of ACLS* • Respiratory Arrest with a Pulse

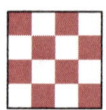

Section 7:
RESPIRATORY CROSSWORD PUZZLE

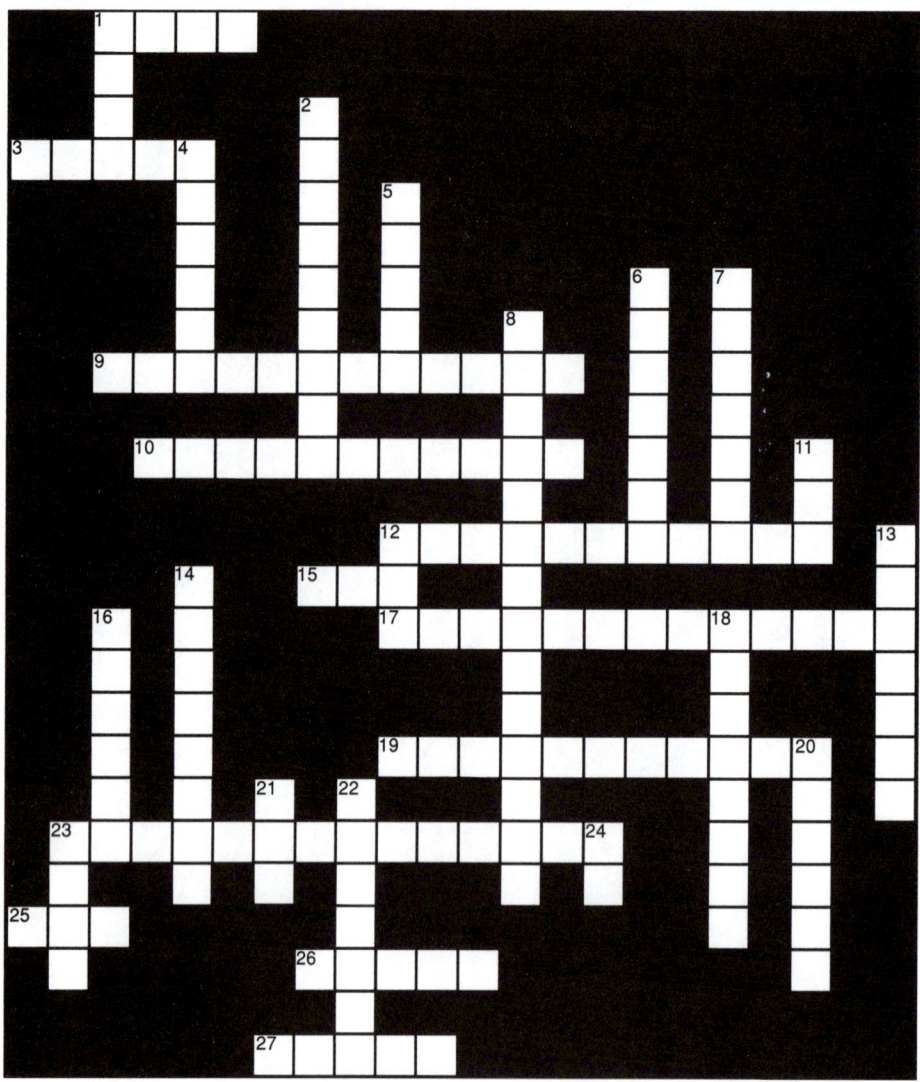

Across

1. A BVM delivers _____ tidal volume than you could with a mouth-to-mask device.
3. The _____ main-stem bronchus is more parallel to the trachea than the opposite main-stem bronchus.
9. A _____, tension or otherwise, may be a reason that breath sounds are not auscultated on the right but are heard clearly on the left.
10. _____ is suspected when an airway is opened using the jaw-thrust maneuver, but ventilation with a BVM does not result in lung inflation.
12. _____ is the cardiovascular response to hypoxia and is defined as a heart rate of more than 100 beats/minute.
15. The mnemonic that uses the first letter of each of the drugs that can be introduced down an ET tube.
17. A passive-flow device for delivering oxygen at rates between 60% and 100%. The name originated from the one-way diaphragm, allowing air to be exhaled out of the face mask while oxygen is inhaled from the oxygen-filled pouch.
19. ET tube placement should be auscultated first over the _____.
23. Clinicians should always _____ before intubating, producing rapid, deep ventilations.
25. When opening the airway, the _____ thrust should be used when trauma is suspected.

26. Even with 15 L/minute of oxygen entering a BVM, without an oxygen reservoir, the greatest oxygen concentration that can be delivered is _____%.

27. Moist crackles or _____ are adventitious lung sounds. Their presence may indicate congestive heart failure.

Down
1. Only the right _____ will be inflated if the tube is pushed too deeply when intubating.
2. A _____, which is a device projecting off the back of a BVM containing oxygen, is necessary for a BVM to achieve a delivered concentration of 100% oxygen. .
4. An oxygen supply rate of _____ to 15 L/minute with a reservoir is necessary to get a BVM to deliver close to 100% oxygen.
5. _____-to-mask ventilation is another form of positive pressure mechanism.
6. This passive-flow oxygen delivery device administers between 21% to 40% delivered oxygen. It is placed in the nares.
7. Pressure on this cartilage prevents air from entering the esophagus when delivering positive-pressure ventilation.
8. This pliable rubber airway is introduced through the nares. Also referred to as a *nasal trumpet,* it makes nasal suctioning easier and less traumatic.
11. The acronym for oropharyngeal airway.
12. ET suctioning should be limited to _____ to 15 seconds before postoxygenating.
13. A piece of plastic preventing mouth-to-mouth contact between patient and rescuer.
14. A rigid-tip pharyngeal suction catheter.
16. If you suspect spinal involvement, the _____ can best be opened using the jaw-thrust technique.
18. Intubation does not guarantee that the patient will not _____ to vomit and then inhale.
20. If you cannot hear the right side of the chest after intubation, a _____ plug may have blocked a bronchus.
21. The acronym for a bag-valve-mask.
22. Intubating a patient should never be the _____ act of securing an airway.
23. Positioning the _____ for intubation is best accomplished by flexing first and then extending it.
24. The acronym for endotracheal.

3 Lethal Arrhythmia Case Studies

- **Ventricular fibrillation and pulseless ventricular tachycardia**
- **Pulseless electrical activity**
- **Asystole**

Often, health care professionals try to memorize each of the following three *lethal arrhythmia* case studies: ventricular fibrillation and pulseless ventricular tachycardia, pulseless electrical activity (PEA), and asystole. Students sometimes think that the best way to retain the information and recall it quickly during an emergency is to memorize it verbatim. This is a mistake. Adults tend to lose short-term memory during stressful situations.

Students are encouraged to look for similarities between these three case studies rather than concentrate on memorizing each independently. Similarities include the following:

- Because each is pulseless, cardiopulmonary resuscitation (CPR) is appropriate.
- Each requires an in-depth primary and secondary assessment, which includes a search for arrest.
- All three have similar etiologies.
- An intravenous lifeline and intubation are instituted in all three.
- Epinephrine is required in all three cases because its vasoconstricting properties allow CPR to be more effective at perfusing both the cerebral and coronary arteries.
- Sodium bicarbonate should be considered in all three whenever an arrest etiology reflects a preexisting bicarbonate responsive situation (e.g., hyperkalemia, aspirin overdose, tricyclic antidepressant overdose).
- Atropine should be administered in any case study in which vagal domination is suspected.

The main difference between the ventricular fibrillation and pulseless ventricular tachycardia protocol and the other two protocols is that the ventricular fibrillation/pulseless ventricular tachycardia protocol is targeted at stopping the fibrillating myocardium by using electrical therapy. Along with defibrillation, the ventricles are extremely irritable; therefore, ventricular tissue-responsive drugs are administered. These drugs can be remembered as the *l*ittle *p*iggy *b*acks: *l*idocaine, *p*rocainamide, and *b*retylium. Neither asystole nor PEA is associated with an irritable myocardium; drugs aimed at decreasing irritability (ventricular antiarrhythmic agents) are not used in these two situations.

In conclusion, look for the therapies that all three share while giving thought to how they differ, rather than attempting to memorize each protocol individually.

Case Studies 2 and 3

Ventricular Fibrillation and Pulseless Ventricular Tachycardia

Because both rhythms represent a myocardium with no organized depolarization, hence no contraction, regardless of which rhythm presents itself, both are treated the same. This case study covers initial defibrillation and subsequent medication therapy.

Section 1: Critical Actions for Student Evaluation

The ACLS instructor checklists for case studies 2 and 3 are shown in Tables 3-1 and 3-2. These forms were designed to guide the faculty when evaluating participants during these particular stations. Refer to them frequently as you read the lecture that follows. *Do not memorize them.* The forms are included only to: (1) show you what the American Heart Association (AHA) considers important during these particular case studies; (2) describe what the faculty are trying to cover in the stations; and (3) provide a summary of the case studies after you have read the lecture.

Table 3-1.
Case Study 2: Ventricular Fibrillation and Pulseless Ventricular Tachycardia

Critical Action	Completed	Not Completed	Comments
Universal algorithm steps			
ABCD survey			
Initiates CPR			
Calls for help			
Calls for defibrillator (AED)			
Delivers shocks			
Appropriate levels			
Defibrillation safety			
Maintains airway and ventilations			
Reassesses for pulse and breathing			
If pulse, checks blood pressure			
Postresuscitation management			

(Reproduced with permission. *Instructor's manual for advanced cardiac life support,* 1997 © Copyright American Heart Association, pp. 6–9.)

Table 3-2.
Case Study 3: Mega Ventricular Fibrillation: Refractory Ventricular Fibrillation and Ventricular Tachycardia

Critical Action	Completed	Not Completed	Comments
Performs ABCs			
Frequent reassessment			
Attaches ECG monitor			
Recognizes ECG rhythms			
Ventricular fibrillation			
Pulseless ventricular tachycardia			
Directs resuscitation effort			
Delivers countershocks			
Sequence OK			
Energy level OK			
Administers drugs			
Resumes shocks after drug administration (rapidly)			
Demonstrates ALS/BLS interface			
Performs IV access			
Attempts intubation			
Proper sequence of pharmacologic agents			
Reassesses patient frequently			
Troubleshoots problems			

(Reproduced with permission. *Instructor's manual for advanced cardiac life support,* 1997 © Copyright American Heart Association, pp. 6–10.)

Section 2: ACLS Algorithm for Ventricular Fibrillation and Pulseless Ventricular Tachycardia

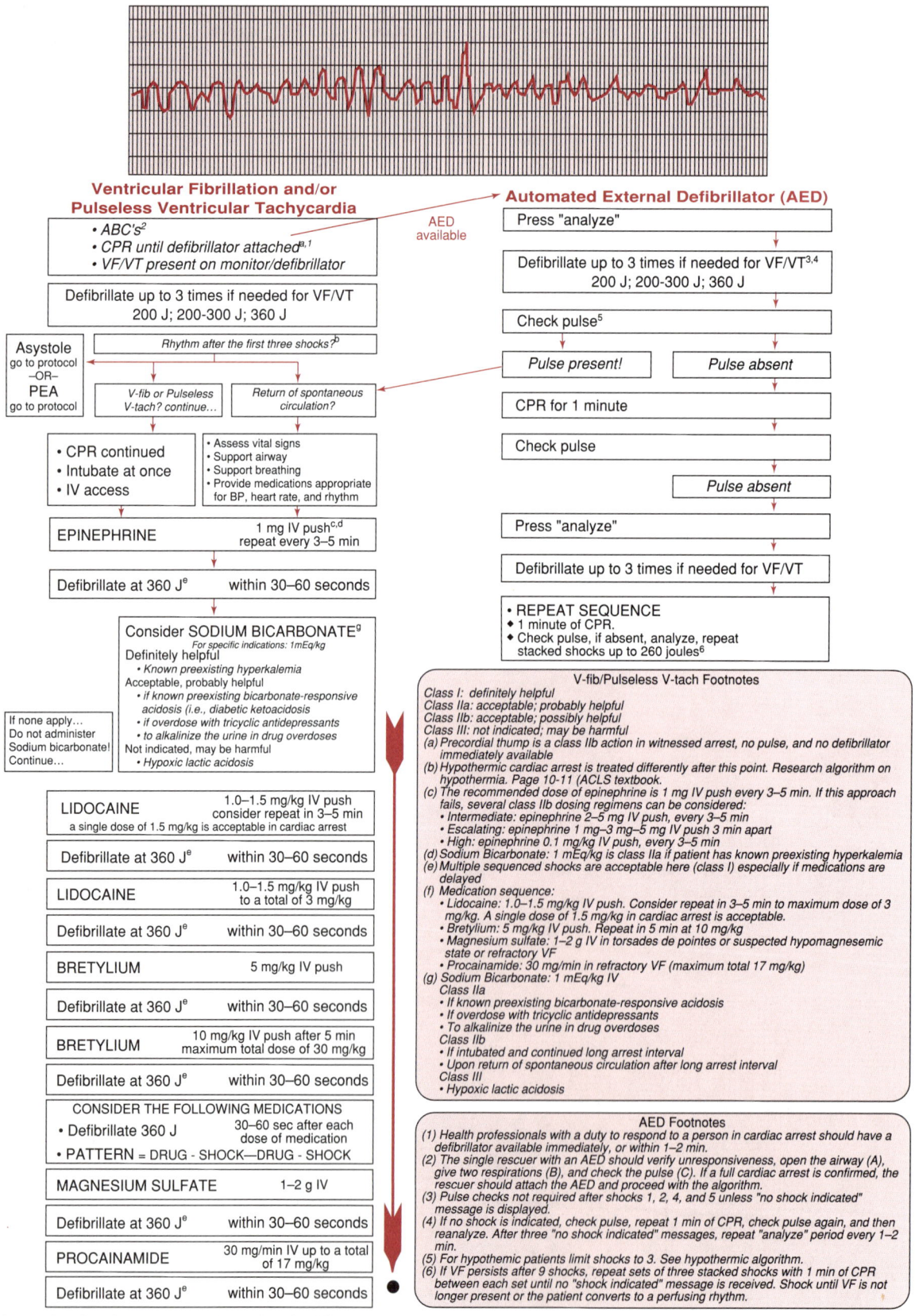

(Reproduced with permission. *Advanced cardiac life support.* Copyright 1997, American Heart Association.)

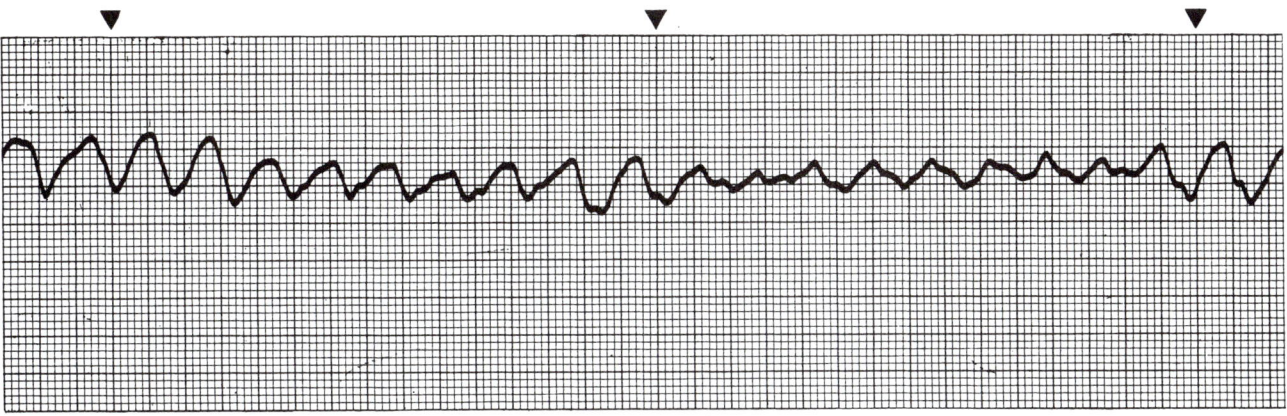

Figure 3-1. Ventricular fibrillation.

Section 3: Identifying Features

Ventricular Fibrillation

Ventricular fibrillation is the most common cause of death in patients with coronary artery disease. The rhythm may be triggered by premature ventricular contractions or by a run of ventricular tachycardia, but may occur spontaneously without any predisposing symptoms. The heart is not responding in any coordinated fashion; hence, there is no associated pulse.

The large number of ectopic pacemakers results in a chaotic, spiked electrocardiogram (ECG) with no specific, observable QRS complexes. The wave deflections vary in height, size and shape. The ECG may appear as in Figure 3-1, with coarse spikes, or it may simply oscillate slightly up and down in an apparently random fashion known as *fine ventricular fibrillation*.

Pulseless Ventricular Tachycardia

Ventricular tachycardia is caused by an ectopic ventricular pacemaker. Because there is generally only one ectopic cell, the rhythm usually fires regularly at a rate between 100 and 250 beats/minute. The ECG appears as a succession of wide QRS complexes. The sinus node may be firing, but it is not initiating the ventricular complex. Any P waves that may evidence themselves are usually obscured by the ventricular beats.

Assuming there is no pulse, ventricular tachycardia is treated like ventricular fibrillation; however, if the patient has a pulse, the cardiac output may be poor to decent. If the ventricular tachycardia has a measurable cardiac output, treat the rhythm with the tachycardia protocol—either stable or unstable, depending on the symptoms (Fig. 3-2).

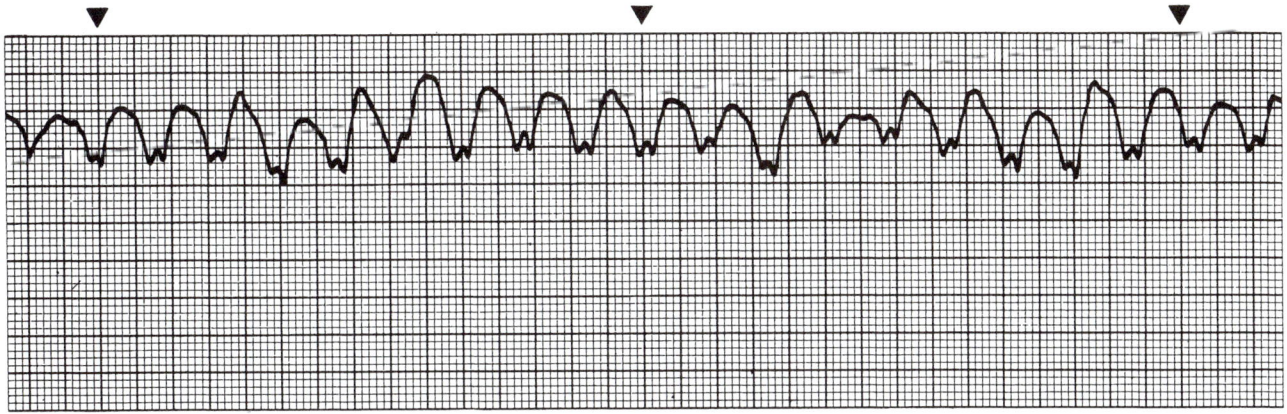

Figure 3-2. Pulseless ventricular tachycardia.

Section 4: Assessment

Primary Assessment

Any assessment should begin with the primary survey noted in the AHA's universal algorithm: the ABCDs—Airway, Breathing, Circulation, and whether or not Defibrillation should be performed. All thoughts about differential diagnoses and possible etiologies leading to the arrest (part of the secondary survey) should be put on hold until the primary survey and any specific life-saving modalities have been instituted. The entire procedure, with the possible exception of defibrillation, should not take more than a few seconds. Always progress in order—ABCD—do not jump to chest compressions when the airway has not been secured. After determining unresponsiveness, activate emergency medical services (EMS), call for a defibrillator, or both.

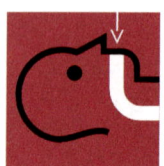

AIRWAY

Immediately inspect the airway. If the airway is open, move on to breathing; however, if there is an obvious obstruction (e.g., chin to chest, blood or vomitus, massive upper airway trauma), correct the problem before moving to breathing by a finger sweep or suctioning. It does not make any difference if the patient is apneic if the airway is occluded. Remember, if trauma is suspected, open the airway with a jaw-thrust maneuver (Fig. 3-3) rather than the spine-compromising, head-tilt and chin-lift technique (Fig. 3-4).

Only after deciding that the airway appears open should you "look, listen, and feel" for breathing attempts. If the patient is adequately ventilating, move to C for circulation. If, however, the patient is apneic or the rate, volume, or effectiveness of the breathing attempts is unacceptable, immediately place an oropharyngeal airway. If this is not *immediately* available, just use the appropriate chin or jaw positioning until you enter the advanced airway portion of the secondary survey.

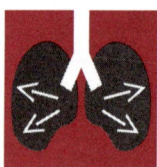

BREATHING

If necessary, attempt to ventilate with a pocket face mask, barrier device, bag-valve-mask (BVM), or demand valve. Give two ventilations spread out over 2 to 4 seconds. This accomplishes two goals: it gives adequate time for the patient to exhale, and discourages forceful breaths that might exceed the esophageal opening pressure, resulting in gastric distention (Fig. 3-5). If other professional health care providers are available, pressure on the cricoid (Sellick's maneuver) during ventilation (mouth-to-mask or BVM) will occlude the esophagus, inhibiting air movement into the stomach and decreasing the chance of aspiration. Readjust the airway if the patient still does not ventilate.

Remember, do not go on to C for circulation if you cannot secure the airway and provide adequate ventilation. Keep trying until you find the problem, and do not proceed further until it is corrected.

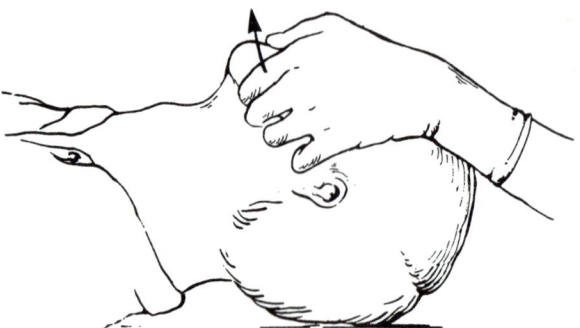

Figure 3-3. The jaw-thrust technique. The hands are placed on either side of the head. The fingers grasp behind the angle of the jaw, bringing it forward, as shown by the *arrow*. (Jones, S.A., et al. [1992] *Advanced emergency care.* Philadelphia: Lippincott-Raven.)

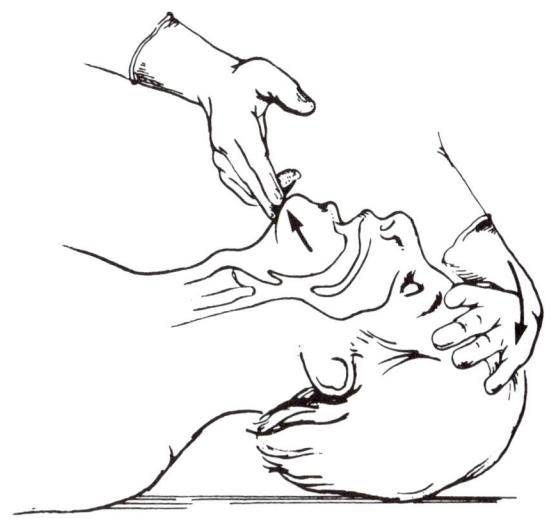

Figure 3-4. The head-tilt and chin-lift technique. The head is tilted backward with one hand (*downward arrow*), while the fingers of the other hand lift the chin forward (*upward arrow*). (Jones, S.A., et al. [1992]. *Advanced emergency care.* Philadelphia: Lippincott-Raven.)

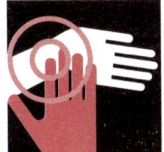

CIRCULATION

After airway and breathing have been secured, check for a carotid pulse. A slow, rapid, or irregular pulse may be difficult to detect; therefore, check the pulse for at least 5 to 10 seconds. If a pulse is present, evaluate its perfusion. If the pulse is absent, begin basic CPR while considering how close the nearest monitor-defibrillator is. It you can reasonably run, bring back a defibrillator, and deliver a shock all within 2 minutes, leave your patient and do so. If the time interval is greater than 2 minutes, continue CPR and call for a defibrillator to be brought to you.

Cardiopulmonary resuscitation should always be started whenever there is no medical or legal reason to withhold it. To prove negligence, the lawyers must prove that the provider failed to act when he should have or administered an improper action. In addition, they must prove that an injury was caused and that there was a definite cause-and-effect relationship between the act and the provider.

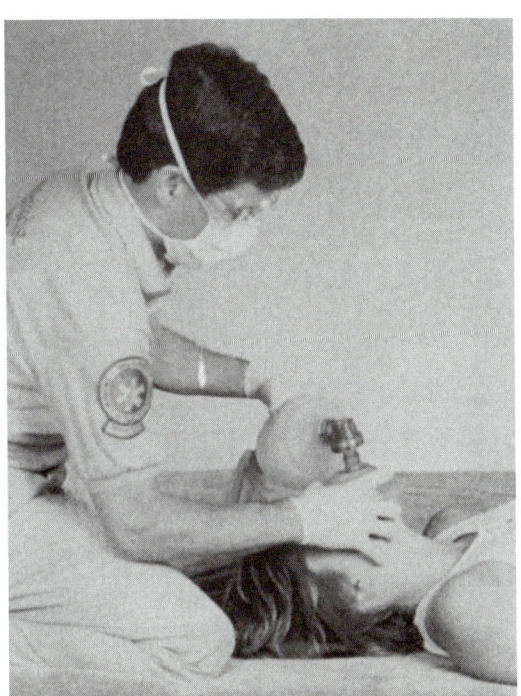

Figure 3-5. Technique for bag-valve-mask ventilation with one health professional. (Jones, S.A., et al. [1992]. *Advanced emergency care.* Philadelphia: Lippincott-Raven.)

DEFIBRILLATION

The last portion of the primary survey, D, stands for defibrillation applicability. A pulseless patient can have only one of the following four rhythms:

- Asystole
- PEA
- Ventricular fibrillation
- Pulseless ventricular tachycardia

In the past, it was common to defibrillate any pulseless rhythm to "stimulate" the heart, assuming that defibrillation could not make it any worse. It is now appreciated that defibrillation does not stimulate the heart; rather, it depolarizes the myocardium, effectively stopping all activity. The prefix *de-* means to remove; *defibrillate* means to remove fibrillation. Therefore, if the rhythm is not fibrillating, there is no need to defibrillate it.

Of the three possible rhythms, the most common initial rhythm in a cardiac arrest is ventricular fibrillation. Research has revealed that most adults (more than 90% in some studies) who have been successfully resuscitated from a sudden nontraumatic cardiac arrest were resuscitated from ventricular fibrillation. The success rate of retrieval is incredibly time dependent.

Success in inducing a viable rhythm is highly dependent on a sufficient amount of high-energy phosphates in the myocardium. Fibrillation decreases these amounts much faster than normal rhythms; hence, the longer someone stays in ventricular fibrillation, the less is the likelihood of success. In fact, studies show that if a patient in ventricular fibrillation has not been shocked within 10 minutes of the arrest, the probability of a successful outcome approaches zero. Research has also shown that rapidly delivered successive countershocks are much more vital to success than standard drug therapy than was previously thought. This is a point to reiterate: *timely defibrillation is more important than most ventricular fibrillation drug therapies.*

▼ *Helpful Hints* for Reducing Resistance to Electric Current

To cease the fibrillatory process, a massive discharge of electrical current is propelled across the thorax through the chest muscle, bone, and sinew. The resistance to this flow of current is referred to as *transthorax impedance.* Anything that the clinician can do to reduce the chest's impedance to the current will increase the chances of success. Reduction of impedance can be accomplished by:

▼ Using liberal conductive medium

▼ Using at least 25 pounds of paddle pressure

▼ Executing the stack of shocks quickly with only minimal time in between (no pulse checks)

   The first shock polarizes the body, reducing the chest's impedance. If the second and third shocks are delivered quickly, the resistance is kept low, maximizing chances of success.

▼ Increasing the joules with each successive shock

▼ Using proper paddle placement

Place the paddles where the flow of current will be maximized across the myocardium—the "sternal" paddle just beneath the right clavicle, lateral to the sternum.

Place the "apex" paddle to the left of the nipple at the left mid-axillary line. If the apex paddle is placed too anteriorly on the chest (i.e., over the apex), the current flow will cross only the anterior surface of the myocardium (the right ventricle), missing the left ventricle.

Manual Defibrillator. When noting the absence of a pulse, use a standard manual defibrillator (Fig. 3-6A) to defibrillate an adult patient starting at 200 joules; if necessary, progressing to 200 to 300 joules; and ultimately, if required, progressing to 360 joules. Pediatric settings are 2 joules/kg initially, and subsequent shocks are 4 joules/kg. Place the paddles over the mid-axilla just lateral to the left nipple and the right sternal border inferior to the clavicle. The paddles can also be attached just to the left of the sternum anteriorly and to the left of the spine posteriorly (see Fig. 3-6B).

Check the monitor after each countershock to determine if the initial ventricular fibrillation pattern has changed. Recharging the defibrillator to the next energy level should begin immediately after each discharge to decrease the time necessary to deliver the next shock.

Although this is an obvious break with tradition, there is no need for interim pulse checks. If a health professional documents ventricular fibrillation initially on the monitor with a pulse check, and finds after shocking that the rhythm is unchanged then it is ventricular fibrillation, and a pulse check is superfluous. Unnecessary delay while checking pulses between the second and the third shocks was determined to be detrimental.

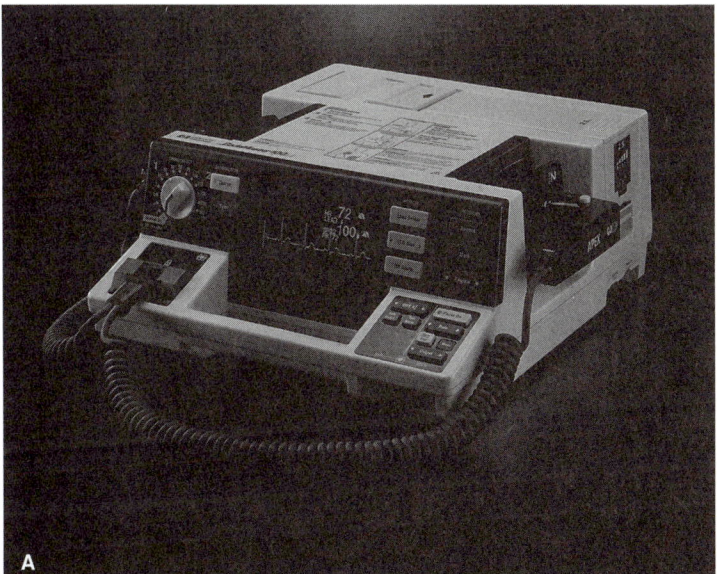

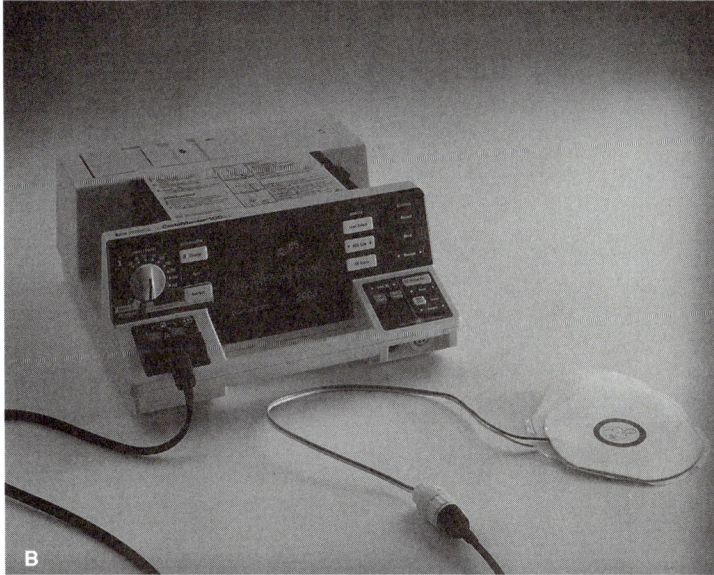

Figure 3-6. (*A*) Standard manual debrillator. The HP CodeMaster 100 Defibrillator/Monitor with pacing, SpO$_2$, and synchronized cardioversion. (*B*) HP shocking through pads—hands-off technique. (Photograph courtesy of Hewlett-Packard Company.)

A phrase to clear the team safely is, "clear the head, clear the feet, clear the head, clear me!" but any phrase that accomplishes this goal is acceptable. The defibrillator team member should clear the head twice because respiratory personnel may not have heard or may be experiencing difficulty removing the BVM from the endotracheal tube adapter. Check for a pulse after all three shocks *or* at any point that the rhythm changes from ventricular fibrillation.

Automated External Defibrillators. Once the province only of health care providers, defibrillation has extended beyond ACLS-trained personnel. With the use of automated external defibrillators (AEDs), basic life support (BLS) personnel, with significantly less training, can quickly deliver the necessary shock sequence before the arrival of EMS personnel. The AED is attached to the patient through adhesive pads similar to pacemaker pads. The placement of the pads is the same as for a manual defibrillator, but they may also be placed to the left of the patient's sternum anteriorly and to the left of hte spine posteriorly. The pads not only deliver the shock but also act as the monitor electrodes for the machine's rhythm input. The AED is technologically sophisticated and can be trusted to differentiate ventricular fibrillation from artifact. Note, however, that any patient movement resulting from CPR, starting an intravenous line, or the vibration from riding in an ambulance may interrupt the machine in the middle of its *analyze* cycle. The machine interprets any movement or vibration as a living patient moving around; thus, do not touch the patient while the machine is in the analyze mode.

There are two main types of AEDs: the fully automated and semiautomated. For the fully automated machine, the simple act of turning it on is sufficient for the machine to diagnose the presence or absence of ventricular fibrillation and, if necessary, charge, clear, and shock the patient without further input from the rescuer. Given the time dependency of successful resuscitation from ventricular fibrillation, this device will save a tremendous number of lives. The AHA advocates that all ACLS providers become familiar with this type of defibrillator and its associated protocol because these devices are being used in hospitals and in lay rescuer units with increasing frequency.

Although the automated models are on the market, the semiautomated models are less expensive and, hence, more prevalent. The semiautomated model requires the operator to push an *analyze* button. The machine checks the rhythm, giving its best advice (whether to deliver or withhold a shock); however, it is necessary for the operator to push the *shock* button to deliver the electricity (Fig. 3-7).

The protocol is to perform CPR while the AED is placed on the patient:

1. Stop CPR and check a pulse.
2. Push analyze button.

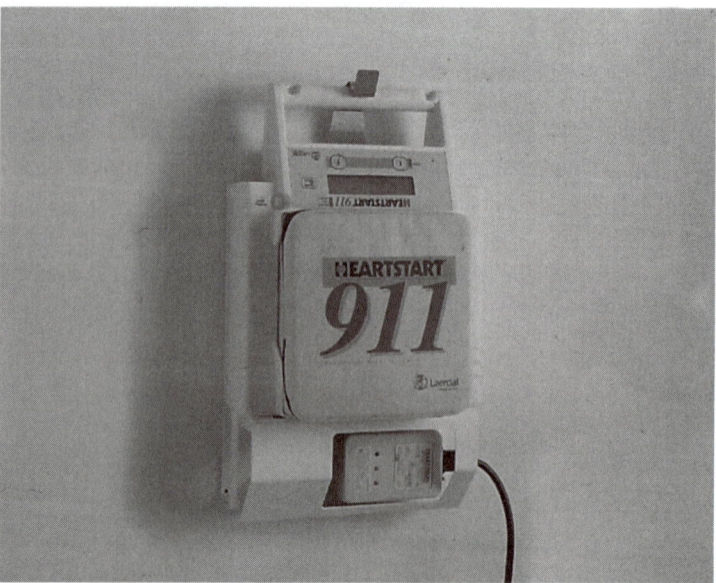

Figure 3-7. Laerdal Heartstart 911 Automated External Defibrillator. (Photograph courtesy of Laerdal Medical Corporation.)

3. Recite "clear" phrase to remove bystanders.
4. Push shock to defibrillate starting at 200 joules, progressing if necessary to 200 to 300 joules, and if required finishing at 360 joules. Push the analyze button again between the first and second shock. As in manual defibrillation, interim pulse checks are not required.
5. After the third shock, check a pulse; if no pulse, perform CPR for 60 seconds. If you only have BLS capability, deliver a "stack" of three shocks every 1 to 2 minutes, with 1 minute of CPR in between, until the machine registers "no shock indicated" or the patient presents with a perfusing rhythm.
6. If you have ACLS capabilities, you can use the AED to shock, or switch over to a manual defibrillator and continue the standard ACLS treatment protocol. In the event that an ACLS provider arrives at the scene to take control, or the AED group arrives at the hospital, do not interrupt in the middle of an AED stacked shock sequence. Take control only after all three stacked shocks have been performed.

Secondary Survey

Only after the primary survey is completed, life-saving maneuvers are instituted, and CPR is begun should the secondary survey—appropriately again called the ABCDs—be performed.

To differentiate between the two sets of ABCDs, the secondary set is referred to as AA, BB, CC, and DD. Luckily, they stand for the same terms as in the primary survey, but at a more advanced level.

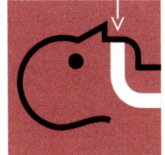

ADVANCED AIRWAY

AA stands for a more *a*dvanced *a*irway—an endotracheal tube. Although intubation is strongly encouraged at this point, use common sense. As long as the airway is secured by other methods (oropharyngeal airway and a BVM in conjunction with cricoid pressure) and acceptable ventilations are being delivered, do not hastily attempt to intubate until you are sufficiently prepared. Initiate an intravenous line in the meantime. Only when you are adequately prepared should you attempt intubation.

Hyperventilate the patient while preparing the equipment, and suction if necessary. Make certain that your attempt does not exceed 30 seconds from ventilation to ventilation. If you are not successful, quickly hyperventilate before making another attempt. After tube placement, listen over the abdomen first to verify that the tube was not placed in the esophagus. Then verify adequate lung sounds by auscultating both lungs during ventilation with a positive-pressure device such as a BVM. Make certain that the lung fields are being inflated equally and that both the rate and the depth are appropriate. Before moving on, make certain that an oropharyngeal airway is inserted next to the tube to protect it and the entire apparatus secured in place. Ensure 100% input with a BVM using an oxygen reservoir coupled with a flow of oxygen of between 12 to 15 liters/minute. Make it a policy to reevaluate airway and breathing on a consistent basis throughout the code because hypoxia can exacerbate the treatment of ventricular fibrillation. Adequate oxygenation, in conjunction with proper epinephrine administration, facilitates myocardial response to defibrillation.

> During any emergency, anything that can go wrong will go wrong.

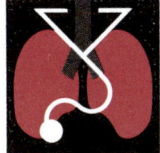

BEWARE BLINDERS

After the advanced airway has been instituted and adequate ventilation verified, consider BB for *b*eware *b*linders. This segment is not a repeat of AA, when breath sounds were verified. It is a combination quick mini-thorax examination and patient history thought pattern. BB reminds the health professional to assess specifically the thorax for any adventitious sounds, such as rales, rhonchi, and wheezing. Checking for those sounds while assessing for muffled heart tones, subcutaneous emphysema, jugular venous distention, and tracheal deviation may be neglected in the chaos of initiating basic life support. Their presence, however, may highlight etiologies that had not yet been considered. For example, if the BB assessment revealed bilateral rales and rhonchi, large amounts of intravenous fluids might be contraindicated. Additionally, if signs of jugular distention were noted, a more in-depth assessment for a possible tension pneumothorax or cardiac tamponade would be in order.

If the history revealed that the patient was a diabetic, cardiac resuscitation would include dextrose or insulin. Likewise, if it revealed that the patient had a preexisting acidosis from an aspirin overdose, sodium bicarbonate would be administered near the beginning of the protocol rather than at the end.

Do not treat BB as simply verifying lung sounds; use it to remember that adequate breathing is not just the presence of equal, bilateral lung excursion. It constitutes a specific assessment for other medical or traumatic pathology that might highlight additional problems or, at the least, point to an etiology of the presenting emergent condition.

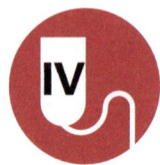

CHOICE CIRCULATION

Only after BB has been completed should the next segment in the secondary survey, CC for *choice circulation*, be considered. CC means to obtain a set of vital signs, initiate an intravenous line, and consider appropriate medications. In a cardiac arrest, the only vital sign that requires mention is the blood pressure.

Historically, clinicians checked for the presence of a pulse during CPR to determine if BLS was effective. Recent research, however, questions this practice. Although the presence of a pulse during CPR does indicate some amount of forward blood flow, it does not give the clinician any information about aortic diastolic or myocardial perfusion pressures.

When scrutinizing the efficacy of the femoral pulse during CPR, it is noted that because the inferior vena cava has no valves, retrograde venous blood flow may be mistakenly taken as a femoral pulse. Capnometry, the measurement of the amount of CO_2 leaving the lungs, also shows promise. Because no reliable criteria assess the adequacy of CPR, the AHA advocates the use of Doppler ultrasound, arterial line measurements, and capnometry rather than solely relying on pulse to determine adequacy of CPR.

Start a peripheral intravenous line with the largest-bore catheter possible using lactated Ringer's or normal saline (NS) solution. The use of D-5-W is discouraged during code situations because high glucose levels may be linked to poor neurologic outcomes. Saline expands the intravascular container better than dextrose solutions and does not appear to cause pulmonary edema as was previously thought. Control the amount of solution by using smaller bags.

The intravenous catheter of choice may be a needle-through-catheter or a catheter-through-needle system, the latter possibly encountering unique complications such as catheter shear. Both systems, however, may easily lead to infection, hematomas, or extravasation. Urgency may preclude strict aseptic technique during insertion. The location of choice is usually the antecubital fossa because it does not interrupt CPR, as do central lines. Central lines have their place, but usually not as the *initial* lifeline in an arrest.

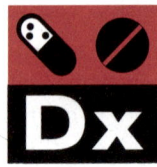

DRUGS AND DIAGNOSIS

The last letters in our secondary survey, DD, provide the mental association to *d*rugs as applicable to *di*agnosis. This is critical. If the patient has not responded after the initial stack of shocks, the patient may have an underlying problem that could be diagnosed and treated if the rescuer takes the time to consider other medical conditions that may have precipitated the arrest. It could be something as simple as volume replacement. Thus, give thought to what could have caused this problem and whether it can be reversed quickly if other treatment modalities are applied (e.g., hyperkalemia, diabetic ketoacidosis).

Although the letters DD help direct the rescuer's thoughts toward the traditional question about what drugs to use in this protocol, the patient would be ill treated if such a narrow course of action were instituted without diligent thought about the reason for the patient's situation. Considering the etiologies of a medical condition is common practice; however, during a cardiac arrest, time is so critical that precipitating events of the arrest may not get the scrutiny they should receive.

Hypothermia

The protocol is altered when encountering a hypothermic patient in ventricular fibrillation. It remains the same up to this point. In the presence of a possible hypothermic condition, however, if after the primary assessment, the resultant three escalating defibrillations are refractory, a temperature should be obtained. If the patient's temperature is above 30°C (86°F), continue with the standard protocol. If the temperature is below 30°C, just continue with CPR; intubate; ventilate with warm, humidified oxygen; and start an intravenous line with warm, NS. Do not continue with defibrillation or perform drug therapy until the core temperature is increased to at least 30°C.

Section 5: Lecture

Treatment

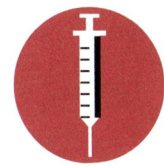

EPINEPHRINE

When considering the possible etiologies of the arrest, it is appropriate to give epinephrine, a class I drug. Studies have shown that no medication has proved superior in improving blood flow, thereby increasing the chance of a favorable outcome. Epinephrine stimulates both α- and β-adrenergic receptors throughout the body. Long revered for its potent β effects (heart and lungs), recent research has demonstrated that its α effects (vasoconstriction) are responsible for the large (up to 15 times) increase in blood flow to the brain and heart during CPR. Thus, it is appropriate to think of epinephrine as making CPR more effective, with the brain and heart profiting from the extra perfusion.

Epinephrine is given every 3 to 5 minutes for the duration of the arrest. After injecting and flushing with 20 mL of NS, raise the extremity containing the intravenous line to enhance delivery. Think of this drug in terms of a stop watch: *regardless of what is going on, when the stop watch ticks past each 3-minute segment, give another dose of epinephrine.*

The standard dose of 1 mg is derived from the dosage given by intracardiac injection in operating rooms. This has carried over to the intravenous dosage. Most medications are based on the patient's weight; however, patients vary in weight, but, within reason, myocardial size does not. Thus, the standard dosage of epinephrine (SDE) advocated by the AHA continues to be 1 mg of a 1:10,000 solution.

A wide variety of studies using high-dose epinephrine (HDE) were presented for review, with some interesting results. In these studies, the rate of patients returned to spontaneous circulation was greater with higher doses of epinephrine; however, the number of these patients who were discharged from the hospital was not significantly different from the number of patients discharged who received the standard 1-mg dose. The data were not conclusive enough to change the standard dose from 1 mg. The AHA, however, did state that, if the clinician chose to use a higher dose of epinephrine after the standard dose had proved refractory, they would neither recommend nor discourage it. Noted HDE dosage regimens are:

Intermediate dose: 2 to 5 mg every 3 to 5 minutes
Escalating dose: 1 mg, then 3 mg, then 5 mg every 3 minutes—"1 mg–3 mg–5 mg"
High dose: 0.1 mg/kg every 3 to 5 minutes

During a cardiac arrest, epinephrine can be given by the intravenous, endotracheal, or intracardiac route. If given endotracheally, the recommended dosage is 2 to 2.5 times the peripheral intravenous dosage diluted in 10 mL of NS. The medication should be introduced as far into the tracheobronchial tree as possible with the assistance of a through-the-needle catheter. Intracardiac injection increases the risk of coronary artery laceration and should be used only during open heart massage or when other routes are not available.

Epinephrine can also be administered during a cardiac arrest through an intravenous drip. This would be easier than having to remember to push the drug at the prescribed times. Put 30 mL of a 1:1000 solution in 250 mL of NS, and run it in at a rate consistent with 1 mg every 3 to 5 minutes, titrating to the desired hemodynamic end-point. Remember, this dilution is only for cardiac arrests; do not confuse it with an epinephrine drip for the treatment of bradycardia because the concentration is 30 times what it should be. Administer the drip by central venous access or a through-the-needle catheter to reduce any problems with extravasation.

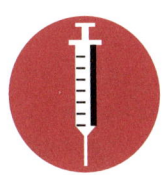

SODIUM BICARBONATE AND MAGNESIUM SULFATE—EARLY ASSESSMENT

During the assessment, if the patient is suspected to have a preexisting hyperkalemia or a preexisting acidosis (diabetic ketoacidosis, aspirin, or tricyclic antidepressant overdose), sodium bicarbonate should be administered as soon as confirmed interventions (e.g., defibrillation, CPR, intubation, ventilation, and more than one trial of epinephrine) have been accomplished. Sodium bicarbonate can be helpful and occasionally life-saving in these situations.

The same is true concerning magnesium sulfate. If the patient is elderly, has signs or symptoms of malnourishment, is a chronic alcoholic, or has a chronic disease process (e.g., chronic obstructive pulmonary disease), consider administering the magnesium sulfate at this juncture rather than waiting until the end of the protocol. Please note the more detailed explanations of each of these two drugs near the end of this case study.

SUBSEQUENT DEFIBRILLATIONS

Timely defibrillation is the single most important modality in treating ventricular fibrillation. After every drug dose, the patient should be defibrillated. In addition, the research data on AEDs point to the fact that defibrillation should be administered about every 1 to 3 minutes and not just after each drug dose. The AHA recommends one shock of 360 joules from this point forward, but notes that because the efficacy of giving a stack of shocks has been proved, it is acceptable to deliver the stack after each drug dose. Do not forget to clear your team before each shock and check for a pulse after each set of shocks.

The AHA's European counterpart—the European Resuscitation Council—advocates four sets of three stacked shocks, with only epinephrine given in between sets. This recommendation indicates that the Council agrees with the AHA in affirming that pharmaceuticals such as lidocaine, procainamide, bretylium, magnesium sulfate, and sodium bicarbonate, previously thought of as highly effective, have not *clearly* been shown to influence the outcome of ventricular fibrillation. The AHA categorizes these medications as acceptable, probably helpful, but not definitely helpful. This information is provided to drive home the point: *health care professionals should give the highest priority to airway ventilation, appropriate CPR, epinephrine administration, and timely defibrillation.*

If the patient has been defibrillated four times, CPR begun, an endotracheal tube placed, an intravenous line started, and a standard dose of epinephrine administered, but is still in ventricular fibrillation, the ventricular fibrillation is considered refractory to initial therapy, and the possibility of successful resuscitation is decreasing.

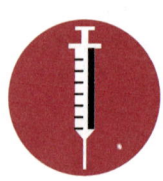

LIDOCAINE

Because the ventricular cells are surrounded by an environment rampant with hypoxia, adrenergic drugs, and acidotic conditions, each cell's fibrillatory threshold is depressed. To elevate the fibrillatory threshold, ventricular antiarrhythmic agents are considered. The antiarrhythmic drug with the fewest side effects is lidocaine, followed closely by bretylium and possibly procainamide.

During ventricular fibrillation, lidocaine is considered a class IIA drug—acceptable, probably helpful—and so is administered at this juncture. The pharmacodynamics of lidocaine are enigmatic and not agreed on by all. Some clinicians believe that two doses of 1.5 mg/kg should be administered with a shock in between. Others recommend a loading dose of 1 to 1.5 mg/kg by intravenous push, repeated with shocks in between in 3 to 5 minutes, with additional doses of 0.5 to 0.75 mg/kg, until a maximum dose of 3 mg/kg is reached. A third group of clinicians believes that one single dose of 1.5 mg/kg is all that is required before moving on to bretylium. Human ventricular fibrillation data are lacking, so any one of these three regimens is both reasonable and acceptable.

If after administration of lidocaine, the patient responds with a viable, perfusing, supraventricular rhythm, it is appropriate to hang a lidocaine drip, 1 g in 250 mL in D-5-W, lactated Ringer's, or NS solution. Start the drip at a rate of 2 to 4 mg/minute (30 to 60 gtt/minute in a micro- or mini-drip). If the patient responds with a ventricular rhythm, withhold the lidocaine because it may decrease automaticity of ventricular pacemakers.

Whatever the lidocaine dosage regimen decided on, shock the patient after each dose. In addition, shock about every 2 to 3 minutes while waiting for successive doses. If lidocaine has been ineffective or ventricular fibrillation or pulseless ventricular tachycardia recurs, take a couple of moments to reassess the endotracheal tube apparatus, quality of ventilations, and efficacy of CPR. Consistent reassessment of the ABCs cannot be stressed enough.

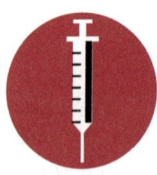

BRETYLIUM

After reevaluating the ABCs and finding that lidocaine was ineffective, consider bretylium. The initial dose is 5 mg/kg given by intravenous bolus. Defibrillate every 2 to 3 minutes while awaiting the dosage interval, and then in 5 minutes repeat bretylium, but at double the dose, or 10 mg/kg. Bretylium can then be repeated two more times at 10 mg/kg at 5- to 30-minute intervals, with defibrillations in between. The initial dose at 5 mg/kg and the other three at 10 mg/kg will maximize the dosage at 30 to 35 mg/kg. Remember that timely defibrillation between giving the drugs is a necessity.

If at any time during the administration of this antifibrillatory agent the patient's vital signs return, consider an immediate maintenance drip of bretylium (1 g in 250 mL of D-5-W, lactated Ringer's, or NS solution) to keep the therapeutic blood level of bretylium stable. Start the infusion at 2 mg/minute

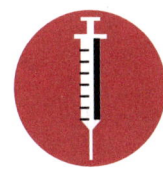

MAGNESIUM SULFATE

After administration of bretylium and subsequent defibrillations, the clinician might think that this would be the time to consider the use of magnesium sulfate. However, magnesium sulfate should have been considered earlier when differential diagnoses were being deliberated (i.e., beware blinders.)

If the patient has a known or suspected hypomagnesemia, is an alcoholic, is elderly, or has a chronic disease, hypomagnesemia should be suspected. Hypomagnesemia can precipitate refractory ventricular fibrillation by interfering with intracellular potassium replacement. Various anecdotal test results are so encouraging, however, that magnesium sulfate is now recommended as a routine prophylactic drug in this protocol.

The dosage is 1 to 2 g given by intravenous push in ventricular fibrillation or pulseless ventricular tachycardia. The drug may be given by diluting 1 g in 10 mL of NS and administering the intravenous push in a cardiac arrest.

Magnesium sulfate is also the treatment of choice in a variation of ventricular tachycardia—torsades de pointes (see case study 9 in Chap. 5).

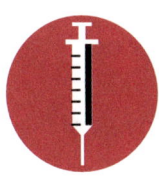

PROCAINAMIDE

Procainamide is the third drug of the antifibrillatory triad. In other protocols, this drug is administered between lidocaine and bretylium. In ventricular fibrillation, however, time is of the essence, and procainamide's inability to be administered quickly resigns this drug to the end of the triad and so is thus rarely administered in a routine arrest.

The dose is 30 mg/minute until a maximum of 17 mg/kg is reached. This means that for an average 70-kg patient, it will take about 40 minutes to administer. Because time is so critical during ventricular fibrillation, consider shocking every 1 to 2 minutes while the procainamide is being administered. Do not wait until the entire maximum dosage is attained before defibrillation.

If at any time during the administration of this antifibrillatory agent the patient's vital signs return, consider an immediate maintenance drip of procainamide (1 g in 250 mL of D-5-W, lactated Ringer's, or NS solution) to keep the therapeutic blood level stable. Start the infusion at 2–4 mg/minute.

Procainamide, like any drug that increases Q-T intervals, is contraindicated in the treatment of torsades de pointes (see case study 9 in Chap. 5).

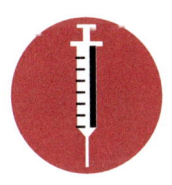

SODIUM BICARBONATE

Sodium bicarbonate was once a routine medication in all cardiac arrest sequences. Since 1986, the AHA has relegated it to a consideration status. However, it is inappropriate to put it out of mind. This drug is classified as *definitely helpful* in the treatment of hyperkalemia. It is also *acceptable, possibly helpful,* in the treatment of the following conditions:

- Known preexisting bicarbonate-responsive acidosis, such as diabetic ketoacidosis
- Tricyclic antidepressant overdoses
- Aspirin overdoses
- To alkalinize the urine in overdoses of drugs such as phenobarbital

When contemplating differential diagnoses, the above clinical states should be considered as possible etiologies in the presenting arrest. If the above etiologies present themselves, sodium bicarbonate should be administered because they represent preexisting acidotic conditions—a metabolic acidosis. If the etiology is found to be metabolic in nature, the dose is 1 mEq/kg. If there are no suspected preexisting bicarbonate-responsive situations, however, sodium bicarbonate is not routinely administered.

On the other hand, the acidosis generated in a routine arrest is generated by retention of carbon dioxide from the patient's failure to breathe. This hypoxic condition is not related to a bicarbonate deficit; it is a failure to remove the carbon dioxide. Thus, in a routine arrest, the etiology of acidosis is respiratory, not metabolic. The mainstay of treatment for acidosis in a routine arrest is hyperventilation in conjunction with appropriate CPR.

Helpful Hints
for Evaluating Refractory Ventricular Fibrillation or Pulseless Ventricular Tachycardia

If at any time a defibrillation results in a successful rhythm, but the rhythm rapidly deteriorates into ventricular fibrillation:

▼ Use common sense and reassesss your ABCs—hypoxia may be the culprit.

▼ Remember that high blood levels of adrenergic agents such as epinephrine may cause tachycardias and increase ventricular automaticity.

▼ If the successful presenting rhythm was a tachycardia before it deteriorated into ventricular fibrillation, withhold epinephrine, especially if you were using the high dosages, and consider the use of β-blockers.

▼ If the successful rhythm was bradycardic, atropine or a transcutaneous pacemaker may be advantageous.

▼ Do not keep defibrillating while giving more and more medications if the rhythm converts initially but rapidly deteriorates. Consider that your drugs or the procedure itself may be precipitating the problem.

▼ Never allow what appears to be a linear ACLS protocol to stop you from considering all of the possibilities and quickly acting on them.

Section 6: Ventricular Fibrillation and Pulseless Ventricular Tachycardia Interim Evaluation

Mark the correct answer.

1. Which of the following drugs should be *considered* in extremely refractory ventricular fibrillation or pulseless ventricular tachycardia (see ACLS text pp. 1–20): (1) magnesium sulfate; (2) sodium bicarbonate; (3) procainamide; (4) morphine sulfate; (5) propranolol? _____

    _____ (a) 1, 3, and 5
    _____ (b) 1, 2, 3, and 5
    _____ (c) 1, 2, and 3
    _____ (d) 2, 4, and 5

2. One should never change the sequence of medications in an ACLS protocol. An example might be giving magnesium sulfate near the beginning of the ventricular fibrillation protocol for a suspected nutritional deficit instead of near the end (see ACLS text pp. 1-4 to 1-20 and pp. 7-14). _____

    _____ (a) True
    _____ (b) False

3. You have arrived at the scene 4 minutes after the cardiac arrest of a 110-pound female. Your monitor-defibrillator displays ventricular fibrillation. There is no pulse. Two rescuers are

performing adequate CPR. A third rescuer has completed an intravenous lifeline. Assuming you have quickly assessed the patient, you would recommend (see ACLS text pp. 1-15 to 1-16): _____

_____ (a) An immediate unsynchronized countershock, up to three times if necessary
_____ (b) Sodium bicarbonate, 100 mEq given by intravenous bolus, and epinephrine 1:10,000, 1 mg given by intravenous bolus, and then defibrillate
_____ (c) Epinephrine 1:10,000, 1 mg given by intravenous bolus, and then administer an unsynchronized countershock
_____ (d) That the patient be oxygenated fully, and perform endotracheal intubation

4. When hooked up to a monitor-defibrillator, a patient is determined to be in pulseless ventricular tachycardia. Which one of the following forms of treatment would you employ initially for this patient (see ACLS text p. 1-17)? _____

_____ (a) Immediate synchronized cardioversion
_____ (b) CPR
_____ (c) Intravenous lidocaine
_____ (d) Immediate defibrillation

5. After delivery of a second ineffective unsynchronized shock of 250 joules in an adult, the next stacked shock should be (see ACLS text pp. 1-15 to 1-17): _____

_____ (a) 100 to 200 joules
_____ (b) 200 to 300 joules
_____ (c) 360 joules
_____ (d) 450 joules

6. Epinephrine has many adrenergic effects. Which one of the following effects serves as the primary reason that it is administered during a cardiac arrest (see ACLS text p. 7-2 to 7-4)? _____

_____ (a) Vasoconstriction (alpha effects)
_____ (b) Increased automaticity (beta effects)
_____ (c) Positive inotropic effects
_____ (d) Positive chronotropic effects

7. The key strategy in the treatment of ventricular fibrillation is (see ACLS text p. 1-15): _____

_____ (a) CPR
_____ (b) Timely defibrillation
_____ (c) Epinephrine administration
_____ (d) Intubation

8. Which of the following represents an ideal situation for an AED to *analyze* a patient properly (see ACLS text pp. 4-8 to 4-14)? _____

_____ (a) Lying in an ambulance moving down the road
_____ (b) While CPR is going on
_____ (c) Lying on the ground with no one touching patient
_____ (d) While attempting to start an intravenous line

9. Automatic defibrillator pads are positioned sternum to apex (see ACLS text p. 4-11). _____

_____ (a) True
_____ (b) False

10. Of the following resuscitative technologies, which is probably going to have the most far-reaching impact for most patients (see ACLS text p. 4-8)? _____

_____ (a) AED
_____ (b) Cryotherapy resuscitation
_____ (c) Surgically implanted defibrillator
_____ (d) External pacemaker capability

11. Sodium bicarbonate therapy (see ACLS text pp. 1-16 to 1-28): (1) may produce metabolic alkalosis; (2) should always be guided by blood gases and pH when available; (3) should only be administered when preexisting bicarbonate-responsive situations are present; (4) is considered class III drug during a hypoxia-related acidosis. _____

    _____ (a) 1, 2, and 3
    _____ (b) 1, 2, and 4
    _____ (c) 2, 3, and 4
    _____ (d) All of the above

12. Present evidence indicates that the recommended first-time dose of epinephrine when injected into the tracheobronchial tree should be (see ACLS text p. 1-10): _____

    _____ (a) 0.5 mg of epinephrine 1:10,000 (5 mL)
    _____ (b) 1.0 mg of 1:10,000 epinephrine (10 mL)
    _____ (c) 2.5 mg. of 1:1000 (2.5 mL)
    _____ (d) 2 to 2.5 mg of 1:1000 epinephrine diluted in NS or distilled water to a total of 10 mL

13. Lidocaine (see ACLS text pp. 7-6 to 7-8): (1) can cause seizures in doses above 3 mg/kg; (2) is frequently given as an initial bolus of 1.5 mg/kg in ventricular fibrillation and repeated at the same dose to a maximum of 3 mg/kg; (3) may be given as a bolus of 1.5 mg/kg (if the rhythm is still refractory, it is acceptable to move directly to the first dose of bretylium); (4) is given as an intravenous infusion at a rate of 1 to 4 mg/minute upon conversion to an idioventricular rhythm. _____

    _____ (a) 2 and 4
    _____ (b) 1, 2, and 3
    _____ (c) 2, 3, and 4
    _____ (d) All the above

14. The main problem when administrating procainamide in refractory ventricular fibrillation is (see ACLS text p. 1-20): _____

    _____ (a) Hypertension
    _____ (b) Excessive length of administration time
    _____ (c) Depression of the fibrillatory threshold
    _____ (d) Increased automaticity

15. In ventricular fibrillation refractory to lidocaine and repeated defibrillation, bretylium is administered in the following dose (see ACLS text p. 1-19): _____

    _____ (a) 10 mg/kg intravenous bolus repeated at 5-minute intervals up to 30 mg/kg
    _____ (b) 10 mg/kg intravenous bolus followed immediately by a continuous infusion at a rate of 5 mg/minute
    _____ (c) 5 mg/kg intravenous bolus, which should not be repeated
    _____ (d) 5 mg/kg intravenous bolus followed by 10 mg/kg in 5 minutes and repeated every 5 minutes to a maximum of 30 to 35 mg/kg

16. Which is the correct way to administer magnesium sulfate when given for ventricular fibrillation or pulseless ventricular tachycardia (see ACLS text p. 1-20)? _____

    _____ (a) 2 g in 500 mL of NS
    _____ (b) 1 mg in 250 mL of NS
    _____ (c) 2 mg/kg in 100 mL of lactated Ringer's solution
    _____ (d) 1 to 2 g diluted in 10 mL of NS and administered by intravenous push

17. The first thing that should be done when encountering a patient with ventricular fibrillation on the monitor but with a palpable pulse is: _____

    _____ (a) Defibrillate immediately with 200 joules
    _____ (b) Administer a precordial thump

_____ (c) Check the ECG leads
_____ (d) Administer a synchronized countershock of 75 joules

18. Which of the following medications are considered class I, *definitely helpful*, in treating ventricular fibrillation? (see ACLS text p. 1-17): (1) magnesium sulfate; (2) epinephrine; (3) oxygen; (4) procainamide? _____

_____ (a) 1 and 2
_____ (b) 2 and 3
_____ (c) 2 and 4
_____ (d) 1 and 4

Section 7
ACLS VENTRICULAR FIBRILLATION AND PULSELESS VENTRICULAR TACHYCARDIA CROSSWORD PUZZLE

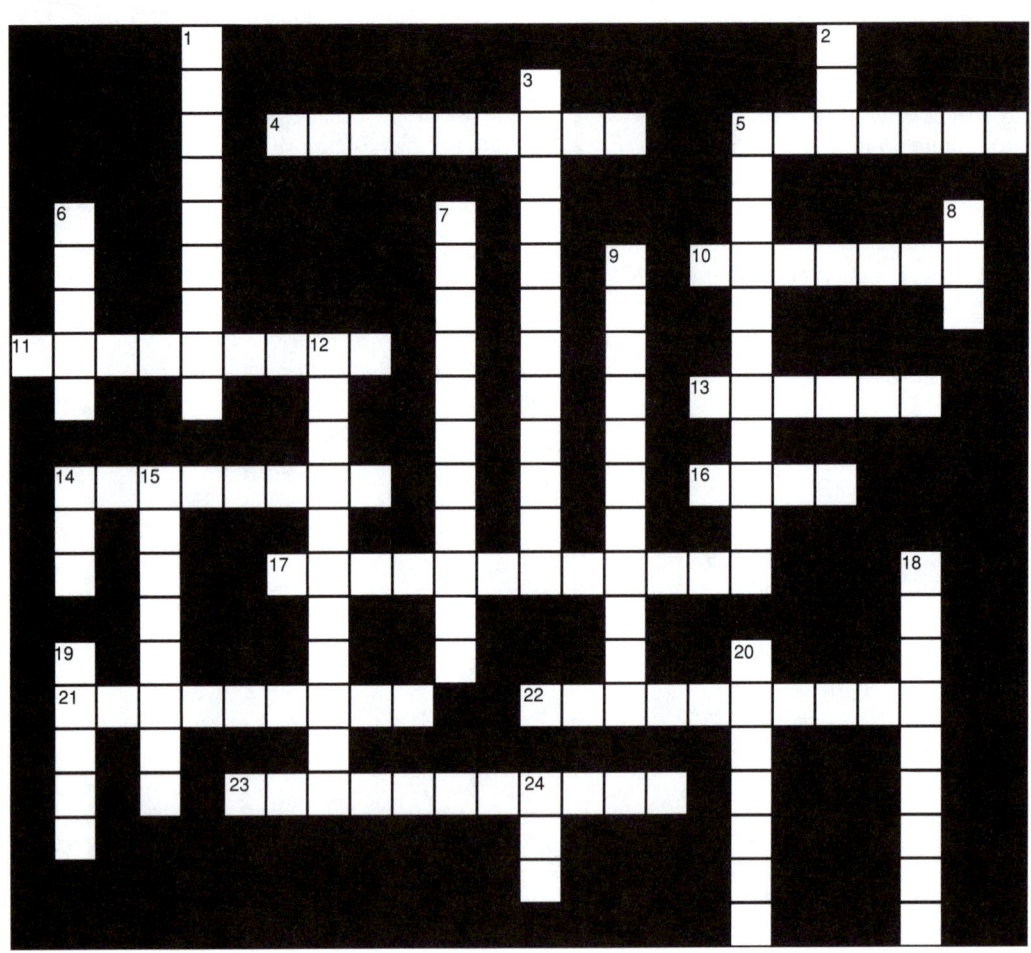

Across

4. This drug is administered immediately if the patient is a long-term alcoholic or presents as apparently malnourished.
5. It is necessary to _____ the extremity containing the intravenous line to assist the introduction of the drug.
10. In a semiautomated external defibrillator, the patient should not be touched or moved during the _____ cycle (the button that is pressed to allow the machine to check the rhythm).
11. _____ ventricular tachycardia is treated the same as ventricular fibrillation (a condition devoid of a heartbeat).
13. No more than _____ to sixty seconds of CPR should follow after administering a drug before defibrillating (number is spelled out).
14. This ECG disturbance is caused by 60-cycle interference (the term ascribing to interference on the monitor).
16. Ventricular fibrillation should be shocked within the first 10 minutes because this protocol is incredibly _____ dependent.
17. Administration of this *considered* medication is rare in most ventricular fibrillations because it takes so long to reach a therapeutic blood level. This drug also increases Q-T intervals.
21. The maximum dose of this drug is 3 mg/kg.
22. Light paddle pressure increases _____ to the flow of defibrillating current (the impedance exerted by the muscle, bone, and sinew to electrical current).
23. This term refers to a class of acidosis that occurs before an arrest and that might be responsive to bicarbonate administration (a general term meaning that the condition was present *before* the arrest).

Down

1. The resistance to flow of defibrillating current will be _____ if the time is taken to check pulses during a set of stacked shocks.
2. The standard milligram dose of epinephrine (the number is spelled out).
3. High-energy phosphates are used up rapidly during ventricular _____ (a condition in which ventricular cells are firing off in an uncoordinated fashion).
5. This drug makes CPR more effective by increasing perfusion to brain and heart.
6. The manner in which all drugs are administered in a cardiac arrest (an older term describing a drug being forced quickly into an intravenous line).
7. This drug assists in driving potassium back into the cell in hyperkalemia.
8. Decrease the transthoracic impedance (resistance) by using a conductive medium such as _____ (rubbed on the paddles).
9. Cardiac _____ are known to result from tricyclic antidepressant overdoses (cardiac rhythm irregularities).
12. The _____ switch should be turned off during defibrillation (the button to push to deliver a shock only on the down slope of an R wave).
14. Acronym denoting the class of automatic defibrillator.
15. Procainamide should not be given in this variation of ventricular tachycardia (this variation is treated with magnesium sulfate or pacemaker override).
18. Lidocaine, procainamide, and bretylium elevate the ventricular fibrillation _____ (the amount of energy necessary to make a cell depolarize).
19. _____ the intravenous tubing with 20 mL of NS to assist in the introduction of the drug.
20. _____ shocks are the key strategy in AEDs (a shock placed right on top of another).
24. The dosage of magnesium sulfate is one to _____ grams intravenous bolus (number is spelled out).

Case Study 4
Pulseless Electrical Activity

Although it has a high mortality rate, rapid assessment and aggressive intervention when encountering PEA may result in a successful resuscitation. This case study demonstrates that an ECG on the monitor does not necessarily imply that the patient has a pulse. Said succinctly: *check the patient, not the monitor*.

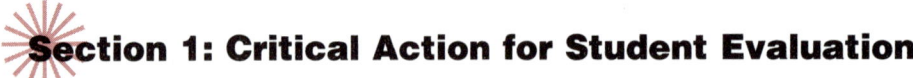

Section 1: Critical Action for Student Evaluation

The ACLS Instruction checklist for case study 4 is show in Table 3-3. This form was designed to guide the faculty when evaluating participants during this particular station. Refer to it frequently as you read the lecture that follows. *Do not memorize it*. The form is only included to: (1) show you what the AHA considers important during this particular case study; (2) describe what the faculty are trying to cover in the station; and (3) provide a summary of the case study after you have read the lecture.

Table 3-3.
Case Study 4: Pulseless Electrical Activity

Critical Action	Completed	Not Completed	Comments
Universal algorithm			
Initiates CPR			
Attaches and operates monitor			
Directs intubation			
Obtains IV access			
Assesses cause			
Pharmacologic support			
Volume expansion if necessary			

(Reproduced with permission. *Instructor's manual for advanced cardiac life support,* 1997 © Copyright American Heart Association, p. 6-11.)

Section 2: ACLS Algorithm for Pulseless Electrical Activity

Pulseless Electrical Activity (PEA)

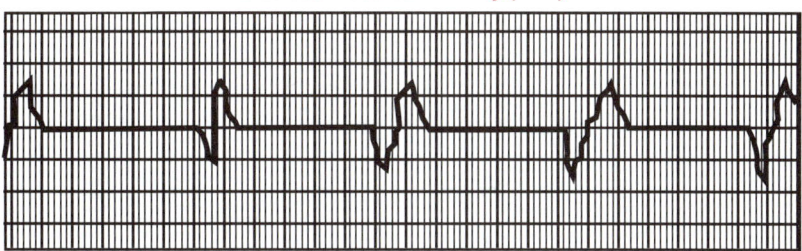

Electromechanical Dissociation (EMD)

Includes
- Electromechanical dissociation (EMD)
- Pseudo-EMD
- Idioventricular rhythms
- Ventricular escape rhythms
- Bradyasystolic rhythms
- Postdefibrillation idioventricular rhythms

- CPR continued
- Intubate at once
- IV access
- Assess blood flow
- (Doppler ultrasound, end-tidal CO_2, (echocardiography, or arterial line)

Consider Possible Causes
(Parenthesis = possible therapies and treatments)
- Hypovolemia (volume infusion)
- Hypoxia (ventilation)
- Hyperkalemia (bicarbonate)
- Tension pneumothorax (needle decompression)
- Hypothermia (see ACLS hypothermia algorithm
- Acidosis[b] (bicarbonate)
- Cardiac tamponade (pericardiocentesis)
- Massive pulmonary embolism (surgery, thrombolytics)
- Massive acute myocardial infarction (see algorithm)
- Drug overdose such as tricyclics, digitalis, beta-blockers, calcium-channel blockers

---

EPINEPHRINE[a,c]   1 mg IV push, repeat 3—5 min

Consider SODIUM BICARBONATE
For specific indications: 1 mEq/kg
Definitely helpful
- Known preexisting hyperkalemia

Acceptable, probably helpful
- If known preexisting bicarbonate-responsive acidosis (i.e., diabetic ketoacidosis)
- If overdose with tricyclic antidepressants
- To alkalinize the urine in drug overdoses

Acceptable, possibly helpful
- If intubated and continued long arrest interval
- Upon return of spontaneous circulation after long arrest interval

Not indicated, may be harmful
- Hypoxic lactic acidosis

ATROPINE[d]   If absolute bradycardia (< 60 beats/min) or relative bradycardia 1 mg IV push repeat every 3—5 min, to a total of 0.03—0.04 mg/kg

---

PEA Footnotes

Class I: definitely helpful
Class IIa: acceptable; probably helpful
Class IIb: acceptable; possibly helpful
Class III: not indicated; may be harmful

(a) Sodium Bicarbonate: 1 mEq/kg:
Class II
- If patient has known preexisting hyperkalemia

(b) Sodium Bicarbonate: 1 mEq/kg:
Class IIa
- If known preexisting bicarbonate-responsive acidosis
- If overdose with tricyclic antidepressants
- To alkalinize the urine in drug overdoses

Class IIb
- If intubated and continued long arrest interval
- Upon return of spontaneous circulation after long arrest interval

Class III
- Hypoxic lactic acidosis

(c) The recommended dose of epinephrine is 1 mg IV push every 3—5 min. If this approach fails, several Class IIb dosing regimens can be considered:
- Intermediate epinephrine 3—5 mg IV push, every 3—5 min
- Escalating: epinephrine 1 mg—3 mg—5 mg IV push, 3 min apart
- High: epinephrine 0.1 mg/kg IV push, every 3—5 min

(d) The shorter atropine dosing interval (3 min) is possibly helpful in cardiac arrest (Class 11b)

(Reproduced with permission. Advanced cardiac life support. Copyright 1997, American Heart Association.)

Section 3: Identifying Features

Pulseless Electrical Activity

Pulseless electrical activity may present with any pulseless ECG rhythm that is not asystole, ventricular fibrillation, or ventricular tachycardia. This rhythm is sinus tachycardia, but without a pulse (Fig. 3-8).

In Figure 3-9, the rhythm is identified as a sinus bradycardia with a second-degree, type II atrioventricular block with a slow ventricular response. Because there is no pulse, but should be, it is PEA.

The rhythm in Figure 3-10 is formally known as a secondary ventricular standstill. It has no sinus beats, and the ventricular response is less than 30 beats/minute. This is an interesting rhythm because a clinician can make a case for treating this pulseless rhythm as either asystole or PEA. Because the drugs are the same, differing only with consideration of a transcutaneous pacemaker (TCP) in the protocol, it is a moot point.

The point to reiterate is: any pulseless rhythm that does not present as asystole, ventricular fibrillation, or ventricular tachycardia should be considered PEA and treated as such.

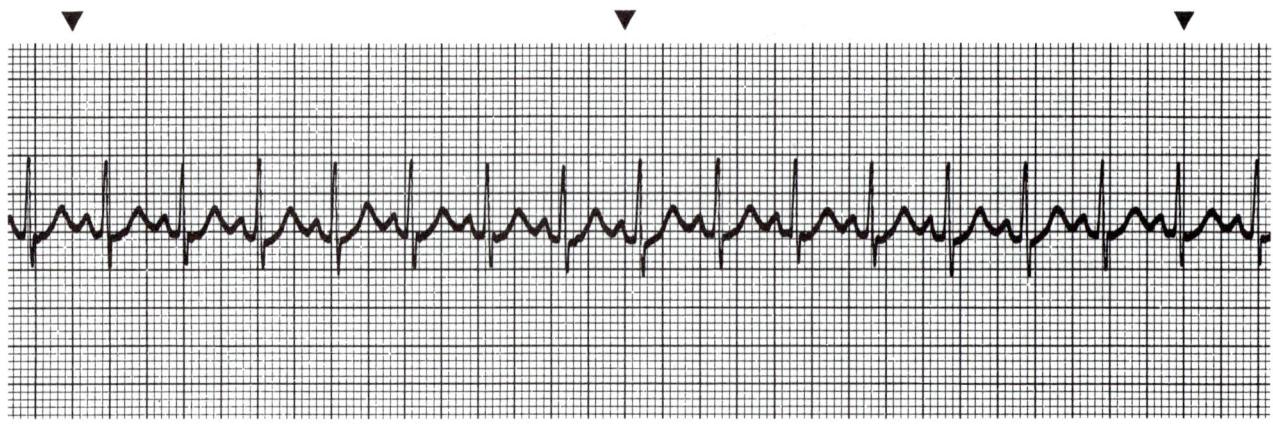

Figure 3-8. A rhythm masquerading as pulseless electrical activity.

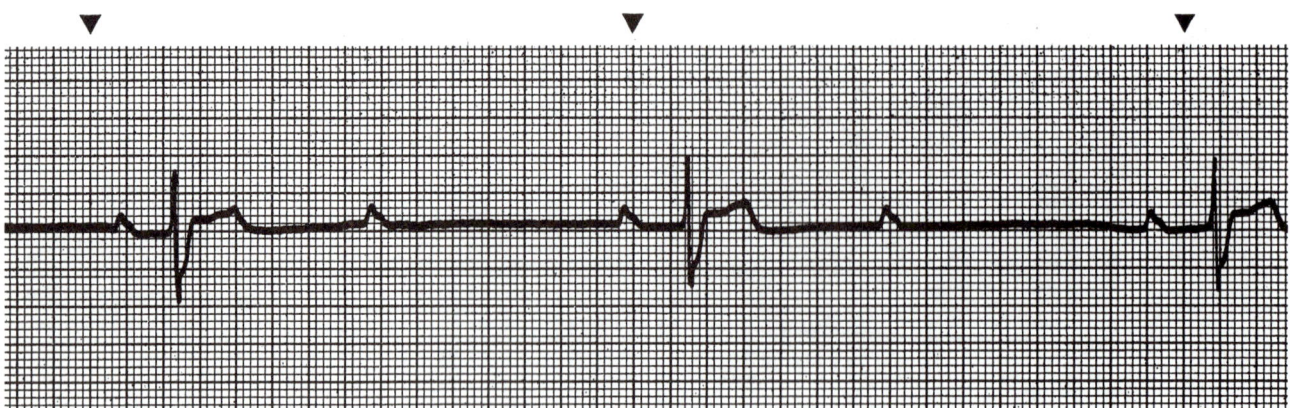

Figure 3-9. A rhythm masquerading as pulseless electrical activity.

Chapter 3 Lethal Arrhythmia Case Studies • Pulseless Electrical Activity

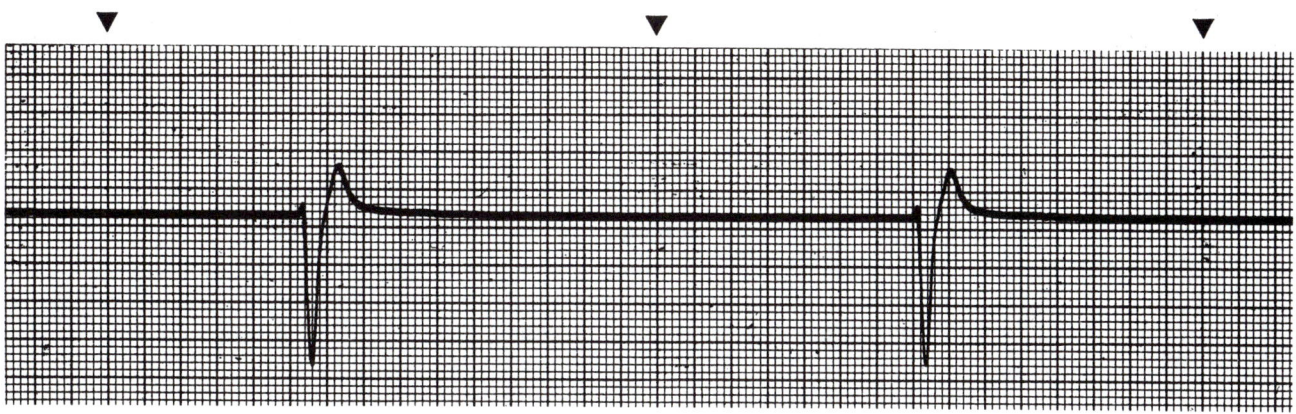

Figure 3-10. A rhythm masquerading as pulseless electrical activity.

Section 4: Assessment

Primary Assessment

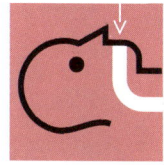 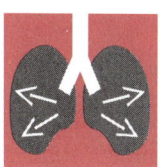

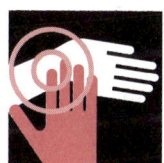 Because this study is concerned with PEA, the pulse will be absent. Immediately begin CPR.

 Because the patient is not in ventricular fibrillation, defibrillation is not an option.

Secondary Assessment

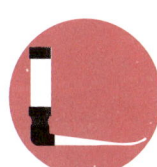 Make it a policy to reevaluate airway and breathing on a consistent basis throughout the code. Remember, hypoxia is a key etiology of PEA.

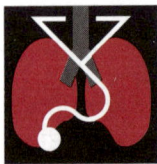

Be sure to inspect the thorax for both medical and traumatic causes of PEA (e.g., cardiac tamponade, tension pneumothorax).

Isotonic solutions, although part of the treatment of any cardiac arrest, bear special examination here. Of all of the etiologies of PEA, the most common one is acute hypovolemia, which also has the best prognoses. Histories of these hypovolemic patients may include nausea, vomiting, gastrointestinal bleeding, trauma, or obvious blood loss. Hypovolemia also commonly presents with flat neck veins, which may be difficult to detect. Therefore, unless the signs and symptoms specifically contraindicate it, all PEAs should receive the first 500 mL bag infused rapidly to rule out hypovolemia. The key strategy is to act quickly and assess for etiologies because mortality is high if no treatable cause is determined. Even then, any prescribed treatments may be too little, too late.

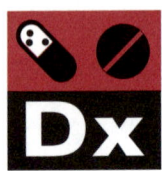

It is crucial in this particular algorithm to check for underlying surgical or medical problems, any condition that could have precipitated the arrest. It could be something simple—hypovolemia or hypoxia. The entire protocol revolves around finding an underlying pathology, then treating it rapidly.

> When treating PEA, he who hesitates is not only lost, but several miles away from the nearest freeway exit.

Section 5: Lecture

Pulseless electrical activity is a curious syndrome in which an ECG rhythm, which would normally be associated with a pulse, presents with the patient in cardiac arrest. The rhythm could be sinus tachycardia, any form of supraventricular bradycardia or an agonal or idioventricular rhythm. Any pulseless rhythm that is not ventricular fibrillation, ventricular tachycardia, or asystole should be assumed to be, and treated as, PEA.

True Versus Pseudo Electromechanical Dissociation. Historically, PEA was thought to have been a problem with the myoneural synapse; depolarization was present, but the heart muscle did not contract. As medical technology improved (e.g., the advent of a Doppler), other medical and surgical conditions were also found to have an apparently normal ECG but no corresponding pulse. The AHA has divided these other PEA-like syndromes into two subsyndromes: true electromechanical dissociation (EMD) and pseudo-EMD. True EMD is the historical EMD: a viable ECG rhythm on the monitor, but no cardiac contraction. Pseudo-EMD marks the other medical or surgical conditions that mimic EMD. These conditions are situations in which poor or inadequate contractions, owing to impaired cardiac output, do not generate an acceptable carotid pulse. With the possibility of an extremely low blood pressure, a Doppler should be employed to detect any subviable cardiac output.

Etiologies

The entire protocol of PEA centers on assessing the patient for a treatable etiology. The refrain, "Hey, Hey, Hey, that's EMD" provides a memorable mnemonic that calls attention to the various known etiologies of PEA.

HEY, HEY, HEY

The first three possible causes begin with the letter H: *h*ypoxia, *h*ypovolemia, and *h*yperkalemia. Hypoxia should always be assumed and therefore treated as part of the cardiac arrest routine. Hypovolemia has been previously discussed and is treated by fluid administration. Hyperkalemia should be suspected in patients receiving potassium, potassium-sparing diuretics, or angiotensin-converting enzyme; in patients with histories of renal failure; in diabetic patients with renal tubular acidosis; and in multisystem trauma or other cell death. Hyperkalemia, when suspected, should be treated with an immediate bolus of calcium chloride along with a combination of sodium bicarbonate, glucose, and insulin in addition to the generic PEA protocol.

THAT'S

That's, or *that,* stands for four additional etiologies. The two T's stand for situations in which venous return to the heart is compromised. With the exception of hypovolemia, these are the next two most obvious pseudo-EMDs: *t*ension pneumothorax and cardiac *t*amponade. These processes interfere with patient oxygenation as well as cardiac output. If your patient develops symptoms of tension pneumothorax or cardiac tamponade, it is helpful to both recognize the condition and verbally demonstrate the treatment. Both require needle placement. The protocol given in this textbook is not meant to be complete but only to provide a brief description. The student is referred to an appropriate text on the subject. The other two etiologies that are recalled are H for *h*ypothermia and A for *a*cidosis. Acidosis will be covered separately when sodium bicarbonate is considered.

Tension Pneumothorax. A patient with a tension pneumothorax might present as PEA or just unexplained hypotension. It presents as pressurized air in the pleural space, causing the involved lung to collapse. The collapsing lung inhibits venous return, kinking the inferior vena cava as it displaces the mediastinum. This displacement causes cardiac output impairment resulting in cardiovascular collapse.

There may not be any specific symptoms except a pulseless, normal-appearing rhythm. However, the following might be in evidence:

- Acute dyspnea if the patient is still breathing spontaneously
- Absent breath sounds on the involved side, demonstrating tympany
- Distended neck veins
- Tachycardia
- Cyanosis
- Depressed level of consciousness

There is no time for radiographic confirmation because this condition is emergent, and in PEA, the alternative is death. Find the second intercostal space of the involved side at the mid-clavicular line, and strike the third rib with a 14-gauge needle, directly in, and sliding just over the top of the rib.

Cardiac Tamponade. The other impaired, venous-return condition is pericardial tamponade, a pericardial effusion that causes enough pressure to impair ventricular diastolic filling. The effusion may be fluid or blood from a medical, surgical, or traumatic condition. Although rare, this condition is treatable if discovered promptly. The key to successful treatment is noting clues in the patient's history. The history may include trauma, recent CPR, an acute MI, prior cardiac surgery, metastatic cancer, recent fever, or viral illness.

In PEA, some or all of the so-called classic symptoms may not be obvious—only cardiac arrest. The following typical symptoms should have been noted before the development of PEA:

- Arterial hypotension combined with venous hypertension as noted by distended neck veins
- Pulsus paradoxus
- Pericardial friction rub
- Anxiety progressing to an altered level of consciousness
- Dyspnea
- Poor pulse, with or without CPR

Cardiac tamponade, even if it does not present as PEA, is an immediate threat to life. Therefore, do not waste time with diagnostic procedures. If you suspect tamponade, treat immediately because the alternative is death. Consider the subxiphoid approach, that is, slow insertion of an intracardiac needle at the left side of the xiphoid at a 30° to 45° angle to the skin, maintaining constant aspiration, angling toward the left shoulder. Advance the needle slowly until the heart is hit. When ectopic beats occur on the ECG, pull back slightly and aspirate the pericardial sac. As little as 10 mL of aspirated fluid should result in immediate improvement.

Hypothermia. Hypothermia should be considered when a patient is cold (electronic thermometer reads 30° to 36°C or less) and has a history of exposure, drugs, alcohol, diabetes, near-drowning, or sepsis. In addition to the normal treatment protocol, aggressive rewarming techniques should be instituted while holding unnecessary movements, procedures, and drugs to a minimum. Treatment is targeted at rewarming the body core, not the periphery. Core rewarming includes warm intravenous fluids, warm humidified oxygen, peritoneal lavage, and warm enemas. Warming of the periphery is not instituted because it dilates blood vessels in the arms and legs, carrying cold, lactic acid–rich blood back to the heart, which may result in ventricular fibrillation.

A patient is usually not declared dead until the core temperature has been increased to near-normal levels. Sometimes, however, trying to raise the core temperature is exceedingly difficult, if not impossible, in the time allowed. Thus, physicians are encouraged to use their best judgment while recognizing that some patients have been successfully resuscitated when the core temperature initially was less than 30°C.

EMD

The last three letters in the mnemonic Hey, Hey, Hey, that's EMD help recall the final three etiologies: *e*mbolism; *m*yocardial infarction, and *d*rug overdose.

Pulmonary Embolism. Although pulmonary embolism is listed as an etiology, it presents as a pulseless condition only rarely and has a poor prognosis; the patient usually does not live to surgery. Clues in this etiology are a history of deep venous thrombosis, hip fracture, trauma, or oral contraceptives.

Acute Myocardial Infarction. Acute MI should be considered in any patient with a history of chest pain. Again, this etiology as a pulseless condition has a poor prognosis. Depending on how much of a cardiac output is being generated with each contraction, a balloon pump might be appropriate if one could be instituted quickly enough and the patient survived the interim.

Drug Overdose. If a drug-induced arrest is suspected, naloxone HCl (Narcan) should be administered at once to rule out an opiate origin. Clues to this etiology are a history of ingestion, empty pill bottles, or a young patient. A generic approach to a suspected overdose is fluids combined with drug-specific remedies. Depending on the capabilities of the medical facility, emergency bypass may be used until the drug is eliminated or otherwise removed. Some drugs may inhibit the cardiac conduction system; therefore, a TCP should be considered in these situations.

Treatment

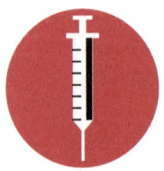

EPINEPHRINE

Important: See the discussion of epinephrine given in section 5 of case studies 2 and 3 (p. 41); the same information is relevant to the patient with PEA in this case study.

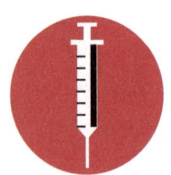

SODIUM BICARBONATE

Important: See the discussion of sodium bicarbonate given in section 5 of case studies 2 and 3 (p. 41); the same information is relevant to the patient with PEA in this case study.

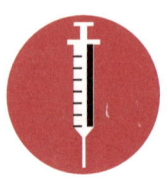

ATROPINE

Actions and Indications. Atropine is classified as a vagal nerve blocker. In a situation in which a relative or absolute bradycardia makes the patient's blood pressure hemodynamically significant, the vagus nerve *may* be the culprit.

An absolute bradycardia is defined as a heart rate of less than 60 beats/minute. A relative bradycardia is a situation in which the heart rate is not below 60 beats/minute, but it is too slow for the individual's cardiovascular status. An example of a relative bradycardia might be a heart rate that plummets to 62 beats/minute due to vagal domination in an elderly man who normally has a heart rate of 92 beats/minute. Although the rate is above 60 beats/minute, the rate for this patient results in a significant drop in blood pressure. A relative bradycardia may have many causes, including β-blockers.

The bradycardic rate, relative or absolute, may not produce a substantial enough cardiac output to generate an effective blood pressure. By accelerating the heart rate, the blood pressure should increase.

If the presenting rhythm in PEA is some form of bradycardia, atropine is given to rule out the possibility of vagal domination. If the heart rate accelerates after administration, the vagus nerve was the cause of the bradycardia; if the rate does not change, the etiology of this particular bradycardia was not vagal. Other etiologies include heart block, ischemia, and trauma.

Dosage. The dosage of atropine in an arrest situation is 1 mg given by intravenous push every 3 to 5 minutes, with the emphasis being on 3 minutes, to a total of 0.04 mg/kg. If the maximum dosage is reached and the rhythm is refractory, the vagus nerve can be effectively ruled out as a cause of the problem.

Because cardiac arrest patients are rarely weighed before treatment, the clinician may wish to make use of the following guidelines:

Small patient (50 kg): (0.04 mg/kg $\times$ 50 kg) = maximum dose of 2 mg
Medium patient (75 kg): (0.04 mg/kg $\times$ 75 kg) = maximum dose of 3 mg
Large patient (100 kg): (0.04 mg/kg $\times$ 100 kg) = maximum dose of 4 mg

▼ *Helpful Hints* for Treating the Patient With Pulseless Electrical Activity

The treatment of a patient with pulseless electrical activity can best be summarized as:

▼ Assess for treatable causes while giving epinephrine to make CPR more effective.

▼ Rule out vagal domination with atropine administration if the presenting rhythm is absolutely or relatively bradycardic.

▼ Consider a fluid challenge because hypovolemia is the most common cause.

Section 6: Pulseless Electrical Activity Interim Evaluation

Mark the correct answer.

1. In PEA, hypoxia can be successfully treated by aggressively hyperventilating the patient; oxygen is not a requirement (see ACLS text pp. 1-21 to 1-22 and 7-1 to 7-2). _____

    _____ (a) True
    _____ (b) False

2. The most common etiology of PEA, _____, is noted by individuals who may exhibit a history of nausea and vomiting, trauma, or upper gastrointestinal bleeding. Which of the following match this etiology (see ACLS text pp. 1-21)? _____

    _____ (a) Pulmonary embolism
    _____ (b) Drug overdose
    _____ (c) Hypokalemia
    _____ (d) Hypovolemia

3. Important interventions that might be considered in the management of PEA are (see ACLS text pp. 1-21 to 1-23): (1) perform a rapid fluid challenge with NS; (2) perform an

abbreviated patient assessment while checking heart sounds for cardiac activity; (3) give epinephrine, 1 mg of 1:10,000 solution by intravenous push; (4) give lidocaine, 1 to 1.5 mg/kg by intravenous push. _____

   _____ (a) 1, 2, and 3
   _____ (b) 1 and 3
   _____ (c) 2 and 4
   _____ (d) 3

4. All of the following are noted as possible noncardiac causes of PEA except (see ACLS text pp. 1-21 to 1-23): _____

   _____ (a) Hypovolemia
   _____ (b) Pulmonary embolism
   _____ (c) Tension pneumothorax
   _____ (d) Ruptured diaphragm

5. While performing a patient assessment on a patient with PEA, you note that he has engorged neck veins. You suspect cardiac tamponade. In a cardiac arrest, the best way to make the diagnosis is (see ACLS text pp. 1-21 to 1-23): _____

   _____ (a) Get a chest radiograph
   _____ (b) Perform a pericardiocentesis
   _____ (c) Institute a TCP
   _____ (d) Perform a cardiac catheterization

6. Which of the following is appropriate treatment for acute hyperkalemia (see ACLS text p. 1-21)? _____

   _____ (a) Calcium chloride and a combination of glucose, sodium bicarbonate, and insulin
   _____ (b) Sodium bicarbonate, lactulose, and calcium chloride
   _____ (c) Dialysis, calcium chloride, sodium bicarbonate, and atropine
   _____ (d) Barbiturates, etomidate, dialysis, and lactulose

7. A patient presents to the emergency department in cardiac arrest. The monitor reveals a sinus tachycardia at 130 beats/minute, although there is neither a pulse nor spontaneous respiration. CPR is in progress. Of the following possible therapies, which is the most appropriate (see ACLS text pg. 1-21 to 1-23)? _____

   _____ (a) Perform a brief patient assessment considering possible causes
   _____ (b) Immediately administer a synchronized countershock at 75 joules
   _____ (c) Give a 500-mL fluid challenge of D-5-W
   _____ (d) Administer verapamil 5 mg slowly through an intravenous line

8. According to AHA guidelines for the management of PEA, at some time in the algorithm, all of the following would be routinely appropriate except (see ACLS text pp. 1-21 to 1-23): _____

   _____ (a) Continue CPR
   _____ (b) Institute a TCP
   _____ (c) Administer epinephrine
   _____ (d) Administer a fluid challenge

9. Acidosis during a cardiac arrest (see ACLS text pp. 7-14 to 7-16): (1) should be treated with increased ventilation; (2) may occur with hypoxia or decreased ventilation; (3) is usually of respiratory origin in an uncomplicated arrest; (4) usually limits itself after perfusion has been restored; (5) is not routinely treated with sodium bicarbonate. _____

   _____ (a) 1 and 4
   _____ (b) 2, 3, and 4
   _____ (c) 1, 2, 4, and 5
   _____ (d) All of the above

10. Using the endotracheal route, the initial dose of atropine in asystole is (see ACLS text pp. 7-4 to 7-6): _____

___ (a) 3 mg diluted to 10 mL total in NS
___ (b) 0.1 mg/kg diluted in 15 mL of NS
___ (c) 1 mg diluted in 20 to 30 mL of NS
___ (d) 2 to 2.5 times the intravenous dosage in 10 ml of NS

11. Atropine is indicated in PEA if a relative or absolute bradycardia is present on the monitor (see ACLS text pp. 7-4 to 7-6). _____
   ___ (a) True
   ___ (b) False

12. All of the following are treatments for severe hypothermia except (see ACLS text pp. 11-1 to 11-3): _____
   ___ (a) Warm intravenous fluids
   ___ (b) Warm blankets
   ___ (c) Warm oxygen
   ___ (d) Peritoneal lavage

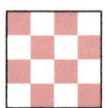

Section 7:
PULSELESS ELECTRICAL ACTIVITY CROSSWORD PUZZLE

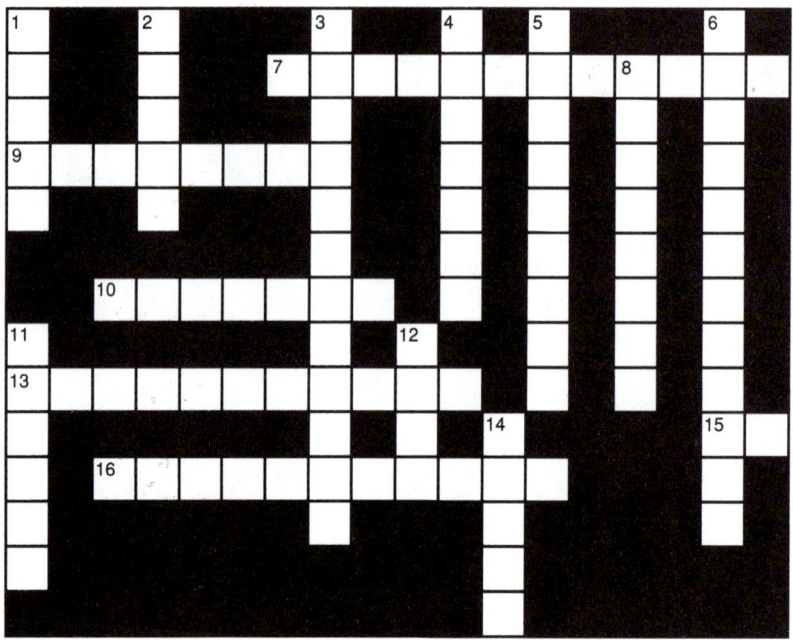

Across

7. A potassium level problem for which calcium and bicarbonate would be especially helpful (think of an etiology of PEA).
9. Atropine is administered in PEA if the presenting rhythm is an _____ or relative bradycardia (heart rate below 60 beats/minute).
10. An electronic device that allows the clinician to measure extremely low blood pressures.
13. Arterial _____ is a key feature of cardiac tamponade (an abnormality in the blood pressure caused by the poor cardiac output in tamponade).
15. Treatment of hypothermia includes infusion of warm _____ (acronym) fluids.
16. The most common etiology of PEA is _____ (may be evidenced by flat neck veins).

Down

1. Failure of this organ system would be associated with high levels of potassium (the organ responsible for altering levels of potassium).
2. The pericardial effusion in cardiac tamponade may present as _____ after an intracardiac injection.
3. Venous _____ is noted in tension pneumothorax (an abnormality in the blood pressure causing jugular distention).
4. A key sign in both tamponade and tension pneumothorax is increased cardiac _____, which is demonstrated by jugular venous distention (the term assigned to the filling tension on the heart or a term meaning the amount of blood returning to the heart).
5. An etiology of PEA associated with fluid under pressure within the pericardial sac.
6. The key strategy in the treatment of PEA is assessing the patient to obtain a _____ diagnosis to guide the treatment (term that implies evaluating different etiologies for an appropriate diagnosis).
8. A pulmonary _____ should be suspected if the patient has a history of deep venous thrombosis or hip fracture (a term for moving clot).
11. A cardiac arrest epinephrine drip contains _____ mg of epinephrine in 250 mL of NS (number is spelled out).
12. The key strategy in the treatment of hypothermia in PEA is to warm the center, or _____, rather than the periphery of the body.
14. A history of _____ illness may be associated with cardiac tamponade (this may be interpreted by the patient as having the "flu").

Case Study 5:
Asystole

This case study is more difficult because a straight line on the monitor is usually taken as confirmation of death. A host of etiologies can result in asystole. This case study emphasizes that, like in PEA, rapid assessment and aggressive intervention may make the difference in correcting what appears at first glance to be evidence of death.

Section 1: Critical Actions for Student Evaluation

The ACLS instructor checklist for case study 5 is shown in Table 3-4. This form was designed to guide the faculty when evaluating participants during this particular station. Refer to it frequently as you read the lecture that follows. *Do not memorize it.* The form is only included to: (1) show you what the AHA considers important during this particular case study; (2) describe what the faculty are trying to cover in the station; and (3) provide a summary of the case study after you have read the lecture.

Table 3-4.
Case Study 5: Asystole

Critical Action	Completed	Not Completed	Comments
Performs primary ABCD			
Initiates CPR			
Recognizes asystole			
Confirms in more than one lead (asystole)			
Recognizes ventilatory support as mainstay of acid-base balance			
Articulates differential diagnosis and management			
Pharmacologic therapy appropriate			
Recognizes need to check pulse with rhythm changes			
Recognizes need to check blood pressure if pulse present			
If transcutaneous pacemaker used, used early			
Articulates indications to terminate efforts			

(Reproduced with permission. *Instructor's manual for advanced cardiac life support,* 1997 © Copyright American Heart Association, p. 6-12.)

Section 2: ACLS Algorithm for Asystole

Asystole

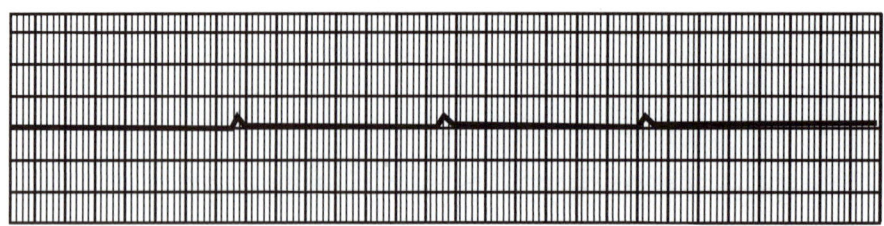

- CPR • Intubate at once
- Intubate at once
- IV access
- Confirm asystole in more than one lead

Consider Possible Causes
- Hypoxia
- Hypokalemia
- Drug overdose
- Hyperkalemia
- Preexisting acidosis
- Hypothermia

TCP[a]   Consider immediate transcutaneous pacing

EPINEPHRINE[b,c]   1 mg IV push, repeat 3–5 min

Consider SODIUM BICARBONATE
For specific indications: 1 mEq/kg
Definitely helpful
- Known preexisting hyperkalemia
Acceptable, probably helpful
- If known preexisting bicarbonate-responsive acidosis (i.e., diabetic ketoacidosis)
- If overdose with tricyclic antidepressants
- To alkalinize the urine in drug overdoses
Acceptable, possibly helpful
- If intubated and continued long arrest interval
- Upon return of spontaneous circulation after long arrest interval
Not indicated, may be harmful
- Hypoxic lactic acidosis

ATROPINE[d,e]
1 mg IV push repeat every 3–5 min,
to a total of 0.03–0.04 mg/kg

Consider termination of efforts[f]

Asystole Footnotes

Class I: definitely helpful
Class IIa: acceptable; probably helpful
Class IIb: acceptable; possibly helpful
Class III: not indicated; may be harmful

(a) TCP is a Class IIb intervention. Lack of success may be due to delays in pacing. To be effective TCP must be performed early, simultaneously with drugs. Evidence does not support routine use of TCP for asystole.

(b) The recommended dose of epinephrine is 1 mg IV push every 3–5 min. If this approach fails, several Class IIb dosing regimens can be considered:
- Intermediate epinephrine 2–5 mg IV push, every 3–5 min
- Escalating: epinephrine 1 mg–3 mg–5 mg IV push, 3 min apart
- High: epinephrine 0.1 mg/kg IV push, every 3–5 min

(c) Sodium Bicarbonate: 1 mEq/kg is Class I
If patient has known preexisting hyperkalemia

(d) The shorter atropine dosing interval (3 min) is Class IIb in asystolic arrest

(e) Sodium Bicarbonate 1 mEq/kg:
Class IIa
- If known preexisting bicarbonate-responsive acidosis
- If overdose with tricyclic antidepressants
Class IIb
- If intubated and continued long arrest interval
- Upon return of spontaneous circulation after long arrest interval
Class III
- Hypoxic lactic acidosis

(f) If patient remains in asystole or other agonal rhythm after successful intubation and initial medications and no reversible causes are identified, consider termination of resuscitative efforts by a physician. Consider interval since arrest.

(Reproduced with permission. *Advanced cardiac life support.* Copyright 1997, American Heart Association.)

Section 3: Identifying Features

Ventricular Asystole

Asystole is an ECG term meaning "without contraction"—the complete absence of ventricular activity. The ECG pattern for asystole may be a perfectly straight line, a straight line with P waves, a wavy line that oscillates slightly up and down, or a cardiac rhythm of less than 30 beats/minute. A wavy line may represent fine ventricular fibrillation; therefore, it is critical that asystole always be verified in more than one lead. Move your lead selector to one of the other leads, usually lead I or III.

Any rhythm presenting with less than 30 beats/minute is referred to as *ventricular standstill*. The ECG in Figure 3-11 is obviously a ventricular standstill (asystole); however, the ECG strip in Figure 3-12 is not so clearcut.

Primary Ventricular Standstill. The formal term for the ECG strip in Figure 3-11 is *primary* ventricular standstill because P waves are present (primary starts with the letter P, making it easy to remember.)

Secondary Ventricular Standstill. In some rare instances, ventricular standstill (asystole) is accompanied by a few erratically spaced, wide ventricular escape beats (agonal beats). The ECG strip in Figure 3-12 is secondary ventricular standstill because the agonal ventricular complexes are beating less than 30 beats/minute, with no P waves present.

It is important to keep in mind that both of these patients present with pulseless rhythms and there-

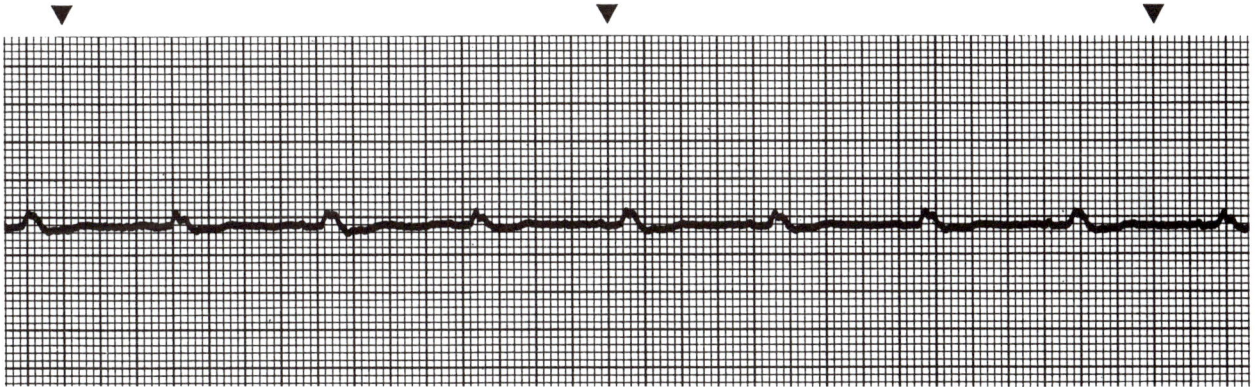

Figure 3-11. Primary ventricular standstill (asystole).

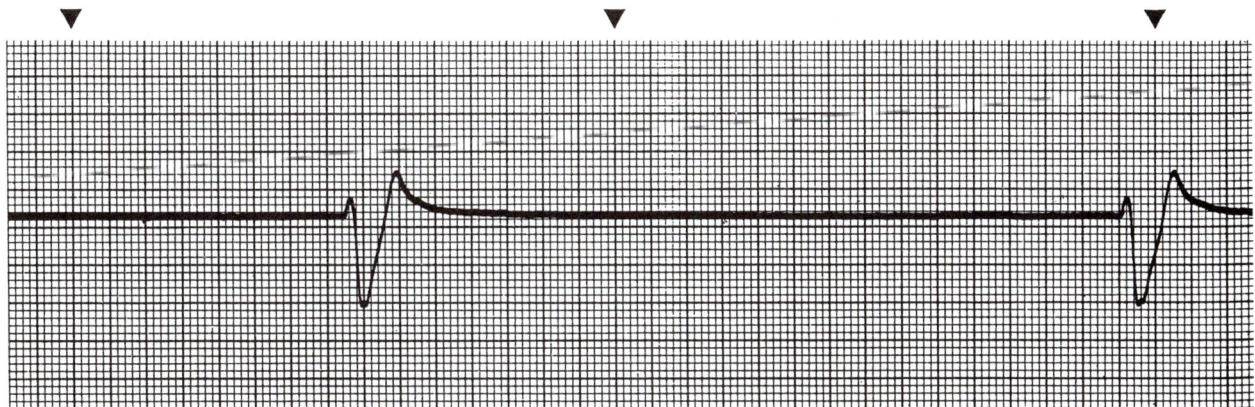

Figure 3-12. Secondary ventricular standstill (asystole).

fore should be treated aggressively. Because these rhythms are pulseless, there is a tendency to call them PEA and treat them as such. These two protocols, PEA and asystole, however, essentially differ only in consideration of a TCP.

Section 4: Assessment

Primary Survey

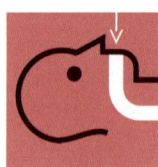 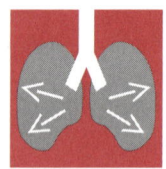 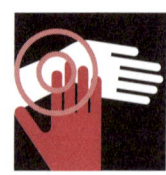

 Defibrillation is not routinely performed in asystole; however, asystole may masquerade as fine ventricular fibrillation, necessitating a change in protocol. Therefore, it is critical that asystole always be verified in more than one lead. If the alternate lead confirms asystole, continue with this protocol. If, however, it appears to be ventricular fibrillation, immediately defibrillate at 200 joules, and proceed with the ventricular fibrillation protocol.

Secondary Survey

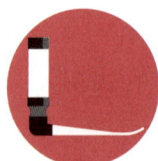 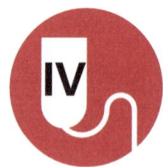

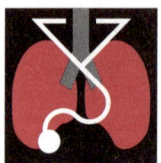 Make it a policy to reevaluate airway and breathing on a consistent basis throughout the code. Remember, hypoxia is a key etiology of asystole.

As in PEA, it is extremely critical in the asystole algorithm to check for underlying surgical or medical problems that could have precipitated the arrest. It could be something simple as hypoxia. The key strategy is to act quickly and assess for etiologies because mortality is high if no treatable cause is determined. Even then, any prescribed treatments may be too little, too late. The entire protocol revolves around finding an underlying pathology and then treating it rapidly.

Section 5: Lecture

The main difficulty in dealing with this rhythm is that it usually implies a confirmation of death rather than a situation to be treated; therefore, the first concern in an asystolic situation is prompt rhythm recognition and confirmation.

A straight line on a monitor may point to a wide variety of situations, none of which involve the patient. Commonly, the power may be off, the leads may not be attached to the chest, the lead wires may become unseated, or, however unlikely, the lead cable was not plugged into the monitor. The most frequent error is that the lead selector was not turned to the proper position.

If you decide to view the patient's ECG through the Quick Look Paddles, do not forget to switch the lead selector to P for Paddles. Wait until the paddle cords have finished bouncing up and down after placing the paddles on the chest as cord movement will give a false reading. Also, do not forget to change the selector switch from P to Lead II when you later place electrodes on the patient.

In the past, asystole was routinely defibrillated as "it might help and could not make it any worse." However, recent research has revealed that electrical shocks, in a true asystolic heart, may produce a "stunned myocardium and a massive parasympathetic discharge." This situation serves to decrease the chances of the return of the heart to spontaneous circulation. Therefore, defibrillation is no longer routinely performed in asystole.

The ECG pattern for asystole may be a perfect straight line, a straight line with P waves, a wavy line that oscillates slightly up and down, or a cardiac rhythm beating less than 30 beats per minute. It is possible that the wavy line represents "fine ventricular fibrillation;" therefore, it is critical that asystole always be verified in more than one lead. Move your lead selector to one of the other leads, usually Lead I or III. If you are visualizing the rhythm through the paddles, change their placement so they are at a 90-degree angle to the one you are presently viewing. If the alternate lead confirms asystole, continue with this protocol. If, however, it appears to be ventricular fibrillation, immediately defibrillate at 200 joules and proceed with the ventricular fibrillation protocol.

If the equipment has been checked and the patient is pulseless and still in asystole, continue with an assessment for treatable etiologies.

Etiologies

The mnemonic, Ho, Ho, Ho, Accidents Do Happen, helps recall the etiologies.

HO, HO, HO

The first three Ho's, *h*ypoxia, *h*yperkalemia, and *h*ypokalemia, are treatable if discovered early enough.

Hypoxia should always be assumed in any cardiac arrest and treated aggressively with ventilation and oxygenation.

Hyperkalemia should be suspected in the following patients:

- All patients receiving potassium
- All patients receiving potassium-sparing diuretics
- All patients receiving angiotensin-converting enzyme
- Patients with histories of renal failure
- Diabetics patients with renal tubular acidosis
- Patients with multisystem trauma or other cell death

When suspected, hyperkalemia should be treated with an immediate bolus of calcium chloride, along with a combination of sodium bicarbonate, glucose, and insulin, to force potassium back into the cell. These should be administered in addition to the generic PEA protocol.

Alternatively, hypokalemia may present in patients with nausea and vomiting, diarrhea, digitalis toxicity, and a history of taking diuretics. Treatment consists of expeditious potassium replacement.

ACCIDENTS DO HAPPEN

The last three words in the mnemonic—"Accidents Do Happen"—help respectively recall *a*cidosis, *d*rug overdoses, and *h*ypothermia. Preexisting types of acidosis (metabolic) are covered separately when sodium bicarbonate is considered.

Drug Overdose. If a drug-induced arrest is suspected, naxolone HCl should be administered at once to rule out an opiate origin. Clues to this etiology are a history of ingestion, empty pill bottles, or a young patient. A generic approach to a suspected overdose is fluids combined with drug-specific remedies. Depending on the capabilities of the medical facility, emergency bypass may be used until the drug is eliminated or otherwise removed. Some drugs may inhibit the cardiac conduction system; therefore, a TCP should be considered in these situations.

Hypothermia. Hypothermia should be considered when a patient is cold (electronic thermometer reads 30 to 36°C or less) and has a history of exposure, drugs, alcohol, diabetes, near-drowning, or sepsis. In addition to the normal treatment protocol, aggressive rewarming techniques should be instituted while holding unnecessary movements, procedures, and drugs to a minimum.

Treatment is targeted at rewarming the body core, not the periphery. Core rewarming includes warm intravenous fluids, warm humidified oxygen, peritoneal lavage, and warm enemas. Warming of the periphery is not instituted because it dilates blood vessels in the arms and legs carrying cold, lactic acid–rich blood back to the heart, which results in ventricular fibrillation.

A patient is usually not declared dead until the core temperature has been increased to near-normal levels. Sometimes, however, trying to raise the core temperature is exceedingly difficult, if not impossible, in the time allowed. Thus, physicians are encouraged to use their best judgment while recognizing that patients have been successfully resuscitated when their core temperatures were less than 30°C.

Treatment

TRANSCUTANEOUS PACEMAKER

Simultaneously with epinephrine administration, a TCP should be considered. *Considered* is the operative term. Routine application of a TCP in all asystolic situations has not been shown to increase survival rates. The time from initiation of asystole to application of a TCP is the critical component necessary to improve outcomes. Research has found that asystole in the prehospital sector almost never responds to pacing because this interval is usually too great. A brief interval is all that appears to be allowed. Therefore, to have any chance of success, a TCP must be applied simultaneously with CPR and medications. A more definitive discourse concerning pacemakers is available in the case study on bradycardia (see case study 7 in Chapter 5).

Pacing is considered a relative contraindication in the patient with hypothermia because the ventricles are paradoxically more resistant to electrical stimulation and more prone to fibrillation.

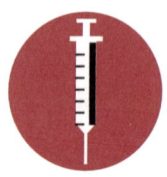

EPINEPHRINE

Important: Epinephrine is the first drug of choice in all pulseless patients and has the same actions, indications, dosage, and precautions in each protocol. See the discussion of epinephrine given in section 5 of case studies 2 and 3 (p. 41); the same information is relevant to the patient with asystole in this case study.

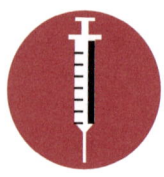

ATROPINE

Important: Atropine is a main drug in two of the three pulseless patient protocols and has the same indications, dosage, and precautions in each. However, the actions of the drug are somewhat different in this case study. I encourage you to read the next paragraph even if you have already read about atropine elsewhere in the text.

Actions and Indications. Atropine is a vagolytic drug. It works by inhibiting the vagus nerve, allowing the sympathetic nerve to dominate. Research has revealed that 25% of all cases of asystole started out as bradycardia but, because of intense vagal domination, they gradually became slower and slower, and eventually became straight-line readings. Atropine is given in asystole to rule out the possibility of vagal domination. If the heart starts up after administration, the vagus nerve was the cause; if the rhythm does not change, the etiology of this asystole was not vagal in nature.

Dosage. The dosage of atropine in an arrest situation is 1 mg given as intravenous push every 3 to 5 minutes, with the emphasis being on 3 minutes, to a total of 0.04 mg/kg. If the maximum dosage is reached and the rhythm is refractory, the vagus nerve can be effectively ruled out as a cause of the problem.

Because cardiac arrest patients are rarely weighed before treatment, the clinician may wish to make use of the following:

Small patient (50 kg): (0.04 mg/kg × 50 kg) = maximum dose of 2 mg
Medium patient (75 kg): (0.04 mg/kg × 75 kg) = maximum dose of 3 mg
Large patient (100 kg): (0.04 mg/kg × 100 kg) = maximum dose of 4 mg

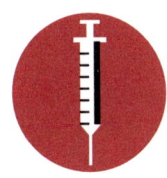

SODIUM BICARBONATE

Important: Sodium bicarbonate should be considered in all pulseless patients and has the same actions, indications, dosage, and precautions in each protocol. See the discussion of sodium bicarbonate given in section 5 of case studies 2 and 3 (p. 41); the same information is relevant to the patient with asystole in this case study.

Termination of Efforts

Because asystole also appears as the rhythm synonymous with death, there must come a time when a halt is called for an unresponsive myocardium that has been without adequate perfusion for a prolonged period. In special situations, such as hypothermia, electrocution, and drug overdoses, resuscitation time may continue in excess. In general, however, the clinician may consider terminating resuscitation when the patient's asystolic rhythm has remained refractory despite being successfully intubated, having an intravenous line established, receiving adequate CPR, and receiving all appropriate medications. There are no hard and fast stopping rules; each physician must use common sense and good clinical judgment.

Section 6: Asystole Interim Evaluation

Mark the correct answer.

1. Clinicians should initially check asystole in more than one ECG lead because (see ACLS text p. 1-23): _____
   - _____ (a) The augmented voltage leads (i.e., aVR, aVL, and aVF) tend to view certain rhythms better than just lead II.
   - _____ (b) The circuitry of a monitor-defibrillator requires that at least two leads be viewed simultaneously to confirm asystole.
   - _____ (c) A significant portion of the human population has a genetic defect in their myocardial tissue that is best viewed from two separate directions.
   - _____ (d) The presenting rhythm might be ventricular fibrillation but may not be clearly visible from only one lead.

2. "Atropine makes the heart go faster" (see ACLS text pp. 7-4 to 7-6). _____
   - _____ (a) True
   - _____ (b) False

3. Hypokalemia might be suspected as an etiology of asystole if the patient had evidence of (see ACLS text p. 8-8): _____
   - _____ (a) A history of potassium infusion
   - _____ (b) Digitalis toxicity
   - _____ (c) Angiotensin-converting enzyme medication intake
   - _____ (d) Renal failure

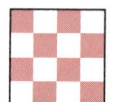

Section 7:
ASYSTOLE CROSSWORD PUZZLE

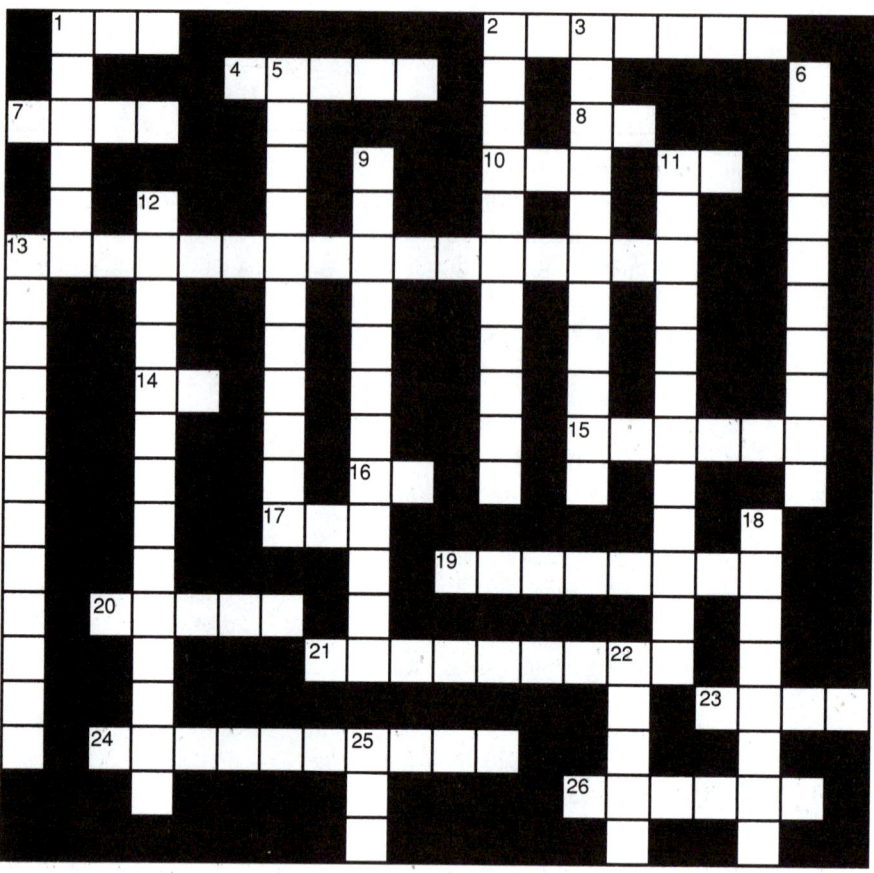

Across

1. Acronym for a transcutaneous pacemaker.
2. Should be treated by aggressive ventilation and oxygenation (shortage of oxygen).
4. Treatment of asystole is complicated by the fact that this rhythm is usually a confirmation of _____.
7. The term for the dosage scheme of epinephrine at 0.1 mg/kg.
8. The abbreviation for the administration route when the dose is 2 to 2.5 times the intravenous dose.
10. The standard dose of epinephrine is _____ mg (number is spelled out).
11. The chemical abbreviation for the drug that is given, along with sodium bicarbonate, in hyperkalemia.
13. The treatment of choice for hypoxia-related acidosis (method of correcting carbon dioxide retention).
14. Initials used for the part of the secondary survey in which a mini-thorax examination is performed.
15. The trade name for the drug administered for all suspected opiate overdoses.
16. The initials standing for the last segment in the secondary survey.
17. Nickname of the drug that makes CPR more effective, improving perfusion to the brain and left ventricle.
19. A generic term for any drug that flushes the kidneys. Hypokalemia should be suspected when this class of drug is given without replacing the ions that are removed from the body.
20. The name of the nerve that is inhibited by atropine (one of the cranial nerves).
21. The name of the survey in which intubation and placement of an intravenous line are considered.
23. The maximum dose of atropine is 0.0 _____ mg/kg (the number is spelled out).
24. Atropine is given whenever the etiology of the arrest is suspected vagal _____.
26. The form of acid generated during any routine cardiac arrest (occurs with increased anaerobic metabolism).

Down

1. In hypothermia, raise the core temp to at least _____ degrees centigrade before declaring the patient nonviable (number is spelled out).
2. An etiology that should be considered if the patient has been on diuretics or has a history of nausea and vomiting (an etiology of asystole).
3. Bicarbonate should be administered for _____ acidosis (term implies that they are in existence before the arrest).
5. Name of drug that improves perfusion to the brain as well as the ventricles.
6. The dosage scheme name for administering epinephrine at 1 mg, then 3 mg, and then 5 mg every 3 to 5 minutes.
9. The dosage scheme for epinephrine noted at 2 to 5 mg every 3 to 5 minutes.
11. When asystole protocol is not specifically linear, initiate a TCP _____ with drug therapy.
12. _____ in asystole may produce a "stunned myocardium" (unsynchronized shock).
13. An etiology that should always be suspected when a patient has a history of renal failure (an etiology of asystole).
18. If preexisting, _____ should be treated with bicarbonate (term for high hydrogen ion concentration).
22. When this organ fails, consider hyperkalemia (failure of this organ would cause potassium imbalances).
25. Acronym for the class of antidepressants that would profit from the administration of bicarbonate (an etiology of asystole).

4 Acute Coronary Syndromes Case Study

David P. Doernbach
Eugene S. Smith III

Case Study 6
Coronary Syndromes

Section 1: Critical Actions for Student Evaluation

The ACLS instructor checklist for case study 6 is shown in Table 4-1. This form was designed to guide the faculty when evaluating participants during this particular station. Refer to it frequently as you read the lecture that follows. *Do not memorize it*. The form is only included to: (1) show you what the American Heart Association (AHA) considers important during this particular case study; (2) describe what the faculty are trying to cover in the station; and (3) provide a summary of the case study after you have read the lecture.

Table 4-1.
Evaluation Checklist—Case 6: Acute Coronary Syndromes

Critical Action	Completed	Not Completed	Comments
Performs immediate assessments in <10 minutes			
Performs immediate general treatments in timely manner			
Assesses 12-lead ECG in a timely manner; classifies patient into one of three algorithm branches			
Recognizes ST-segment elevation or depression as indications for reperfusion therapy and adjunctive therapy			
Applies indications and exclusion criteria for use of thrombolytics			
Understands use of major adjunctive agents			
Understands basic approach to infarct localization			

(Reproduced with permission. *Instructor's manual for advanced cardiac life support,* 1997 © Copyright American Heart Association, p. 6-13.)

Section 2: ACLS Algorithm for Acute Coronary Syndromes

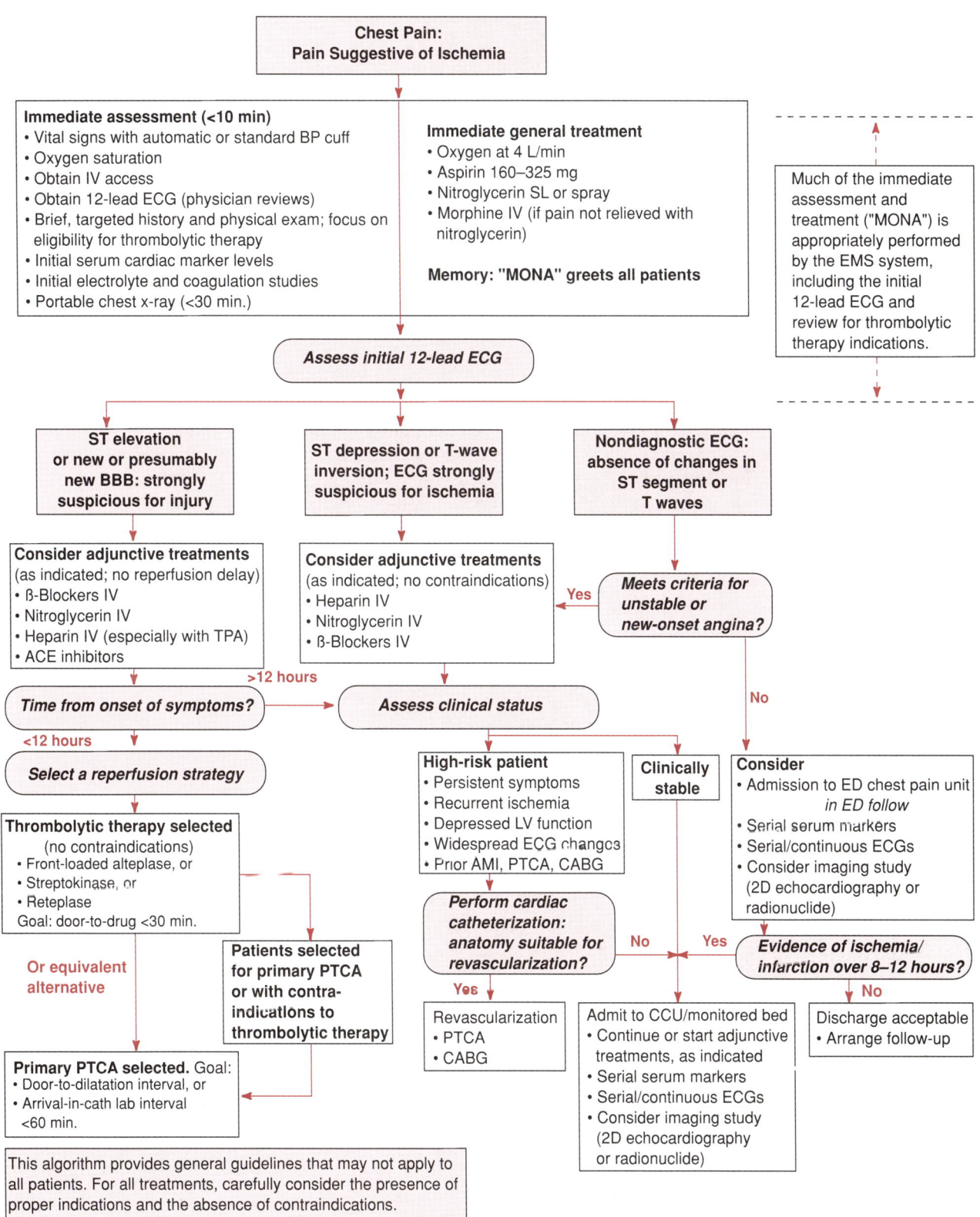

(Reproduced with permission. *Advanced cardiac life support.* Copyright 1997, American Heart Association.)

Section 3: Identifying Features

Pathophysiologic Features

A myocardial infarction (MI) is a change in a coronary artery lumen brought about by an acute thrombotic incident. The climatic event occurs owing to the formation of a thrombus as plaque ruptures away from the walls. The enlarging thrombus fills the arterial lumen and instantly blocks all perfusion distal to the blockage. With the exception of any preexisting collateral circulation, any distal myocardial tissue quickly becomes hypoxic, with resultant ischemia. If the ischemic area is not reperfused within 1 to 4 hours, the myocardial cells begin to die.

If the involved tissue does not drastically interfere with cardiac output, the patient may survive the initial insult. The infarcted tissue dies and is replaced with scar tissue in about 14 days. The heart then begins to change internally in response to the initial insult—the process of *remodeling*. Remodeling is the tendency of a ventricle to change its shape and form in response to the damage caused by an MI. This is analogous to hypertrophy that occurs in response to pathology or exercise. During remodeling, however, not only the muscle thickness but also the actual structure is changed; this occurs in noninfarcted tissues as well as scar tissues. As remodeling proceeds, the involved area balloons out, reducing the overall ejection fraction. Although scar tissue forms in about 14 days, the remainder of the myocardium may continue to undergo changes for 6 to 12 months and even beyond. The remodeling process explains why some post-MI patients appear to be healthy for a period of time and yet carry a greater incidence of developing congestive heart failure remote from the initial incident.

Common signs and symptoms of an acute MI include the following:

- Chest pain, commonly described as crushing or viselike. The patient's history and physical examination continue to be the most important tools when making a diagnosis involving chest pain. The clinician should maintain a high index of suspicion when evaluating patients with chest pain; patients may have difficulty describing the pain, and atypical features are common.
- Radiation of pain to one or both shoulders, arms, neck, lower jaw, and back
- Prolonged indigestion
- Known angina unrelieved by three nitroglycerin tablets taken over a period of 10 minutes
- Shortness of breath, diaphoresis, and cool skin

Electrocardiographic Features

When a patient is experiencing chest pain from a cardiac etiology, the heart undergoes depolarization and repolarization changes that are commonly captured in a 12-lead electrocardiogram (ECG). The key term is *commonly*. Some changes show up immediately, whereas others may not appear for hours or days, and some may never show up. Therefore, relying only on changes in the ECG to diagnose an MI is dangerous and foolhardy because in some patients ECG changes are completely absent or atypical.

If ECG changes do appear, myocardial injury is in evidence when the ST-segment elevates (Fig. 4-1). The ST segment is the straight line between the end of the S wave and the beginning of the T wave. This segment represents the completion of ventricular depolarization to the initiation of ventricular repolarization. Normally, this segment is even with the baseline (isoelectric line). Elevation of the ST segment more than 1 mm (one little tiny box on the ECG paper) usually indicates myocardial injury (Fig. 4-2).

If the segment is elevated, note which ECG leads are involved because changes in these leads indicate that they are monitoring the injured area.

If the clinician thinks of an ECG machine as a camera, it is easy to see that ECG changes can be photographed only if you point the lens toward the involved area. That is why a 12-lead is always ordered im-

Chapter 4 *Acute Coronary Syndromes Case Study* • Coronary Syndromes

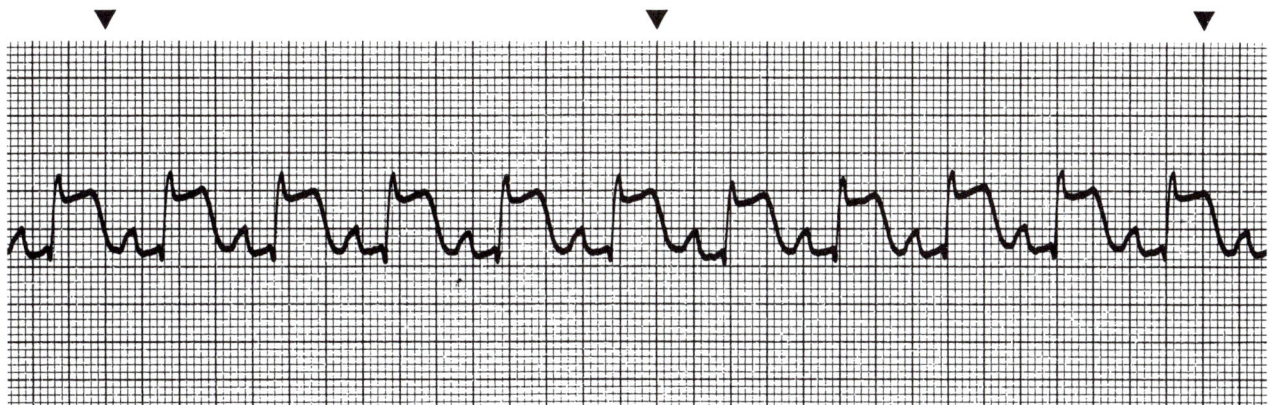

Figure 4-1. Myocardial infarction ECG demonstrating elevated ST-segment changes.

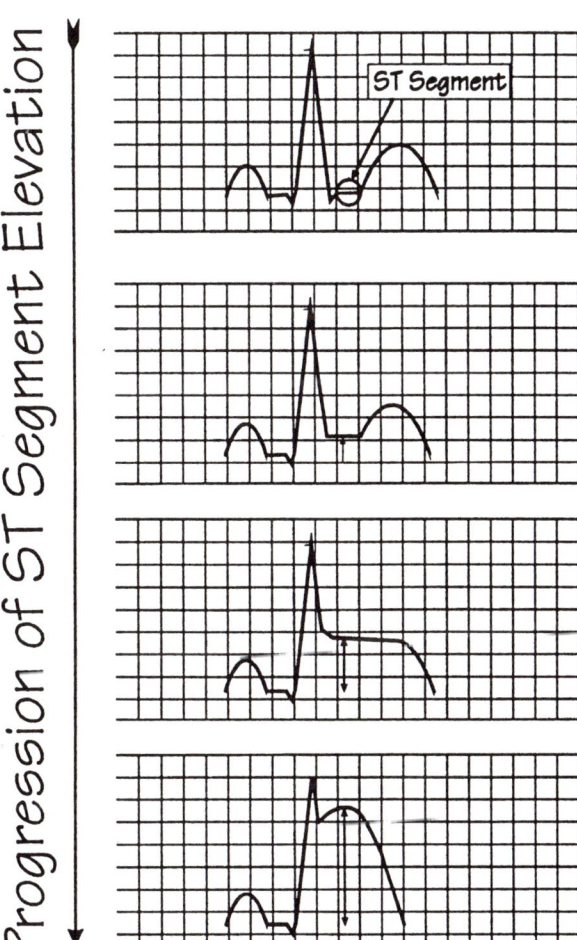

Figure 4-2. Progression of ST-segment elevation, indicating myocardial injury.

mediately so that the heart may be seen from angles other than what can be seen by one lead. If all you use is lead II, the only spot visible is the inferior aspect of the heart; other areas of the heart are invisible.

If ST elevation appears in leads II, III, or aVF, consider inferior involvement. ST elevation in leads V_1 and V_6 indicates septal involvement. ST elevations in leads I, aVL, and V_5 and V_6 indicate a left lateral problem. Anterior infarction is noted in leads V_1 through V_4. Posterior involvement is noted by depression, not elevation in leads V_1 through V_3.

Section 4: Assessment

Primary Survey

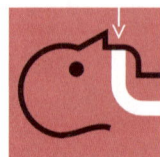

Even though the patient is supposed to be stable for this case study, the clinician should reevaluate his airway and breathing on a consistent basis. If the patient is alert and coherent, the primary ABCDs are obvious. However, a flippant diagnosis of stability is premature because the patient is 15 times more likely to develop ventricular fibrillation in the first hour than in the succeeding 12 hours.

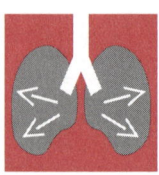

Because the patient is not in ventricular fibrillation, defibrillation is not an option. Coming at a conscious patient with charged paddles may cause the patient to arrest.

Secondary Survey

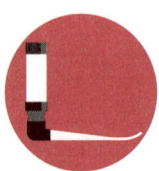

This patient would profit from oxygen by standard face mask or nonrebreather mask.

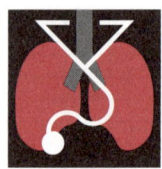

Check for pertinent history.

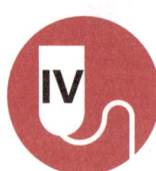

Start peripheral intravenous line because central lines are contraindicated if thrombolytic agents are considered later on.

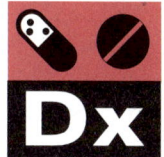

Pain relief is paramount to decrease effects of circulating catecholamines. Consider nitroglycerin and morphine.

> In MI treatment, delay is the deadliest form of denial.

Section 5: Lecture

This case study details the principles of early management and treatment of acute MI patients. No treatment principle is more important, however, than knowing that the shorter the time between the onset of cardiac symptoms and competent medical assistance, the greater is the likelihood of survival. Studies show that ventricular fibrillation is 15 times more apt to occur during the first hour than during the succeeding 12 hours after cardiac insult.

Patients experiencing acute MI often deny it, especially those who are aware of their condition and are taking medication. On average, a patient allows 2 to 4 hours to elapse before seeking medical attention. Keep in mind that tissue death occurs after 1 to 4 hours. This patient decision-making time period must be aggressively reduced if medical care is to be successful. Community involvement, through public education and a community-wide 911 telephone system, can increase the likelihood that, when faced with a cardiac situation, emergency medical services (EMS) would be called immediately and competent medical assistance would be delivered.

The best case scenario would be that all communities had paramedics on their ambulances; however, that is not the case for most of the nation. Depending on the size and location of your community, EMS prehospital training may range anywhere from volunteer first-aid providers to advanced life support (ALS) paramedics. As opposed to other EMS professionals, paramedics have the training to assess and administer lifesaving medications at the scene and during transport. Therefore, scrutinize your community's EMS capabilities before the need arises. If the EMS staff are not trained to the paramedic level, seek to implement training for them. When a community lacks a paramedically staffed EMS system, lay people are more apt to transport the patient themselves. With few exceptions, it is dangerous, as well as medically and legally detrimental, to put someone in your private car and madly speed to the hospital.

Treatment

While obtaining a brief targeted history and physical examination, paramedics would normally administer oxygen, start an intravenous line, attach the cardiac monitor, and obtain a quick set of vital signs. Remember that a normal ECG does not exclude the diagnosis of an MI. The changes may not have shown up yet, or the lead from which you are looking may not be viewing the involved portion of the myocardium. The foregoing procedures should be performed in any cardiac emergency and should be considered as a single word: *oxygen–IV–monitor–vital signs*.

Start the intravenous line peripherally using normal saline (NS), lactated Ringer's solution, or D-5-W. Although NS is less expensive, has a longer shelf life, expands the intravascular container better than dextrose solutions, and does not throw the patient into pulmonary edema as was originally thought, D-5-W may be given if the clinician desires. Note that although glucose-containing solutions are discouraged during a cardiac arrest, if the clinician wishes, D-5-W may still be used in the routine MI protocol. Start the intravenous line in a peripheral arm vein because central lines are contraindicated in thrombolytic therapy.

The ECG monitor should be attached with haste because 50% of all MI patients who die will do so before they reach the hospital. The majority of these will have ventricular fibrillation as the initial rhythm in the arrest. Recognition of any arrhythmias and their subsequent treatment should begin as soon as possible.

Serial vital signs are necessary to establish a baseline. Some medications may adversely affect the blood pressure or are contraindicated if the patient is hypotensive.

All these steps should be accomplished in an minimal amount of time and patient transportation begun. Getting the patient to the emergency room quickly and quietly, while continuing with the treatment phase, greatly increases the patient's chances of survival.

PREHOSPITAL TREATMENT

Advanced life support paramedical personnel are an extension of the hospital and as such can provide emergency medications that historically have not been available in the prehospital sector. Because control of pain is of prime concern in the uncomplicated MI, the emergency room physician may order the following medications en route (the mnemonic MONA—"Mona greets all patients"—can be employed): morphine, oxygen, nitroglycerin, and aspirin.

Oxygen

Oxygen is given to all suspected cardiac patients, even with a normal PaO_2. There is evidence that slight elevation of PaO_2 may limit the size of the infarct. Routine flows vary from 4 to 6 L/minute.

Nitroglycerin

Sublingual or spray nitroglycerin can be initiated if the patient's blood pressure is not below 90 mmHg. The dose of 0.3 to 0.4 mg by pill or spray inhaler may be repeated every 5 minutes. If the patient responds to the nitroglycerin, infarction is less likely. The clinician is cautioned, however, that responses to nitroglycerin are not unique to angina; other situations (e.g., esophageal spasm) can be relieved as well.

In general, nitroglycerin has been shown to reduce infarct size and areas of ischemia while relieving pain. Nitroglycerin achieves most of its advantages when administered intravenously; oral nitrates appear to have no long-standing survival benefit. The oral preparation is useful for symptoms only. Use with caution because the medication reduces preload and hypotension may develop. Prolonged attempts to give multiple doses of nitroglycerin are inappropriate because nitroglycerin alone may not be adequate to relieve pain and should not delay additional treatment.

Aspirin

In the double-blind ISIS-2 study, patients presenting with symptoms of an MI were randomly given one or more medications packaged in nondescript boxes. Neither the patient nor the clinician knew what the box contained before opening it. Upon breaking the seal, the clinician found either: (1) a 30-day regimen of aspirin placebos or a single streptokinase placebo, (2) a 30-day regimen of aspirin, (3) a single dose of streptokinase, or (4) a combination thereof. Incredibly, the ISIS-2 researchers noted that patients who received the daily regimen of aspirin had the same decrease in mortality as the patients receiving streptokinase. The isolated placebo achieved a baseline of 14% mortality, whereas streptokinase and aspirin—when used individually—reduced the mortality of each of their patient groups to 11%. Furthermore, when both agents—streptokinase and aspirin—were administered together, an apparent cumulative effect reduced the overall morality to 8% (Second International Study of Infarct Survival Collaborative Group [ISIS-2], 1988.)

Aspirin has proven utility across the range of coronary syndromes. Its action of decreasing platelet aggregation reduces risk in myocardial infarctions and unstable angina. Since a single dose is well tolerated in almost everyone, current recommendations advise giving a dose of aspirin to anyone with chest pain unless he or she has an absolute contraindication. Some EMS systems routinely administer aspirin to patients with chest pain with no specific contraindications, and others should be encouraged to do so.

The recommended dose of aspirin is 325 mg initially. Some studies have used 162 mg, but less than one-half an adult aspirin should be discouraged. Since an adult aspirin is difficult to both chew and swallow, two tablets of children's flavored aspirin are often substituted; one is chewed while the other is swallowed.

Another option of using Alka-Seltzer may be of benefit, because each tablet contains 325 mg of aspirin. For some patients, swallowing fluid is much easier than swallowing crushed aspirin. This method has the additional benefits of being absorbed more quickly and of neutralizing stomach acid if the patient becomes nauseated, vomits, and aspirates. The patient should continue taking an aspirin each day for at least 1 month following the initial insult.

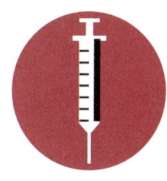

Morphine Sulfate

Morphine sulfate is the analgesic of choice in acute MI. Morphine also has some coexistent hemodynamic effects. It reduces both preload and afterload, thereby giving the heart a chance to reduce its myocardial oxygen demand. It also reduces anxiety, with a concurrent decrease in vasoconstricting adrenaline.

Small doses of 1 to 3 mg given slowly intravenously may be administered until pain is relieved. Watch for respiratory depression. Nausea and vomiting are common side effects. Any untoward respiratory effects can be reversed with naloxone (Narcan).

Thrombolytic Screening

Advanced life support personnel should also begin to gather data to prescreen patients who might benefit from thrombolytic therapy. Some ALS units are equipped with a computerized 12-lead ECG to alert the emergency room that an acute MI is en route. Prescreening through a targeted history and the transmission of a 12-lead ECG decrease the *door-to-drug interval:* the time after the patient enters the emergency room until the initiation of thrombolytic therapy. Currently, few ALS systems administer thrombolytic agents in the field. Systems with long patient transport times would reap the most benefit, while those with a short transport time would not significantly increase the patient survival rates.

Although some clinical benefits occur if an acute MI patient is treated within 12 hours, the greatest benefit occurs when the patient is treated within 90 minutes from the onset of symptoms. Thus, it is the goal of the entire community medical system to get possible MI patients to call EMS quickly so they can be treated for an acute MI within 90 minutes from onset of symptoms. The door-to-drug interval (30 to 60 minutes in the emergency room) must be kept low for maximal thrombolytic benefits.

A system-wide approach to reduce mortality and morbidity in cardiac patients necessitates that ALS companies, emergency departments, and hospital medical staff meet in advance and agree to a specific patient management plan that would reduce the door-to-drug time interval. The strategy should specify who will be the decision maker (e.g., emergency room physician, cardiologist) and detail what laboratory work, radiographs, analgesia, consults, and, if appropriate, what thrombolytic therapy should be ordered. Even though it is a necessary part of the treatment plan, do not tolerate delays to thrombolytic therapy when obtaining radiographs, laboratory studies, or ECGs. The hospital should seek to resolve all potential internal issues among primary care givers that might result in a delay. A sense of urgency should be communicated to all because "time is tissue." Seek to keep the time to potential thrombolytic therapy to less than 60 minutes.

As an integral part of the plan, ALS units should alert the hospital to potential cardiac patients. Once notified, the staff and necessary equipment can be mobilized to minimize delays. On arrival, the patient is quickly reassessed and the treatment plan initiated. If the patient arrives by private car, or the ambulance transporting the patient is not staffed with paramedics, the treatment plan should include all of the specific treatments (oxygen–IV–monitor–vital signs, analgesia, thrombolytic screening, and so forth).

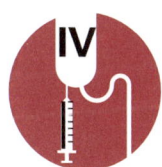

TREATMENT MODALITIES OF *CLEAR* BENEFIT

Intravenous Nitroglycerin

Although oral or spray nitroglycerin may have been administered by ALS personnel, intravenous nitroglycerin has been shown in studies to reduce morbidity and mortality in acute MI (Yusuf et al., 1988). Most of these studies were conducted before the era of thrombolytic therapy. Nitroglycerin is still frequently ordered for patients suspected of having an MI. In addition to suspected ischemic chest pain, intravenous nitroglycerin would be of benefit in the following situations:

- Unstable angina
- Acute pulmonary edema (if systolic blood pressure is greater than 100 mmHg)
- Hypertension in the acute MI setting

In the treatment of MI, nitroglycerin is used not only for pain relief but also for its hemodynamic effects. The drug should be titrated to the amount necessary to reduce the mean blood pressure. This serves to diminish the myocardial oxygen requirement by unloading the heart-reducing preload and afterload. The lowering of the blood pressure indicates that the drug is having the solicited effect. Too much of a good thing is undesirable, however, so monitor the blood pressure carefully, especially in right ventricular infarcts, which are extremely preload dependent and may suffer inordinately from nitroglycerin administration.

The drip should be initiated within the first 24 hours and continued for 2 to 3 days. The dosage of intravenous nitroglycerin is 10 to 20 mcg/minute, increased by 5 to 10 mcg/minute every 5 to 10 minutes, titrating to hemodynamic end point. Be extremely cautious if blood pressure is less than 100 mmHg because hypotension is a major side effect. Because your goal is to reduce the mean blood pressure, expect a decrease and endeavor to titrate the drug so that the systolic drop is no more than 10% to 15% in a normotensive patient or 30% in a patient who is initially hypertensive. Endeavor to keep the mean arterial pressure above 80 mmHg. If you reduce the blood pressure too low, the resulting hypotension causes its own problems.

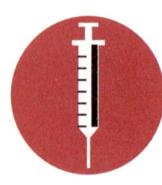

Reperfusion Therapy

Thrombolytic Agents. If the blocked vessel can be cleared within the first hour after insult, almost all involved tissue can be salvaged. The longer the hypoxia lasts, however, the smaller the amount of redeemable tissue. Because patients routinely deny their chest pain for the first few hours, medical attention is delayed and time becomes a critical factor. Thrombolytic therapy should be considered in all potential candidates up to 12 hours after the onset of pain.

More tissue can be salvaged and subsequent mortality decreased if thrombolytic agents are employed as early as possible. The greatest amount of myocardial salvage occurs if thrombolytic agents are administered within the first 4 hours. If treatment is delayed longer than 4 hours, the ability to salvage much myocardium is lost. After this time, opening up the artery probably just assists perfusion in the border zone—the area adjacent to the infarcted tissue. Reperfusion of this area salvages slightly more tissue that otherwise would have died. Even though the amount salvaged is not extensive, thrombolytic therapy is encouraged after 4 hours; survival can be improved even as late as 12 hours after the onset of chest pain (Late Assessment of Thrombolytic Efficacy Study Group, 1993).

Although thrombolytic treatment after 12 hours, but before 24 hours, has exhibited benefits in some studies, it has not been clearly demonstrated in all studies (ISIS-2, 1988). Therefore, during this interval, clinicians are encouraged to select only patients in whom the possible benefits of thrombolytic therapy outweighs the inherent risks.

The decision to order thrombolytic agents is based on a number of variables: the patient's history, age, ECG findings of two or more leads with ST elevation, infarction location, symptom duration, and an estimate of risks versus benefits. Thrombolytic agents were engineered to break down any thrombus. They are not selective for a coronary thrombus—any clot will be dissolved, including an old cerebrovascular accident, gum disease, or an ulcer. Thrombolytic agents have no effect on the layered material on the inner wall of the lumen–cholesterol plaque. Essentially, they are analogous to a commode plunger: they remove the immediate blockage but have no effect on the rusted or deteriorating pipe walls.

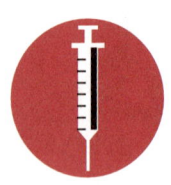

Streptokinase or Alteplase. Although both streptokinase (Kabikinase, Streptase) and alteplase (tPA, Activase) have reduced mortality in acute MI, a front-loaded regimen of alteplase showed a clear advantage over streptokinase (GUSTO Investigators, 1993). This advance was most pronounced in patients with:

- An infarction time less than 4 hours
- Age less than 75 years
- Anterior infarctions

Because alteplase is significantly more expensive and is associated with a higher rate of intracranial hemorrhage, some have suggested using it in subgroups in whom its benefits are more pronounced and using streptokinase in all others.

Reteplase has recently come onto the market. It is more easily administered than the other thrombolytic agents; whether it is as clinically effective as alteplase remains to be determined.

▼ *Helpful Hints* for Assessing Thrombolytic Therapy Candidates

Because thrombolytic agents act on all blood clots, regardless of where they are, patients are gauged as candidates for therapy based on whether they have a high likelihood of bleeding or a moderate likelihood of bleeding following thrombolytic therapy.

High Likelihood of Bleeding (Absolute Contraindications)
▼ Active internal bleeding

▼ Suspected aortic dissection

▼ Known traumatic CPR

▼ Severe persistent hypertension despite pain relief and initial drugs (>180 mmHg systolic or >110 mmHg diastolic blood pressure)

▼ Recent head trauma or known intracranial neoplasm

▼ History of cerebrovascular accident in past 6 months

Moderate Likelihood of Bleeding (Relative Contraindications)
▼ Recent trauma or major surgery in the past 2 months

▼ Initial blood pressure >180 mmHg systolic or >110 mmHg diastolic controlled by medical treatment

▼ Active peptic ulcer or guaiac-positive stools

▼ Remote history of cerebrovascular accident, tumor, injury, or brain surgery

▼ Known bleeding disorder or current use of warfarin

▼ Signficant liver dysfunction or renal failure

▼ Known cancer or illness with possible thoracic, abdominal, or intracranial abnormalities

▼ Prolonged CPR

In the past, excessive patient age was cited as an absolute contraindication. This is no longer the case—there is no age limit. Elderly patients should receive thrombolytic therapy if the benefits to that patient outweigh the risks.

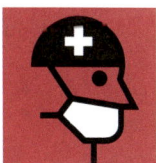

Acute Angioplasty. In centers where cardiac interventions are performed routinely, percutaneous transluminal coronary angioplasty (PTCA) is a valuable alternative to thrombolytic therapy. Mechanically opening the occluded artery rather than using thrombolytic agents is the most direct way to handle an MI. New data clearly show that PTCA can be superior to thrombolytic therapy (Angioplasty Substudy Investigators [GUSTO IIb], 1997). However, PTCA must be done in a facility that has rapid access to a catheterization laboratory and personnel trained to carry out the procedure within 1 hour. If your facility does not have this capability, consider referring the following types of patients immediately!

- Patients in whom thrombolytic agents are contraindicated
- Patients who do not respond to thrombolytic therapy within 60 to 90 minutes
- Patients who show signs and symptoms of cardiogenic shock

Because direct PTCA is associated with fewer complications, it may be a cost-effective alternative to thrombolytic therapy (Gibbons et al., 1993). Therefore, PTCA should be considered not only for thrombolytic candidate rejects but also as another competitive therapy equally as effective. Nevertheless, it

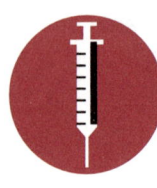

should not be performed as an adjunctive procedure if the patient responds initially to thrombolytic therapy.

Heparin

Thrombolytic agents break up the thrombus, but the surfaces still remain "fresh," encouraging more thrombus formation. Heparin helps discourage the reformation of new thrombi. In addition, it specifically decreases the incidence of ventricular thrombi and thus is indicated in all anterior MIs.

Heparin has long been thought of as a fundamental part of the thrombolytic "package"; however, although its use is essential with the short-acting thrombolytic alteplase (tissue plasminogen activator), it offers no advantage with longer-acting agents, such as streptokinase or anisoylated plasminogen streptokinase activator complex, and may increase bleeding complications (Ridker et al., 1993).

Heparin can be given with or after thrombolytic administration. Give a bolus of 5000 units intravenously, and then continue with 1000 units/hour for 24 to 48 hours. Titrate to maintain 1.5 to 2 times the control values of the activated partial thromboplastin time (PTT). Some clinicians recommend obtaining a baseline PTT value before the initial dosing. Specific criteria and treatment protocols should be developed for the use of this medication.

Heparin has similar contraindications as thrombolytic agents. Therefore, the patient who qualifies for thrombolytic therapy also qualifies for heparin administration.

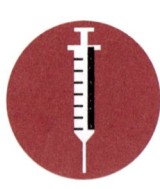

β-Blockers

When considering treatment of an MI, it is difficult to know exactly how β-blockers work because they possess a multitude of diverse effects. β-Blockers have been shown to reduce myocardial oxygen consumption by:

- Lowering myocardial contractility (negative inotropic effect)
- Reducing heart rate (negative chronotropic effect)
- Blocking catecholamine stimulation
- Lowering the blood pressure

Traditionally, β-blockers were employed in catecholamine-driven tachycardias. During an MI, the heart is stimulated by excess sympathetic activity, causing tachycardias, which usually precipitate an elevation in blood pressure. Recent research suggests, however, that their effectiveness may not require the patient to be tachycardic to obtain benefit. β-Blockers block catecholamine stimulation, which, depending on the patient, may not produce tachycardia.

Several large trials of β-blockers in MIs demonstrated a clear benefit by reducing mortality rates by 25% (Hjalmarson and Osson, 1991). This reduction in mortality may be due to a reduction of arrhythmias, reduction in infarct size, or some other beneficial effect to the myocardial tissue. Therefore, β-blockers should always be considered immediately when patients present with symptoms of MI in the emergency department.

Common β-blockers include metoprolol (Lopressor), atenolol (Tenormin), and propranolol (Inderal). Some institutions prefer esmolol (Brevibloc) because its half-life is less than 10 minutes; if problems occur, the drug is metabolized and its effects neutralized quickly. A specific classification of β-blockers, intrinsic sympathomimetic activity (ISA) β-blockers, bears closer scrutiny. Studies suggested that ISA β-blockers were not as helpful in MI treatment because their β blockade appeared incomplete.

Administration of β-blockers in the emergency room should be aggressively considered **unless** the MI patient presents with any of the following contraindications:

- Systolic blood pressure less than 100 mmHg
- Pulse rate less than 50 beats/minute
- Rales covering *greater than* one third of the lungs
- Reactive airway disease (asthma or chronic obstructive pulmonary disease)
- Second- or third-degree AV heart block

Diabetes is not a contraindication to β blockade.

Traditionally, clinicians have been overly anxious about the potential side effects of β-blocker administration. Images of precipitous drops in blood pressures or initiation of atrioventricular blocks have long dominated their thoughts. This inordinate concern for disastrous side effects is not warranted because the safety of β-blockers has been well documented in the literature. In a fresh infarct, potential benefits of β-blockers outweigh the possible risks because these patients really do better. Caution should always be exercised, however, and careful monitoring of the patient is recommended.

Angiotensin-Converting Enzyme Inhibitors

Angiotensin-converting enzyme (ACE) inhibitors, including captopril (Capoten), enalapril (Vasotec), lisinopril (Zestril, Prinivil), and ramipril (Altace), should be considered in all MI patients. ACE inhibitors should be initiated within 24 hours in all patients who have a systolic blood pressure of greater than 100 mmHg. Other factors may be involved, but the use of ACE inhibitors appears to block or limit the remodeling process. The worse the pump failure after an MI, the more likely it is that ACE inhibitors will be of benefit.

ACE inhibitors appear to have unquestioned benefit in patients with impaired left ventricles, that is, with ejection fractions of less than 40% (Pfeffer, 1995). Nevertheless, large studies, totaling well over 100,000 patients, indicate that *almost anybody who has had an MI* may benefit from ACE inhibitors. These studies average a 20% reduction in overall mortality rate (Fourth International Study of Infarct Survival Collaborative Group [ISIS-4], 1995).

Consider administration early in the treatment process because many of the remodeling changes may occur within the first week or two. ACE inhibitors are given long-term. The trials that used them employed them for at least 1 month post-MI, and some of the trials have gone far beyond that.

TREATMENT MODALITIES OF *LIMITED* BENEFIT

Calcium-Channel Blockers

Although proven efficacious in the treatment of many cardiovascular disorders, calcium-channel blockers have not demonstrated any specific survival benefits in the acute MI setting. If employed at all, they should be used in the subacute setting. Common calcium-channel blockers include diltiazem (Cardizem), verapamil (Calan, Isoptin), and nifedipine (Procardia, or Adalat).

Although the foregoing medications are all classified as calcium-channel blockers, they are not interchangeable in the treatment of MIs. Specifically, nifedipine does not appear to have any long-term benefit. On the other hand, both verapamil and diltiazem have demonstrated specific instances in which their use in the *sub*acute setting might improve the outcome of an acute MI.

With no signs of heart failure by day 8, initiating a verapamil regimen within 1 to 2 weeks post-MI has been shown to decrease overall mortality rates by 25% (*American Journal of Cardiology*, 1990). The patients who receive the most benefit are probably those unable to take β-blockers because of a contraindication such as restrictive airway disease.

As long as no signs of diminished heart function exist, diltiazem appears to have a special niche in the treatment of patients with a different species of infarct known as non Q-wave MI. Non Q-wave MIs represent all infarcts in which diagnostic Q waves fail to evolve within 48 to 72 hours of an infarct. This type of infarction has a much greater tendency for reinfarction in the 12 months following the initial event. Diltiazem reduces the rate of reinfarction. β-Blockers have not really been shown to be beneficial in that subset of MI patients who do not have Q waves. Therefore, if Q waves fail to develop within 3 days (i.e., time enough for a Q wave to form), the β-blockers should be discontinued and the patient placed on diltiazem (Gibson et al., 1986).

Although some calcium-channel blockers have been shown to have an impact on acute MI survival rates, β-blockers have shown an advantage in the treatment process by reducing early mortality. Because it is unwise to use calcium blockers until the acute stage has passed, β-blockers are preferred unless specifically contraindicated.

Warfarin

Because the contraction is no longer exactly the same after an extensive MI, damaged myocardial muscle may promote stagnant areas within the left ventricular cavity that allow blood pooling. This pooling can increase the incidence of developing a thrombus with possible concurrent reinfarction or stroke. Warfarin is a long-term anticoagulant. A 3-month regimen should be started in any patient with severe myocardial tissue destruction, with particular emphasis on anterior wall infarcts and severe left ventricular dysfunction. Any person with an MI might develop a thrombus, but those with anterior involvement and left ventricular dysfunction have a much greater incidence of developing a thrombus in the left ventricle (Nordrehaug, 1985).

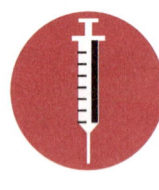

Magnesium Sulfate

Interest in the use of magnesium sulfate in the treatment of acute MI has increased. The antiarrhythmic qualities of magnesium sulfate are clear; however, its routine use in acute MI is controversial.

Since the 1997 publication of the ACLS textbook, conflicting studies concerning magnesium's role in acute MI have surfaced in the literature. An English investigation, the LIMIT-2 study, demonstrated a 25% overall decrease in mortality rates of patients (ISIS-2, 1988). A more recent study, the multicenter ISIS-4, did not document any significant decrease in mortality rates in patients given magnesium sulfate (ISIS-4, 1995). On one level, this contradiction might appear baffling; however, if these two studies and one more recent one are closely examined, some particulars may shed light on this discrepancy.

When the ISIS-4 study failed to establish a clear benefit for magnesium, the door appeared to close on its use. This study has been criticized, however, for inadequacies in its design. In ISIS-4, magnesium was only administered *after* thrombolytic therapy. A more recent Israeli study noted that patients *who did not receive thrombolytic therapy* and were given magnesium again showed the strong benefit that other trials had shown (Shechter, 1995). Therefore, proponents of magnesium's use still press for its employment in those patients who are not candidates for thrombolytic therapy but who are seen early in the course of their infarction. It gives no survival advantage if administered later.

In summary, on the basis of all the available research data, magnesium has not demonstrated any clear survival benefit if the patient will shortly undergo PTCA or thrombolytic therapy. However, *in those patients who are at high risk (especially those who are not candidates for either therapy), the clinician should consider magnesium*, given the facts that these patients have an otherwise high mortality rate and that some studies suggest a powerful benefit. Although not documented by research studies, should a clinician wish to administer magnesium sulfate in addition to thrombolytic therapy or PCTA, its advantages appear to accrue only if it is employed *before* opening the vessel with the designated therapy or if the patient has a magnesium deficit.

In the first 24 hours after an MI, magnesium sulfate is administered with an intravenous loading dose of 1 to 2 g of 50% magnesium sulfate ($MgSO_4$) diluted in 50 to 100 mL of D-5-W, over 5 to 60 minutes. This is followed with 0.5 to 1 g/hour for as long as 24 hours. Watch for hyporeflexia, hypotension, diaphoresis, and drowsiness. Although the first dose is well tolerated, adjust subsequent dosing for patients with renal failure.

In addition to its other uses, magnesium sulfate is the drug of choice for a variation of ventricular tachycardia—torsades de pointes. When treating torsades, give 1 to 2 g and administer it over 1 to 2 minutes. It has demonstrated efficacy in other arrhythmias as well. See case study 9 in Chapter 5 for a more in-depth discussion.

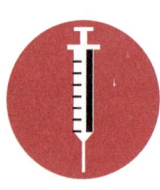

TREATMENT MODALITY OF *NO* BENEFIT

Lidocaine

When employed in primary ventricular fibrillation or ventricular tachycardia or after successful defibrillation, lidocaine clearly demonstrates its effectiveness in reducing mortality and is the treatment of choice. However, if administered to suppress dangerous arrhythmias that *might occur* in the acute MI, lidocaine is considered prophylactic and has no benefit.

Traditionally, ventricular ectopic beats were thought to be the harbinger of ventricular tachycardia or fibrillation and were looked on with dread and anxiety. Clinicians were taught to extinguish all ventricular ectopic beats that fell into the following categories: more than six per minute; multiformed; exhibiting the R on T phenomenon; or exhibiting bursts, salvos, or runs of ventricular tachycardia. Lidocaine was routinely administered to patients with these phenomena who were being treated for something totally unrelated such as a fractured hip.

Lidocaine administration is not considered prophylactic when administered to halt an emergent cardiovascular episode. Guidelines for emergent use of lidocaine are not agreed on by all, but a consensus is reached when the patient is actively infarcting: most clinicians would employ lidocaine immediately for *significant* ectopic rhythms—runs or bursts of ventricular tachycardia. Less severe ventricular ectopy frequently goes untreated. For example, some clinicians treat multiformed ectopic beats, but some do not. This is a gray area, and clinician judgment is required. Nevertheless, lidocaine only treats the symptom. Give thought to what could be causing the ventricular irritability—treat the myocardium. Proper attention to the patient's status—oxygenation, blood pressure, and heart rate—is much more valuable than just giving lidocaine without thought to the cause of the irritability. Remember, treating ventricular ectopic beats with lidocaine is like treating fever with aspirin—it only treats the symptom, not the cause.

Studies have not only questioned the continued use of prophylactic lidocaine in the treatment of acute MI, but also have equated it to an *increase* in fatal asystolic events. A meta-analysis of six trials of prophylactic use of lidocaine in patients with acute MI found that the mortality rate was slightly higher in the lidocaine group (MacMahon et al., 1988). The evidence suggests that the central nervous system and cardiovascular side effects inherent in prophylactic lidocaine therapy have an associated greater mortality rate than is seen with treatment of only those patients who evidence ventricular fibrillation or ventricular tachycardia. Emergency personnel and critical care nurses have become so proficient in treating these lethal arrhythmias that the associated mortality is not as high as the side effects of lidocaine intended to suppress their incidence. *The risks of fatal asystolic episodes and neurologic dysfunction associated with prophylactic lidocaine therapy outweigh its benefits.*

If ventricular ectopic beats are significant and require treatment, the recommended dose is 1 to 1.5 mg/kg given by intravenous push. The lower dose is for more stable situations in which time is not a concern. If the patient is beginning to decompensate, consider the higher dose because it can be maximized quickly. A second bolus of 0.5 to 0.75 mg/kg is required afer 10 minutes to prevent subtherapeutic levels after the first bolus. This can be repeated if necessary every 5 to 10 minutes with additional doses of 0.5 to 0.75 mg/kg until a maximum dose of 3 mg/kg is reached.

Because the half-life of lidocaine is fairly short, it is necessary to hang a lidocaine drip, 1 G in 250 mL of NS or D-5-W, to keep up a therapeutic blood level. Start the drip between 2 and 4 mg/minute (30 to 60 gtt/minute a microdrip or minidrip).

Because lidocaine is metabolized by the liver, use lower doses and longer intervals in patients in whom the liver could be impaired; in those who have congestive heart failure, bradycardias, or conduction disturbances; and in the elderly. Lidocaine is contraindicated in ventricular escape rhythms and complete heart blocks because it may stop the heart completely. Watch for clinical signs of toxicity, which is usually evidenced as central nervous system problems (e.g., altered consciousness, tinnitus, seizures).

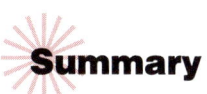

Summary

See Figure 4-3 for a summary of the treatment of an acute MI. When a patient presents with chest pain, immediately administer 325 mg of aspirin (or equivalent), assuming there are no contraindications. Administer oxygen by mask, obtain a 12-lead ECG, and administer morphine sulfate and sublingual nitroglycerin, assuming there are no contraindications.

If the 12-lead ECG suggests acute MI, observe the patient's vital signs. If the patient is not bradycardic, hypotensive, or showing signs and symptoms of congestive heart failure, consider administering an intravenous β-blocker. The β-blocker is then continued orally through at least the first year. If the patient has signs of cardiovascular compromise, consider correcting the underlying problem. This could entail using either, both, or a combination of the bradycardia protocol and the shock, pulmonary edema, and congestive heart failure protocol.

If the patient's blood pressure is still above a mean arterial pressure of 80 mmHg, consider intravenous nitroglycerin. Use with caution in right ventricular infarcts after administration of a β-blocker. If the patient remains or becomes hypotensive, bypass nitroglycerin administration.

Administer heparin unless a contraindication exists or the patient is receiving a long-acting thrombolytic agent. Make a decision about whether magnesium sulfate will be of benefit. Magnesium appeared to be helpful only when given before thrombolytic agents or PCTA; however, data are lacking about whether it significantly increases the patient's chances if thrombolytic therapy or PCTA is promptly car-

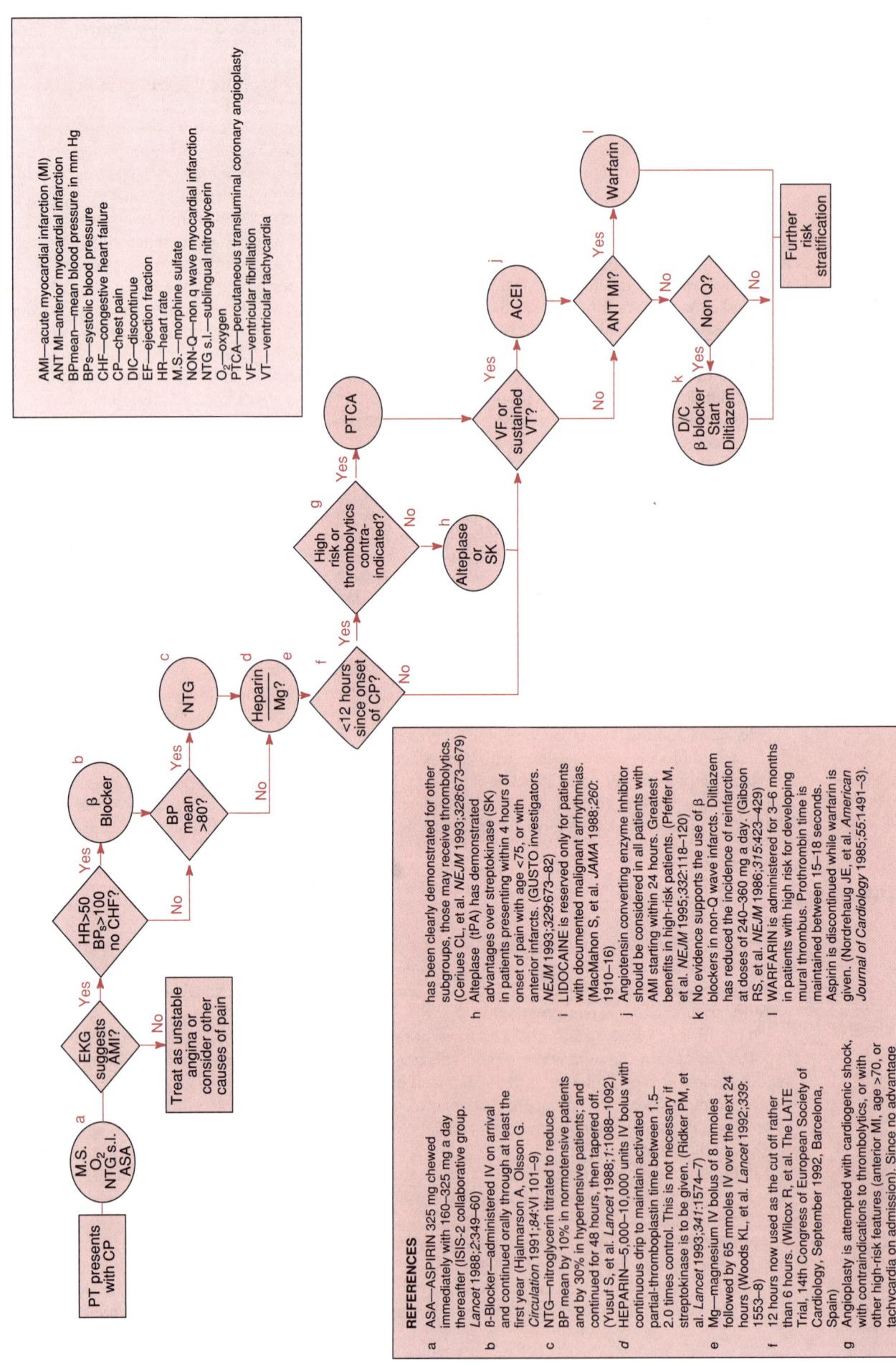

Figure 4-3. Acute myocardial infarction algorithm.

ried out. Magnesium appears to reach its maximum benefit when administered to patients who are not acceptable candidates for either therapy.

For patients presenting with an acute MI that occurred within the past 12 hours, the clinician should decide whether to use thrombolytic agents or PCTA. The reader is referred to the Inclusion and Exclusion Criteria for thrombolytic therapy versus PCTA. Although thrombolytic therapy or PCTA might have some limited benefit past the first 12 hours, routine thrombolytic therapy or PCTA for infarcts after 12 to 24 hours should be based on relative benefits gained versus obvious risks incurred for each patient.

If at any point the patient presents with a life-threatening ventricular arrhythmia, lidocaine may be employed. It is considered an emergent drug for malignant arrhythmias; however, it is no longer given to ward off ectopic "demons."

Assuming the patient has survived the initial insult, ACE inhibitors should be considered within the first 24 hours. ACE inhibitors limit or inhibit the remodeling process. Research has shown that its greatest benefits lie in treating high-risk patients.

If the patient has an anterior infarction, consider the use of warfarin before discharge to inhibit the formation of fresh thrombi. If the patient does not exhibit a Q wave after the infarction, discontinue the β-blockers because diltiazem probably has a greater chance of improving the survival rate by inhibiting the possibility of reinfarction.

Treatment of an acute MI is remarkably time dependent. A community-wide system composed of lay-public medical education, a 911 system, EMS involvement, and emergency room guidelines and hospital policies is necessary to achieve rapid access to the medical support team. The door-to-drug interval—the time from the opening of the emergency room doors until thrombolytic therapy is administered or PCTA is initiated—should not be greater than 30 minutes to 1 hour (Fig. 4-3).

References

Angioplasty Substudy Investigators (GUSTO IIb). (1997). The global use of strategies to open coronary arteries in acute coronary syndromes. *New England Journal of Medicine, 336,* 1621–1628. (See Fig. 4-3, reference g.)

Fourth International Study of Infarct Survival Collaborative Group (ISIS-4). (1995). A randomized factorial trial assessing early oral captopril, oral mononitrate, and intravenous magnesium sulphate in 58,050 patients with suspected acute myocardial infarction. *Lancet, 345,* 669–685. (See Fig. 4-3, reference e.)

Gibbons, R., Holmes, D.R., Reeder, G.S., et al. (1993). Immediate angioplasty compared with the administration of a thrombolytic agent followed by conservative treatment for myocardial infarction. *New England Journal of Medicine, 328,* 685–691.

Gibson, R.S., Boden, W.E., Theroux, P., & the Diltiazem Reinfarction Study Group. (1986). Diltiazem and reinfarction in patients with non-Q-wave myocardial infarction: Results of a double-blind, randomized, multi center trail. *New England Journal of Medicine, 315,* 423–429. (See Fig. 4-3, reference j.)

Grines, C.L., Browne, K.F., Marco, J., et al. (1993). A comparison of immediate angioplasty with thrombolytic therapy for acute myocardial infarction. *New England Journal of Medicine, 328,* 673–679.

The GUSTO Investigators. (1993). GUSTO: An international trial comparing thrombolytic strategies for acute myocardial infarction. *New England Journal of Medicine, 329,* 673–682. (See Fig. 4-3, reference h.)

Hjalmarson, A., & Osson, G. (1991). Myocardial infarction: Effects of beta-blockade. *Circulation, 84,* 101–107. (See Fig. 4-3, reference b.)

Late Assessment of Thrombolytic Efficacy Study Group (LATE). (1993). Late assessment of thrombolytic efficacy study with alteplase 6–24 hours after onset of acute myocardial infarction. *Lancet, 342,* 759–766. (See Fig. 4-3, reference f.)

MacMahon, S., Collins, R., Peto, R., et al. (1988). Effects of prophylactic lidocaine in suspected acute myocardial infarction: An overview of results from the randomized, controlled trials. *Journal of the American Medical Association, 260,* 1910–1916. (See Fig. 4-3, reference i.)

Nordrehaug, J.E., Johannessen, K.A., & von der Lippe, G. (1985). Usefulness of high-dose anticoagulants in preventing left ventricular thrombus in acute myocardial infarction. *American Journal of Cardiology, 55,* 1491–1493. (See Fig. 4-3, reference k.)

Pfeffer, M.A. (1995). ACE inhibition in acute myocardial infarction. *New England Journal of Medicine, 332,* 118–120.

Ridker, P.M., Hebert, P.R., Fuster, V., & Hennekens, C.H. (1993). Are both aspirin and heparin justified as adjuncts to thrombolytic therapy for acute myocardial infarction? *Lancet, 341,* 1574–1577. (See Fig. 4-3, reference d.)

Second International Study of Infarct Survival Collaborative Group (ISIS-2). (1988). A randomized trial of intravenous streptokinase, oral aspirin, both, or neither amount in 7,187 cases of suspected acute myocardial infarction. *Lancet, 2,* 349–360. (See Fig. 4-3, reference a.)

Shechter, M., Hanoch, H., Chouraqui, P., et al. (1995). Magnesium therapy in acute myocardial infarction when patients are not candidates for thrombolytic therapy. *American Journal of Cardiology, 75,* 321–323.

Staff. (1990). Effect of verapamil on mortality and major events after acute myocardial infarction (the Danish Verapamil Infarction Trial II—DAVIT II). *American Journal of Cardiology, 66,* 779–785.

Woods, K.L., Fletcher, S., Roffe, C., & Haider, Y. (1992). Intravenous magnesium sulphate in suspected acute myocardial infarction: Results of the second Leicester Intravenous Magnesium Intervention Trial (LIMIT-2). *Lancet, 339,* 1553–1558.

Yusuf, S., Collins, R., MacMahon, S., & Peto, R. (1988). Effect of intravenous nitrates on mortality in acute myocardial infarction: An overview of the randomized trials. *Lancet, 1,* 1088–1092. (See Fig. 4-3, reference *c*.)

Section 6: Acute Myocardial Infarction Interim Evaluation

Mark the correct answer.

1. A normal ECG excludes the diagnosis of MI (see ACLS text pp. 1-5 to 9-9). _____

   _____ (a) True
   _____ (b) False

2. A diaphoretic patient with chest pain radiating to the neck and arms should be (see ACLS text pp. 9-1 to 9-12): (1) monitored for cardiac arrhythmias; (2) given prophylactic propranolol 5 mg orally; (3) given intravenous isoproterenol; (4) given supplemental oxygen. _____

   _____ (a) 3 and 4
   _____ (b) 2 and 3
   _____ (c) 1 and 2
   _____ (d) 1 and 4

3. A 150-pound patient walks into the emergency room with his wife. He relates that he has had severe, crushing, mid-chest pain that has been present for 30 minutes with no relief with nitroglycerin. He has a history of angina on two other separate occasions. His pulse is 98; blood pressure is 110/70 mmHg. His ECG shows a sinus rhythm. Of the selection below, the *first* drug and dosage is (see ACLS text pp. 9-1 to 9-13): _____

   _____ (a) Furosemide, 20 to 40 mg given intravenously
   _____ (b) Morphine sulfate, 2 to 10 mg given intravenously
   _____ (c) Atropine, 0.5 mg given intravenously
   _____ (d) Procainamide, 20 mg/minute

4. The percentage of deaths from MI outside the hospital is (see ACLS text p. 9-4): _____

   _____ (a) 10%
   _____ (b) 30%
   _____ (c) 50%
   _____ (d) 75%

5. A substantial impact on survival from prehospital cardiac arrest can be achieved in a community when (see ACLS text p. 9-5): _____

   _____ (a) Lay persons are trained in cardiopulmonary resuscitation
   _____ (b) Rapidly responsive basic rescue units are available
   _____ (c) Advanced life support is rapidly available (within 8 to 10 minutes)
   _____ (d) All of the above

6. According to the ISIS-2 study, if administered within the first 24 hours, aspirin may achieve the same decrease in mortality as streptokinase (see ACLS text p. 9-30). _____

   _____ (a) True
   _____ (b) False

7. Which of the following statements is false regarding MIs (see ACLS text pp. 9-1 to 9-3)? _____

   _____ (a) Most occur during heavy physical exercise
   _____ (b) Many occur during sleep

_____ (c) Severe exertion, excessive fatigue, and unusual emotional stress have been incriminated as a combination likely to precipitate MI.

_____ (d) Most individuals who die due from MI do so before reaching the hospital.

8. The diagnosis of suspected acute MI should be primarily based on the patient's history (see ACLS text pp. 9-1 to 9-13). _____

_____ (a) True
_____ (b) False

9. In the presence of crushing chest pain, even though premature ventricular contractions are absent, it is appropriate to administer lidocaine prophylactically (see ACLS text p. 9-34).

_____

_____ (a) True
_____ (b) False

10. Magnesium sulfate may be administered for all except (see ACLS text p. 7-14): _____

_____ (a) Torsades de pointes
_____ (b) High-risk MIs
_____ (c) In patients with eclampsia
_____ (d) None of the above

11. Which of the following drugs, used in therapeutic doses, directly depresses the pumping function of the heart muscle (negative inotropic effects) (see ACLS text pp. 8-11 to 8-12): (1) atropine; (2) lidocaine; (3) propanol; (4) isoproterenol? _____

_____ (a) 1, 2, and 4
_____ (b) 2 and 3
_____ (c) 1 and 3
_____ (d) 3

12. Propranolol may be useful in the treatment of (see ACLS text pp. 8-11 to 8-12): _____

_____ (a) Atrial fibrillation with ventricular rate of 80/min after MI
_____ (b) Congestive heart failure
_____ (c) Narrow complex tachydysrhythmias refractory to adenosine and verapamil
_____ (d) Third-degree heart block

13. Sublingual nitroglycerin is the initial treatment of choice for most forms of ischemic cardiac pain (see ACLS text p. 8-10). _____

_____ (a) True
_____ (b) False

14. Nitroglycerin (see ACLS text pp. 8-9 to 8-11): (1) may be given sublingually; (2) may be useful in relieving pain in acute MI; (3) may produce hypotension; (4) should only be given as a single dose and not repeated. _____

_____ (a) 1, 2, and 4
    (b) 1, 2, and 3
_____ (c) 2 and 4
_____ (d) All of the above

90 Unit 1 *Fundamental Concepts of ACLS* • Coronary Syndromes

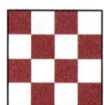

Section 7
ACUTE MYOCARDIAL INFARCTION CROSSWORD PUZZLE

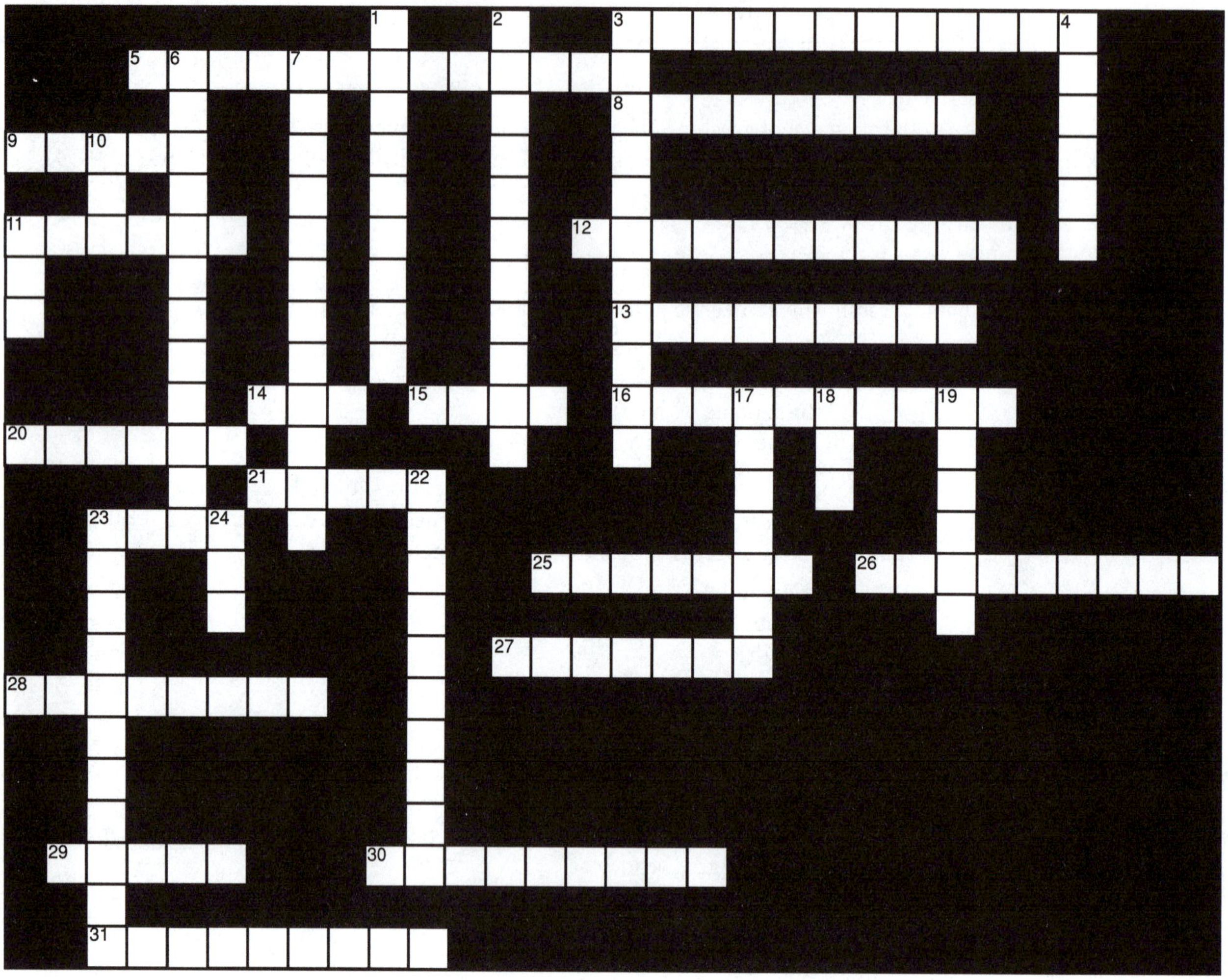

Across

3. High blood pressure. Depending on severity, it can be relatively or absolutely contraindicated when considering thrombolytic therapy.
5. One of the two major thrombolytic agents.
8. This drug might be considered helpful in treating MIs. Although literature sources conflict, this drug may serve to decrease mortality levels in that subset of patients who cannot undergo thrombolytic therapy or PCTA.
9. An open sore or lesion. An active stomach open sore or lesion is considered a relative contraindication to the use of thrombolytic therapy.
11. A physical injury or wound. A history of this is an absolute contraindication to the use of thrombolytic agents.
12. Low blood pressure. This condition can complicate the treatment of an MI. This condition may be a major side effect of sublingual nitroglycerin.
13. The drug classification of morphine. Necessary for relief of pain and apprehension in an MI. Pain relief classification only.
14. A normal 12-lead _____ does not preclude the diagnosis of an MI.
15. The name of an adrenergic receptor that, when stimulated, is responsible for both positive chronotropic and inotropic activity in the heart. Propanolol blocks this receptor.
16. The term for the condition downstream from a coronary artery occlusion.
20. The greatest clinical benefits in thrombolytic therapy occur if the drug is administered within _____ minutes of onset of the infarct.
21. These must be balanced against the benefits when confronting a patient who presents with a relative contraindication to thrombolytic therapy.

23. The abbreviation for percutaneous transluminal coronary angioplasty.
25. Operative procedures for correction of deformities and defects. Recent history of this is considered an absolute contraindication to the use of thrombolytic agents.
26. In the past, women who presented with this status were considered to have an absolute contraindication to the administration of thrombolytic agents. However, available data suggest that thrombolytics may be safely administered to women with this condition; of course, controlled studies for this group are impossible. A condition that results in a person who is adorable initially but unfortunately grows up to become a teenager.
27. A drug given in conjunction with some thrombolytic agents to keep clots from reforming on freshly vacated sites.
28. The generic name for Coumadin. An anticoagulant drug.
29. The possibility that a patient may _____ from old injuries, medical conditions, or surgeries is a main factor in deciding whether a patient is a candidate for thrombolytic therapy. The term for the situation in which fluid leaves a blood vessel.
30. _____ of the ST segment in an ECG means myocardial injury. Opposite of depression.
31. This drug is no longer administered prophylactically. It is only indicated for occurrences of significant situations (i.e., runs of ventricular tachycardia).

Down
1. Term meaning death rate. Reduction of this result is accomplished by decreasing the door-to-drug time.
2. A form of invasive coronary artery surgery chosen if an MI patient is not a candidate for thrombolytic administration.
3. The forces involved in circulating through the body. It is commonly used when describing a bradycardia that is causing hypotension and an altered level of consciousness. The bradycardia is termed _____ (-ally) significant.
4. The tonicity of _____ saline is 0.9%. This fluid can be given to cardiac patients because it has not been shown to cause pulmonary edema as originally thought.
6. A class of medication that breaks up blood clots.
7. A term meaning "in case of." Lidocaine is no longer administered in this manner. Oxygen is usually given in this manner to all patients with MI regardless of their current oxygen saturation.
10. A recent _____ is an absolute contraindication to the use of thrombolytic therapy. Abbreviation for an intracranial event.
11. Abbreviation of one of the two major thrombolytic agents.
17. In the ISIS-2 study, this drug, if administered within 24 hours of an MI, has the same reduction in mortality as the administration of streptokinase.
18. Trauma from _____ during cardiac arrest is an absolute contraindication to the use of thrombolytic agents. (The abbreviation for cardiopulmonary resuscitation.)
19. This drug has been shown to limit infarcts. It should never be withheld from patients who present with symptoms of hypoxia.
22. Nitroglycerin is commonly given in this manner. The medical term for a medication given underneath the tongue.
23. The generic name for Inderal.
24. The abbreviation for the class of inhibitors used to block or limit ventricular remodeling in post-MI patients.

5 Rate-Driven Case Studies

- **Bradycardias**
- **Unstable tachycardias**
- **Stable tachycardias**

In the following rate-related case studies on bradycardias, unstable tachycardias, and stable tachycardias, it is important to provide some general rules to assist in treatment. If the heart rate is the clinician's only consideration, the patient may be mistreated. A tachycardic or bradycardic heart is not always a cardiovascular response to an underlying pathology. The heart rate may be only a sympathetic reaction to stress or exercise, a mirror of the body's response to a fluid deficit, or a response to excessive vagal domination. The point to reiterate is: *all fast or slow rhythms are not treated by reversing the rates*.

The clinician must be aware that with such diverse causes of bradycardia and tachycardia, it is too simplistic to administer the tachycardia protocol when the heart rate is too fast or to administer the bradycardia protocol when the rate is too slow. These protocols do not take into account patients who present with tachycardia in whom the heart rate is not causing the problem. In these patients, the heart rate may be an overt sign of an underlying pathology (e.g., hypovolemia, heart block, myocardial infarction [MI], drugs, or congestive heart failure [CHF]).

> **One statement holds true for all of the rate protocols:**
> Consider the tachycardia or bradycardia protocol if the heart rate specifically is responsible for the patient's signs and symptoms. If the rate isn't causing the problem, consider other possibilities and hence other treatments.

How can the clinician tell the difference between a rate-related rhythm and one that is compensating for an underlying condition? How should these patients be treated? The clinician first needs to decide if the presenting signs and symptoms are abnormal for the patient. Some people have slower than normal heart rates because they are athletic or on medication. Others may have slight tachycardia due to high-pressure, high-stress lifestyles. Again, treat the patient, not the monitor.

A patient is generally considered cardiovascularly compromised, or *hemodynamically significant*, when some or all of the following signs and symptoms are in evidence:

- Altered level of consciousness
- Hypotension (systolic blood pressure less than 90 mmHg)

- Cool extremities
- Diaphoresis

The reason for the hemodynamic significance may not be rate related. When a tachycardia is not rate related, it is termed *compensatory*. The heart is speeding up to compensate for an underlying situation. The patient may be hypovolemic, or the heart may be trying to maintain an adequate cardiac output during heart failure. The tachycardia is not causing the problem; the heart is responding to an underlying pathology. Likewise, a slow rate may be a response to ischemia of the conduction system from an MI.

A generalized approach to this quandary is *rate—volume—pump. The heart rate can be instrumental in revealing the cause of the problem. Assuming that the patient's vital signs reflect hemodynamic significance*, but are not absent, consider the heart rate first.

Consider the Heart Rate First

If the heart rate is less than 60, consider the bradycardia protocol (Fig. 5-1). Normally, if the patient exhibits symptoms of shock, you would expect a tachycardic, not a bradycardic, heart. This happens frequently; a slow pacemaker is usually not a volume problem, but there are exceptions to this rule. In some inferior or right ventricular MIs, the involved myocardial tissue may manifest enhanced parasympathetic tone, resulting in bradycardia with resultant hypotension. A careful fluid challenge may be life-saving in providing the necessary increase in right ventricular filling pressure. Always maintain a high index of suspicion if your initial treatment does not correct the problem. With the exception of case-specific inferior or right ventricular MIs, most hemodynamically significant bradycardias should be treated with the bradycardia protocol (increasing heart rate), not with pushing fluids.

If the heart rate is excessively fast (more than 170), consider the tachycardia protocol (Fig. 5-2). Regardless of the origin of the ectopic cell (i.e., supraventricular or ventricular, wide or narrow), this rapid rate is usually indicative of an ectopic pacemaker cell problem rather than fluid deficit. Luckily, pulse rates in hypovolemic shock and CHF are rarely above 160 to 170. Usually, a response to fluid loss, even a documented 50% blood loss, does not push the pulse to more than 160 beats/minute. CHF compensatory pulse rates are usually in the 120 to 140 range. Thus, in a narrow complex tachycardia, if the pulse is greater than 160 to 170, an ectopic pacemaker cell usually is the cause of the presenting problem, not tachycardia compensating for a volume deficit. Close attention to any trauma or cardiac history is a necessity, however, when narrowing down the choices of treatment.

In supraventricular tachycardia (SVT), also known as *atrial tachycardia,* the heart rate may range from 140 to 270 beats/minute. Although occasionally the rate may be as low as 140, it is usually noted above 160 to 170. With the exception of aberrantly conducted SVTs (which may appear wide), most wide complex tachycardias are normally treated with the tachycardia protocol from as low as 100 beats/minute.

The two main exceptions to the rate rule are atrial fibrillation and atrial flutter. These two narrow complex arrhythmias are treated in the tachycardia protocol but do not usually result in excessively fast heart rates (i.e., greater than 170). It is necessary for the clinician to recognize these two rhythms so that the patient can be referred to the tachycardia protocol for treatment. If these rhythms are not recognized, they could be falsely identified as compensatory and treated with fluids or the pump failure protocol.

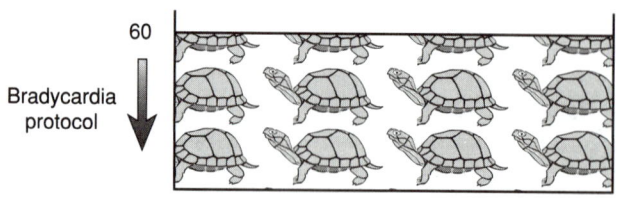

Figure 5-1. Consider bradycardic heart rate.

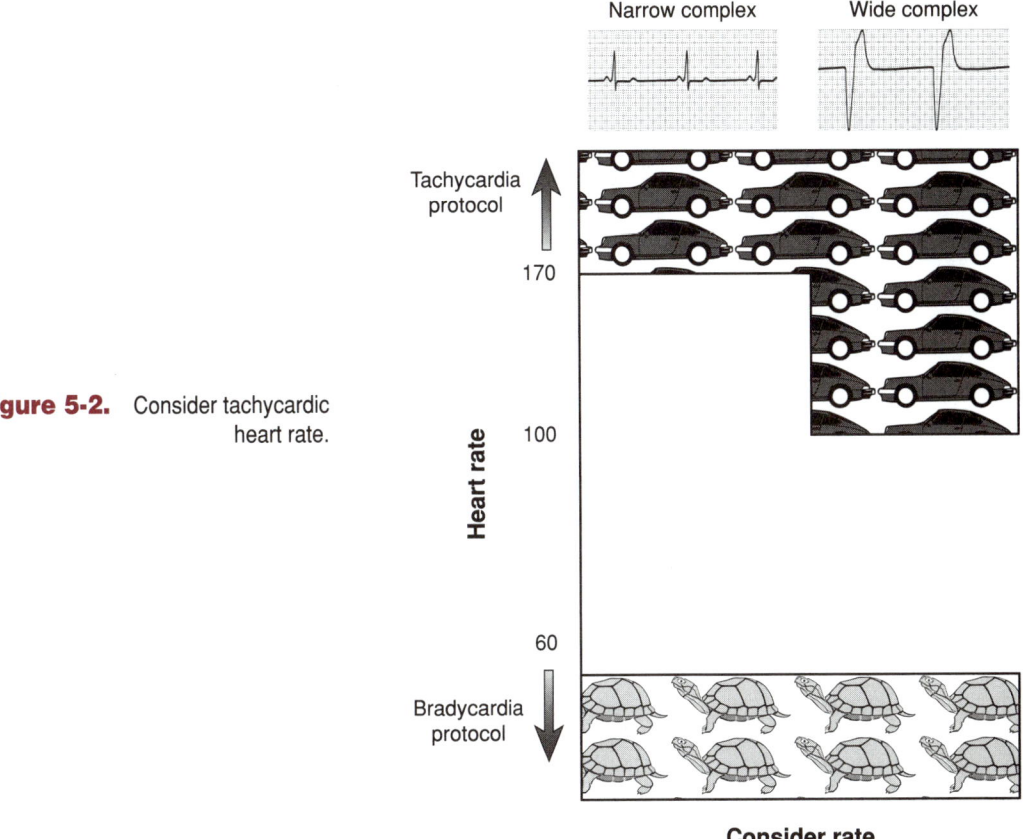

Figure 5-2. Consider tachycardic heart rate.

In summary, assuming the patient is hemodynamically significant, but not pulseless, with the exception of atrial fibrillation and flutter, treat narrow complex tachycardias with heart rates above 170 and any wide complex tachycardias with heart rates above 100 with either the stable or unstable tachycardia protocol. Pick the protocol that matches the patient's stability status. (See case study 9 on stable tachycardias for a more detailed discourse on how to determine if a QRS complex is wide or narrow.) If the patient's heart rate is not too fast and is not atrial fibrillation or flutter, consider the possibility that the patient's symptoms may reflect a volume deficit.

Consider Volume

With the exception of atrial fibrillation or flutter, narrow complex tachycardias with rates of more than 60 but less than 170, with the exception of SVT with aberrancy (which may appear wide), and most wide complex tachycardias with rates of more than 60 but less than 100, should prompt fluid volume deficit consideration (Fig. 5-3). The key term is *consideration*. This does not mean that all patients with assumed compensatory tachycardias should be given fluid; it means that fluid loss should always be considered before progressing to other treatments.

If you decide to administer a fluid challenge of 500 mL of normal saline (NS) or lactated Ringer's solution, and the patient's status does not improve, or if you decide that fluid would not be appropriate (e.g., because of symptoms of CHF), consider that the presenting tachycardia may be a response to a pump problem (e.g., cardiogenic shock or CHF).

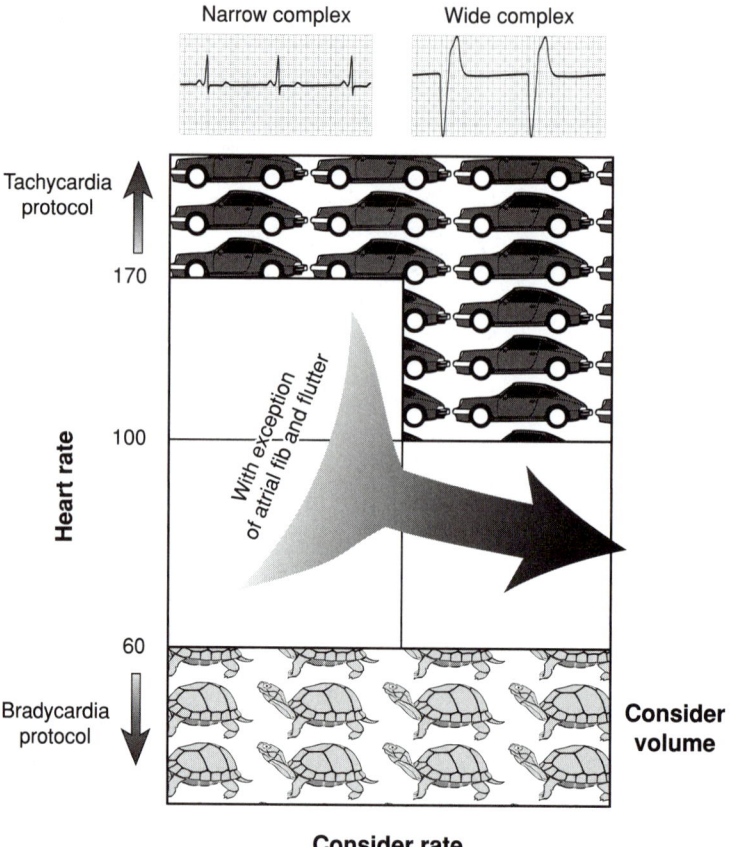

Figure 5-3. Consider volume.

Consider Pump

The medications of choice that help support the blood pressure in nonhypovolemic patients are dopamine and norepinephrine (Fig. 5-4). Dopamine is acceptable for most hypotensive crises, but if the blood pressure is moderately low (e.g., less than 70 mmHg systolic), norepinephrine should be employed. Norepinephrine does not stimulate the dopaminergic receptors on the kidneys; hence, it is common to switch to dopamine when norepinephrine has succeeded in raising the blood pressure to more than 70 mmHg systolic to keep the kidneys perfused.

Again, *do not even consider a vasopressor before deciding if the situation would profit from a fluid challenge* because these drugs exacerbate hypovolemic shock. Always progress in order: rate–volume—pump (Fig. 5-5).

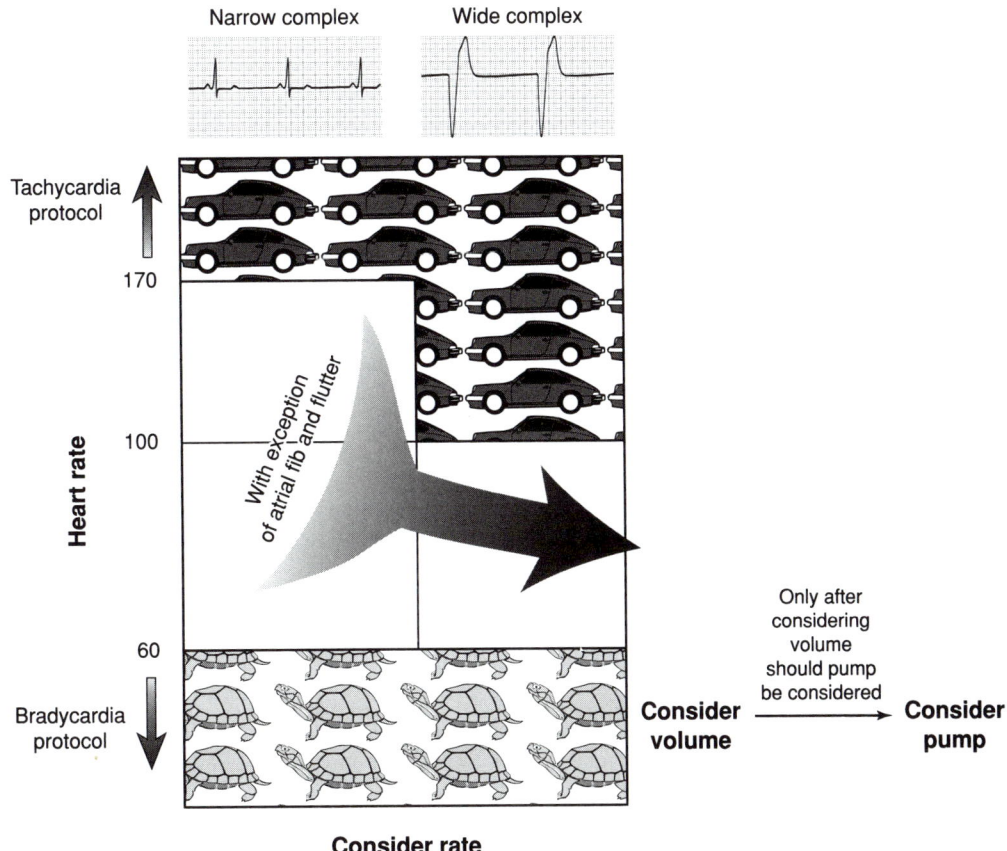

Figure 5-4. Consider pump.

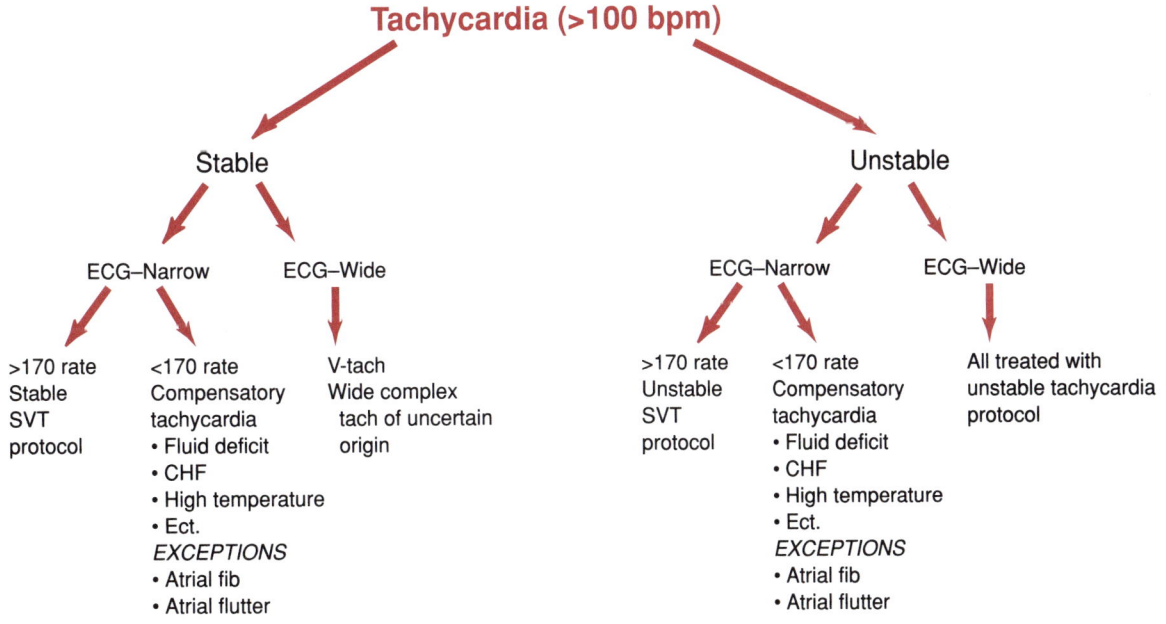

Figure 5-5. Tachycardia flow chart.

Case Study 7
Bradycardias

Heart rate is a key factor when considering cardiac function. This case study demonstrates that simultaneous mechanical and pharmacologic intervention may be required for a patient exhibiting a hemodynamically significant decompensating rate.

Section 1: Critical Actions for Student Evaluation

The ACLS instructor checklist for case study 7 is shown in Table 5-1. This form was designed to guide the faculty when evaluating participants during this particular station. Refer to it frequently as you read the lecture that follows. *Do not memorize it.* The form is only included to: (1) show you what the American Heart Association (AHA) considers important during this particular case study; (2) describe what the faculty are trying to cover in the station; and (3) provide a summary of the case study after you have read the lecture.

Table 5-1.
Evaluation Checklist—Case 7: Bradycardias

Critical Action	Completed	Not Completed	Comments
Recognizes signs and symptoms of bradycardia with hemodynamic compromise			
Obtains intravenous access			
Gives oxygen as needed			
Attaches monitor			
Applies transcutaneous pacemaker when indicated			
Is knowledgeable about atropine dosing			
Recognizes			
Second-degree AV Block			
Type I			
Type II			
Third-degree AV Block			
Recognizes need for transvenous pacing after stabilized			
Recognizes other pharmacologic support			
Recognizes need for thrombolytic therapy in acute MI			
Orders 12-lead ECG			

(Reproduced with permission. *Instructor's manual for advanced cardiac life support,* 1997 © Copyright American Heart Association, p. 6-14.)

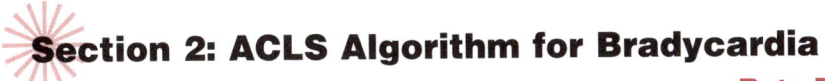

Section 2: ACLS Algorithm for Bradycardia

**Rate Problems:
(Patient is not in Cardiac Arrest)**

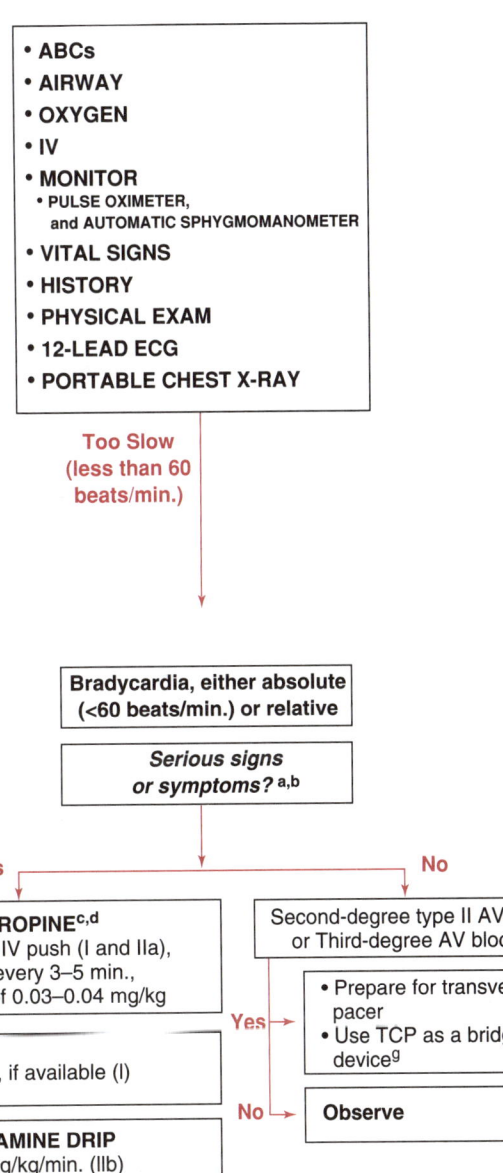

Bradycardia Footnotes

(a) Serious signs or symptoms must be related to the slow rate. Clinical manifestations include:
 • symptoms (chest pain, shortness of breath, decreased level of consciousness)
 • signs (low BP, shock, pulmonary congestion, CHF, acute MI)
(b) Do not delay TCP while awaiting IV access or for atropine to take effect if patient has symptoms.
(c) Denervated transplanted hearts will not respond to atropine. Go at once to pacing, catecholamine infusion, or both.
(d) Atropine should be given in repeat doses every 3–5 min. up to total of 0.03–0.04 mg/kg. Use the shorter dosing interval (3 min.) in severe clinical conditions. It has been suggested that atropine should be used with caution in atrioventricular (AV) block at the His-Purkinje level (type II AV block and new third-degree block with wide QRS complexes) (class IIb).
(e) Never treat third-degree heart blocks plus ventricular escape beats with lidocaine.
(f) Isoproterenol should be used, if at all, with extreme caution. At low doses, it is class IIb (possibly helpful); at higher doses, it is class III (harmful).
(g) Verify patient tolerance and mechanical capture. Use analgesia and sedation as needed.

(Reproduced with permission. *Advanced cardiac life support.* Copyright 1997, American Heart Association.)

Section 3: Identifying Features

Bradycardia

Bradycardia is a nonspecific clinical term referring to any electrocardiogram (ECG) rhythm with a ventricular response of less than 60. The rhythm could originate from any portion of the heart (sinus, junctional, or ventricular), or it could originate from a heart block; origin is not the issue, just the rate.

Clinicians do not treat bradycardias as a class; they only treat *significant* bradycardias. Any bradycardic rhythm is considered significant when it causes any or all of the following symptoms of cardiovascular compromise: altered level of consciousness concurrent with hypotension (blood pressure usually less than 90 mmHg), pulmonary edema, ventricular ectopy, diaphoresis, chest pain, shortness of breath, or weakness.

Sinus Bradycardia. The ECG strip in Figure 5-6 is a sinus bradycardia. This rhythm is treated only if the patient's symptoms are significant. The rhythm is easily identified; each QRS complex is preceded by a sinus P wave. The ventricular rate is slightly less than 60.

High Junctional Rhythm. A bradycardic rhythm could arise from anywhere. In the ECG strip in Figure 5-7, the origin is from the atrioventricular (AV) junction. The origin is not the point; the rate is! This rhythm is identified as a high junctional rhythm operating at a ventricular response of about 50 beats/minute. The rhythm is regular, and the P waves are inverted in front of each QRS complex seen. In lead II, these features point to a junction rhythm.

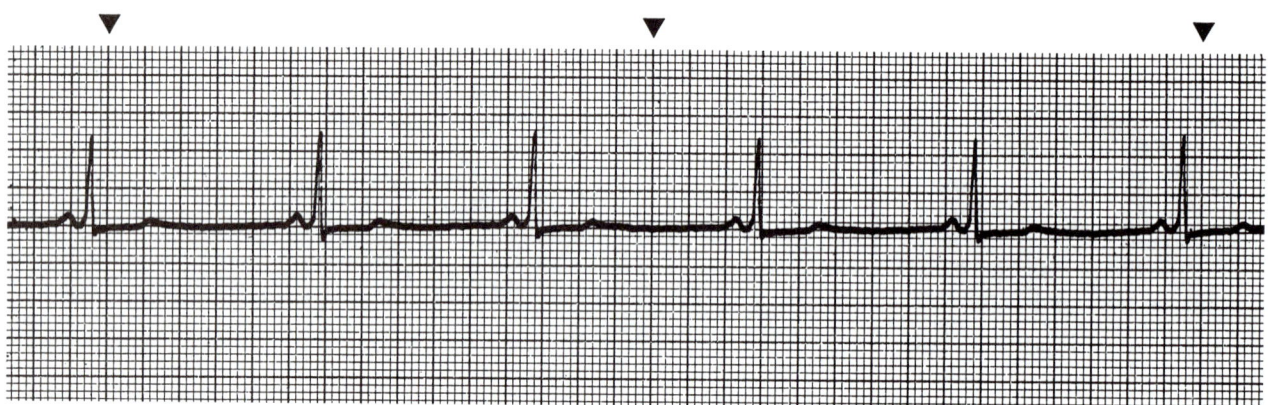

Figure 5-6. Sinus bradycardia.

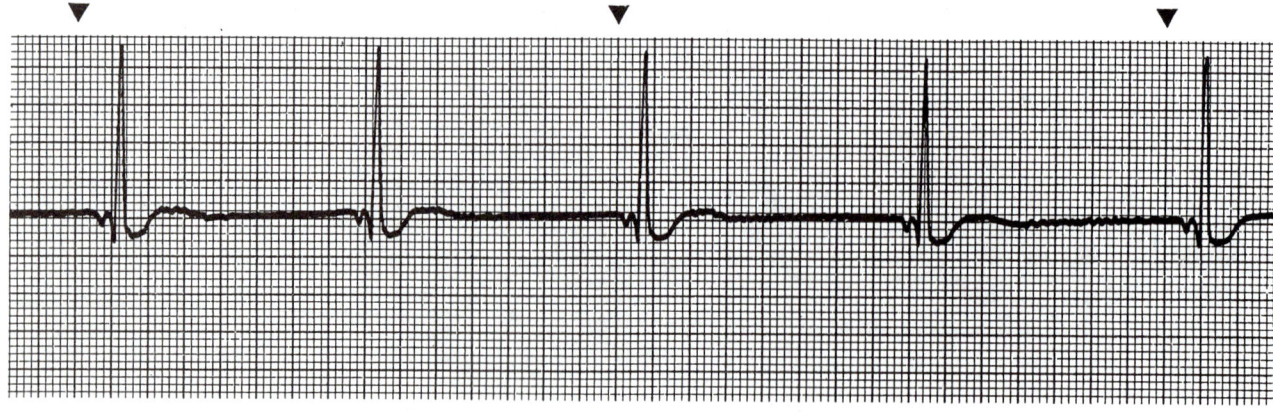

Figure 5-7. High junctional rhythm.

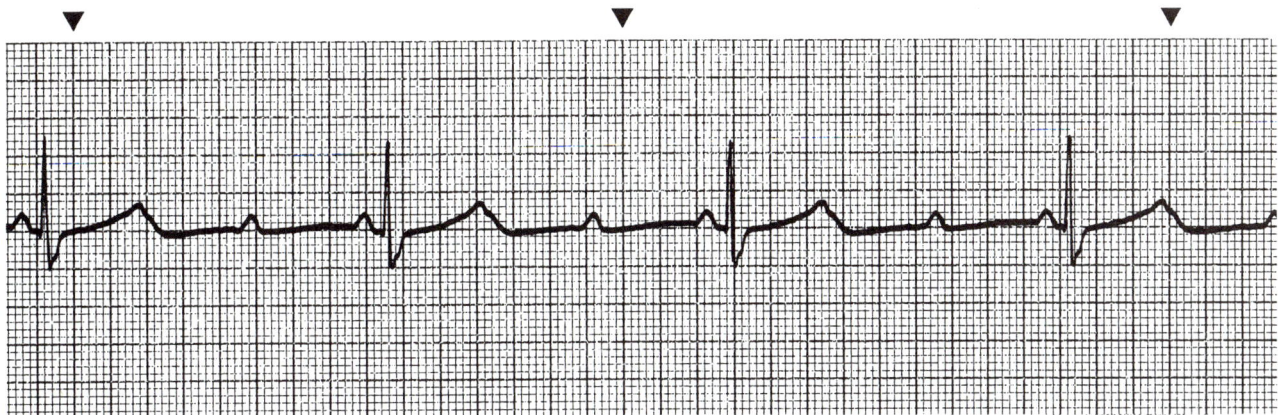

Figure 5-8. Sinus rhythm with a second-degree, Type II AV block.

Sinus Rhythm With a Second-Degree Type II Atrioventricular Block. The strip in Figure 5-8 is a sinus rhythm with a second-degree, Type II AV block. Again, this rhythm generally would not be treated unless the patient's symptoms were significant. In this situation, however, this statement is too simplistic. Even though patients with this form of block may not always exhibit acute symptoms, they need transvenous pacemaker implantation without delay because this form of AV block tends to progress to a complete heart block.

The underlying rhythm is identified by the presence of P waves depolarizing at a rate of about 90 (sinus rhythm), whereas the ventricular response is about 40. All QRS complexes do not have P waves preceding them; however, for all those that do, the PR intervals appear equal. P waves with occasional absent QRS complexes, combined with consistent PR intervals (for those with P waves and QRS complexes together), confirm the diagnosis of a sinus rhythm with a second-degree, type II AV block bradycardic ventricular response. The underlying rhythm is *sinus;* the AV block is only an abnormality to the underlying sinus rhythm.

Sinus Rhythm With a Third-Degree Atrioventricular Block. The ECG strip in Figure 5-9 is a sinus rhythm with a third-degree AV block (also referred to as a *complete heart block*). Although one might expect a third-degree block to be the worst of all the blocks, that is not always the case. It depends on the ventricular response and hemodynamic status of the patient. A patient with a second-degree, type II AV block with a ventricular response of 30 usually has a worse prognosis than a patient with a complete heart block with a ventricular response of 60. The clinician should concentrate on the rhythm's cardiac output rather than the degree of the block.

Even though patients with this form of block may not exhibit acute symptoms, they need to be watched carefully and should be treated aggressively only when appropriate. A complete heart block resulting from an anterior MI should be paced immediately. These tend to be escape ventricular rhythms with poor ventricular responses. When a complete heart block is noted in conjunction with an inferior MI,

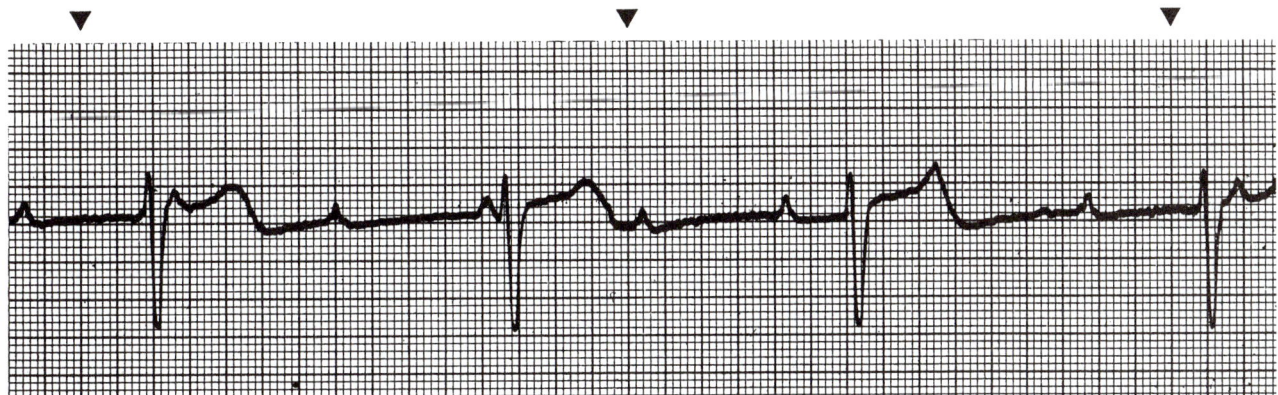

Figure 5-9. Sinus rhythm with a third-degree AV block.

however, treatment may not necessarily be as aggressive. Inferior MI–related complete heart blocks may respond to standard therapy, such as atropine administration, because the mechanism of the block is usually increased transient parasympathetic activity.

The rhythm is identified by the presence of P waves depolarizing at a rate of about 70 (sinus rhythm), whereas the regular ventricular response was only 40. All QRS complexes do not have P waves preceding them, and none of the PR intervals appears equal (i.e., the atria and the ventricles are beating but not in synchronization with each other). P waves with occasionally absent QRS complexes, combined with inconsistent PR intervals (for those with P waves and QRS complexes that appear in close proximity) and a regular ventricular response, confirm the diagnosis of a sinus rhythm with a third-degree AV block.

Section 4: Assessment

Primary Survey

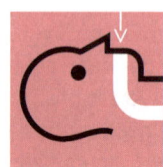

Even though the patient is not in arrest, a compromised cardiovascular status should prompt the clinician to reevaluate airway and breathing on a consistent basis.

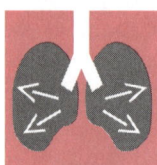 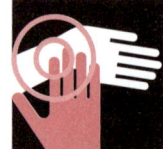

Because the patient is not in ventricular fibrillation, defibrillation is not an option.

Secondary Survey

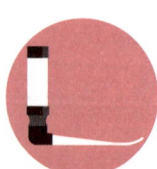

This patient would profit from oxygen and an oropharyngeal airway (OPA) if required. Administer each in a manner dependent on the patient's ventilatory and consciousness status (passive or positive pressure for the oxygen and level of consciousness for the OPA).

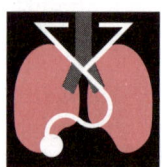 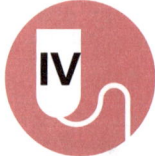

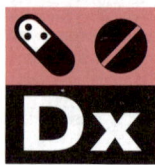

Assuming that this is an emergency, it is critical in this particular algorithm to perform a focused history. The time sequence should be elicited for any predisposing symptoms before deciding on a specific treatment. Chest pain that occurred before the presenting situation could suggest an acute MI and therefore would necessitate consideration of thrombolytic therapy. When there is no history of chest pain and the patient presents with hypotension of an undetermined cause, consider **rate–volume–pump**.

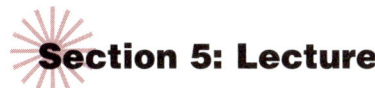
Section 5: Lecture

Assuming there is time, obtain a 12-lead ECG, hook the patient to a pulse oximeter, and order a chest radiograph. These tests will yield valuable data during the assessment.

While you are preparing to intervene with medications, send for the transcutaneous pacemaker (TCP). A TCP is the definitive therapy for a significant bradycardia. The medications should only be viewed as stop-gap measures until a transcutaneous or transvenous pacemaker can be instituted.

If the patient assessment reflects a bradycardia that appears hemodynamically significant, aggressive action is required. Significant hemodynamic symptoms are defined as a blood pressure less than 90 mmHg, signs and symptoms of depressed levels of consciousness, and other signs of cardiovascular compromise. These might include pulmonary edema, ventricular ectopy, diaphoresis, chest pain, shortness of breath, and weakness. If the patient's status is not emergent, however, proceed with a more relaxed assessment. It is critical that the *patient* be treated, not the *heart rate*. Many people have heart rates that are bradycardic but are not compromised, such as elderly people, who have adjusted to a slower heart rate, or training athletes.

The term bradycardia usually refers to *absolute bradycardia*—a heart rate of less than 60; however, a patient may have *relative bradycardia*. This condition exists when the patient has a heart rate in excess of 60 but not an acceptable cardiac output. This could happen in a normally hypertensive person with slight tachycardia whose heart rate, owing to some vagal pathology, plummeted to 65, with resultant hypotension. β-Blockers can also cause a relative bradycardia by competing with the sympathetic neurotransmitters, resulting in a lower pulse rate.

Treatment

Treating hypotensive patients with fluids is common. Except in cases of right ventricular MI, however, which can present with bradycardia, the heart responds to fluid loss by becoming tachycardic. In patients with right ventricular MI, a careful fluid challenge might prove life-saving by providing an increase in right ventricular filling pressure. In most other cases, however, a bradycardic patient with hypotension should be considered to have a slow pacemaker cell problem rather than fluid volume deficit. Thus, with the exception of right ventricular infarction, most hypotensive patients with bradycardias should be treated with the bradycardia protocol, not fluids.

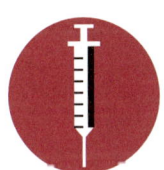

ATROPINE

The information in this section is different from other case studies using atropine. Do not skip this section!

Atropine is the first and most benign medication in the bradycardia protocol. It should be administered while initiating a TCP. Do not wait to find out how atropine fared—call for or institute the TCP immediately. The only exception to this rule is transient sinus bradycardia in a patient with an inferior MI, in which case atropine alone usually suffices.

Atropine inhibits the vagus nerve. In a situation in which a relative or absolute bradycardia makes the patient's blood pressure hemodynamically significant, the vagus nerve may be the culprit. The bradycardic rate may not produce a substantial enough cardiac output to generate an effective blood pressure. Accelerating the heart rate should increase the blood pressure. Essentially, atropine is given to rule out the possibility of vagal domination. If the heart rate accelerates after administration, the vagus nerve was the cause of the bradycardia; if the rate does not change, the cause of this particular bradycardia was not vagal. Because the atria are more heavily enervated by the vagus nerve than the ventricles, look for atropine to have a more pronounced effect when administered for atrial bradycardia than for ventricular bradycardia.

Anytime that you increase the heart rate, myocardial oxygenation demand goes up, increasing the heart's tendency to respond with ventricular tachycardia or ventricular fibrillation. Atropine should be tried in all cases; but in new infranodal blocks, such as second-degree, type II or third-degree AV blocks, atropine may cause an increase in the atrial rate, with the AV node becoming more selective (a higher block). Both these conditions may result in a slower ventricular rate. Because the hypotension that can ensue is a clinical rarity, do not perform a detailed ECG analysis before administering atropine. Atropine should still be employed initially because its side effects are rare and it is the most benign drug in the bradycardia armamentarium.

Dosage. The dosage of atropine in a symptomatic bradycardia is 0.5 to 1.0 mg/kg given intravenously every 3 to 5 minutes, to a total of 0.04 mg/kg. Consider decreasing the time interval to 3 minutes if the patient is moderately unstable. If the maximum dosage is reached and the rhythm is still refractory, the vagus nerve can be effectively ruled out as a cause of the bradycardia.

TRANSCUTANEOUS PACEMAKER

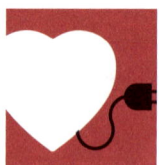

Emphasis should be made on calling for or instituting a TCP simultaneously with atropine administration. A TCP is both easy and quick to place. The anterior pacing pad is placed on the patient's thorax to the left of the sternum centered over the point of maximal cardiac impulse. The posterior pad is placed on the identical spot of the anterior pad but on the posterior thorax.

A TCP does not have the disadvantage of invasive catecholamines, such as dopamine and epinephrine, in maintaining therapeutic blood levels. Its chief advantage lies in its ease of use while preparing for a more definitive transvenous pacemaker.

Helpful Hints for the Use of a Transcutaneous Pacemaker

Use of a transcutaneous pacemaker (TCP) is indicated in the following patients with bradycardia:

▼ Those patients with cardiac problems, such as heart block, that *might* progress, causing hemodynamic compensation. The TCP would act as a "bridge device" until a more definitive pacemaker could be implanted.

▼ Cardiovascularly compromised patients who have hemodynamically significant bradycardia that may or may not be refractory to medications. Speed in correcting the problem is the issue. The TCP may be started simultaneously with medications to stabilize the patient's status as rapidly as possible.

▼ Bradycardic patients in whom the heart rate is so slow that *ventricular escape beats* are in evidence. These rhythms may not respond to rate medications and have a high incidence of deteriorating into ventricular tachycardia or ventricular fibrillation.

Although lidocaine is normally contraindicated in heart blocks, with the use of a TCP, treating significant ventricular ectopic beats may be accomplished without fear of losing the only remaining pacemaker. Special attention should be paid to ventricular ectopic beats that do not come prematurely but come as late–escape beats. Patients with escape beats should not receive lidocaine because these beats represent an attempt by the heart to continue when the normal pacing sites fail to fire. Increasing the heart rate usually decreases or eliminates these beats.

Pacemaker Settings. There are two modes by which the pacemaker may operate: fixed or demand. The demand setting does not compete with the patient's own heartbeat, as does the fixed. For the most part, the demand setting is preferred, but if there is too much artifact, the fixed mode is better suited. The fixed mode would be better in the back of a bouncing ambulance or when a patient's movement interferes with the sensing capability of the TCP.

The pacemaker wires are attached to the pads, and the machine's pacer dial is set anywhere between 60 and 80 beats/minute. The dial delineating the milliamperage (the resistance) is slowly increased from zero milliamperes to a point at which capture is achieved. Normally, in a conscious patient, the dialing speed is slow because the pacing process is painful. The monitor shows a small pacing spike, quickly followed by a wide QRS complex. The dialing speed should be increased if the patient is failing fast. In asystole, consider starting at the maximal milliamperage setting to achieve capture because pain is not an issue.

Once the captured beat is noted, *it must generate a pulse*. Check the femoral pulse rather than the carotid because muscle twitching in the thorax may obscure the palpation. Patient size, pad location, and the presence of a large pericardial effusion may be responsible for noncapture. Continuous monitoring is necessary because capture ceases if the patient goes into ventricular fibrillation. Pacing is usually painful, and an analgesic or a sedative is appropriate if the patient is conscious.

> It is impossible to make any ACLS algorithm foolproof, because fools are so ingenious.

DOPAMINE DRIP

If the patient is still symptomatically bradycardic, a catecholamine infusion should be used if a TCP is not available or is unsuccessful. Note that few, if any, of the ACLS protocols are perfectly linear. They are not meant to progress only when the one step proves refractory. Although they appear to be given in order—from top to bottom—this is not the case. It may be appropriate to administer the first dose of atropine, call for a TCP, and hang a dopamine drip simultaneously if the patient is rapidly decompensating.

Dopamine affects three different adrenergic drug receptors: α, β, and dopaminergic. It does not affect all of them at the same time (Fig. 5-10).

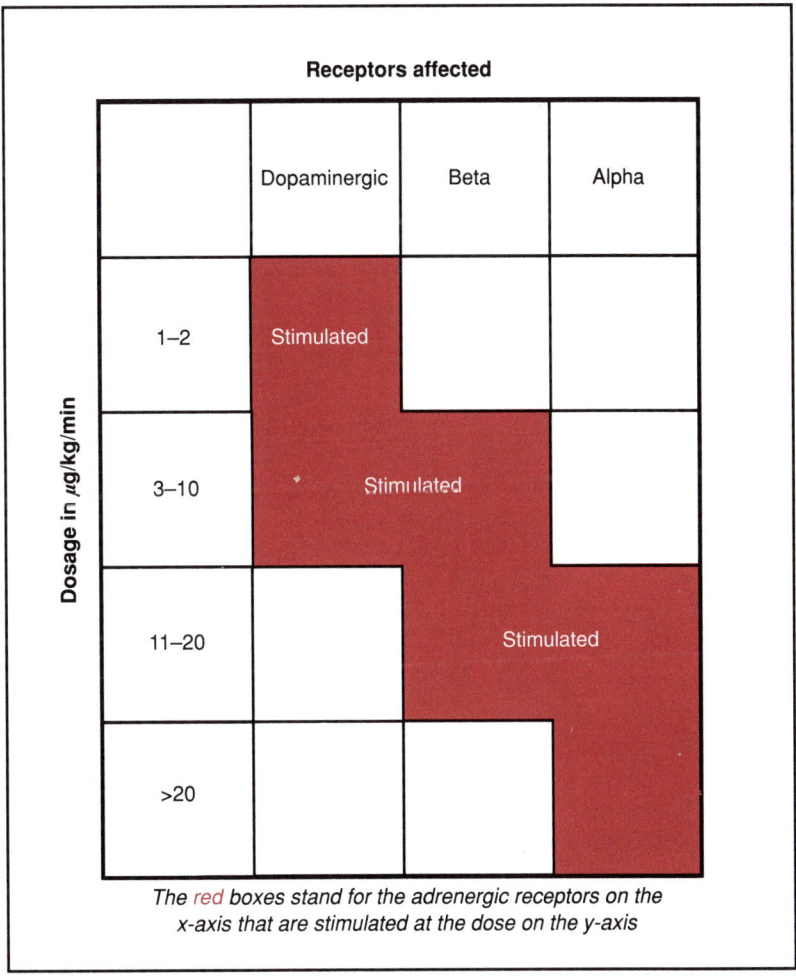

Figure 5-10. Adrenergic drug receptors affected by dopamine.

- At low doses, 1 to 2 mcg/kg/min, dopamine causes diuresis and mesenteric vasodilation.
- At moderate ranges, 2 to 10 mcg/kg/min, dopamine causes diuresis, mesenteric vasodilation, a more rapid and forceful heart beat, and only mild, if any, α-adrenergic receptor stimulation. Thus, in moderate doses, by sheer contractility and rate alone, the blood pressure begins to elevate.
- At high ranges, 11 to 20 mcg/kg/min, dopamine no longer stimulates the kidneys. The positive inotropic and chronotropic effects on the heart (the increased rate and contractility) continue, but pronounced α-adrenergic receptor stimulation is noted, resulting in vasoconstriction.
- At extremely high dosages, 20 mcg/kg/min or more, only α-adrenergic receptors are stimulated.

A drip is created by mixing 400 mg of dopamine (1 ampere) in 250 mL of NS or D-5-W, creating a concentration of 1600 mcg/mL. Adjust the rate from 2 to 20 mcg/kg/min, titrating the drip rate to elevate the heart rate above 60. Remember, the drug is being employed for its rate-enhancing qualities only; thus rate, not blood pressure per se, is the object here. Taper the drug off slowly when discontinuing it; do not just turn it off because hypotension will ensue.

Dopamine is the chemical precursor to norepinephrine, which is a potent vasoconstrictor. Therefore, any dopamine that is introduced affects the amount of norepinephrine. Side effects of dopamine are related to this fact and include: excessive vasoconstriction, arrhythmias, possible fall in blood pressure initially, nausea and vomiting, and tissue sloughing if it extravasates. Dopamine is discouraged with patients with pheochromocytoma and those taking monoamine oxidase inhibitors because these conditions dramatically enhance its effect.

EPINEPHRINE DRIP

If either a TCP or dopamine, separately or together, fail to elevate the patient's rate, employ an epinephrine drip. Note that this is not an intravenous push situation, as in a cardiac arrest, in which epinephrine is introduced directly by intravenous bolus. The bradycardia protocol employs this drug specifically for its positive chronotropic effects and thus is given as an intravenous drip administered over time.

The drip is mixed by introducing 1 mg of epinephrine (1:1000 dilution) in 250 or 500 mL of NS or D-5-W. Run it at a rate of 2 to 10 mcg/min, titrating the drip rate to elevate the heart rate above 60 beats/minute. Watch for signs of tachycardia.

ISOPROTERENOL DRIP

Isoproterenol (Isuprel) is a pure β-adrenergic receptor–stimulating drug. It is classified as both a positive inotropic and a chronotropic agent. It is ominously effective because it definitely increases the heart rate but also both increases the myocardial oxygen demand and causes vasodilation, resulting in myocardial ischemia and hypotension. This is obviously a problem because patients who have hemodynamically significant bradycardias usually present with hypotension. Therefore, if nothing else works, a low infusion rate of isoproterenol, at a rate that does not exacerbate the hypotension, may be effective. In this instance, isoproterenol is a class IIb drug (possibly helpful), but in higher doses, it is considered class III (harmful).

A drip is created by mixing 1 mg of isoproterenol in 250 mL of NS or D-5-W, making a concentration of 4 mcg/mL. Run it at a rate of 2 to 10 mcg/min, titrating the drip rate to elevate the heart rate above 60.

TRANSVENOUS PACEMAKER

Even if the patient does not have symptoms, second-degree, type II blocks are serious arrhythmias, often associated with anteroseptal MIs. These blocks can rapidly progress to a complete heart block without warning. Therefore, for both mildly symptomatic or asymptomatic third-degree (complete heart blocks) and second-degree, type II AV blocks, the clinician should prepare for the definitive transvenous pacemaker.

The TCP pads should be placed on the patient and the equipment hooked up but not turned on. This prophylactic measure allows the TCP to act as a bridge device if the patient's condition deteriorates before the transvenous pacemaker is introduced. Remember: *do not treat the rate, treat the patient.*

Section 6: Bradycardia Interim Evaluation

1. A patient presents to you after successful resuscitation. The patient's rhythm is sinus bradycardia at 34 beats/minute, generating a systolic blood pressure of 70 mmHg. Although this protocol is not necessarily linear, which of the following is an acceptable order of progression necessary to correct the situation (see ACLS text pp. 1-28 to 1-32): (1) external pacemaker; (2) oxygenation; (3) dopamine drip; (4) epinephrine drip; (5) atropine?

    _____ (a) 2, 3, 5, 1, and 4
    _____ (b) 5, 3, 4, 1, and 2
    _____ (c) 2, 5, 1, 3, and 4
    _____ (d) 5, 4, 2, 3, and 1

2. Epinephrine, when administered as part of the bradycardia protocol, is employed primarily for which of its following effects (see ACLS text pp. 1-30 to 1-31 and 7-2 to 7-4)?

    _____ (a) inotropic
    _____ (b) chronotropic
    _____ (c) dopaminergic
    _____ (d) α-adrenergic

3. In conjunction with hypotension, which of the following rhythms or situations might profit from a fluid challenge (see ACLS text pp. 1-28 to 1-32): (1) sinus tachycardia at rate of 130 beats/minute; (2) sinus bradycardia at rate of 46 beats/minute; (3) right ventricular infarct at a heart rate of 40 beats/minute; (4) SVT at rate of 190 beats/minute?

    _____ (a) 1 and 3
    _____ (b) 1 and 4
    _____ (c) 1, 3, and 4
    _____ (d) 2 and 4

4. In which of the following cases should an external TCP be considered (see ACLS text pp. 1-28 to 1-32)?

    _____ (a) Sinus rhythm with a first-degree block
    _____ (b) Hemodynamically significant ventricular tachycardia
    _____ (c) Pulseless electrical activity
    _____ (d) Any form of hemodynamically significant bradycardia

5. All of the following are reasons for noncapture of a TCP *except* (see ACLS text p. 1-31):

    _____ (a) Patient size
    _____ (b) Sex of the patient
    _____ (c) Pad location
    _____ (d) Pericardial effusion

6. When treating a patient for hypotension, which of the following is the dosage range for dopamine that will raise the blood pressure but still keep the kidneys perfusing (see ACLS text p. 8-3)?

    _____ (a) 1 to 2 mcg/kg/min
    _____ (b) 3 to 10 mcg/kg/min
    _____ (c) 11 to 20 mcg/kg/min
    _____ (d) 20 mcg/kg/min or more

7. In rare instances, atropine administration may cause hypotension in the presence of infranodal blocks, such as second-degree, type II AV blocks or complete heart blocks (see ACLS text p. 7-4).

_____ (a) True
_____ (b) False

8. A 45-year-old, 220-pound man arrives at the emergency department complaining of dizziness concurrent with crushing substernal chest pain. His pulse is 42 beats/minute, and blood pressure is 72/40 mmHg. Your monitor exhibits a sinus bradycardia with sporadic premature ventricular contractions (PVCs). Which of the following is indicated initially (see ACLS text pp. 1-29 to 1-32)?

_____ (a) Propranolol, 1 to 3 mg given intravenously
_____ (b) Atropine, 0.5 mg to 1.0 mg given intravenously
_____ (c) Lidocaine, 100 to 150 mg given intravenously
_____ (d) Synchronized cardioversion at 50 joules

9. Isoproterenol in an adult patient (see ACLS text p. 8-6): (1) is only administered with extreme caution and then only if necessary; (2) should initially be given sublingually; (3) decreases cardiac oxygen consumption; (4) may increase the amount of myocardial ischemia during MI.

_____ (a) 1 and 3
_____ (b) 1 and 4
_____ (c) 2 and 3
_____ (d) 2 and 4

10. If a hemodynamically significant bradycardia with PVCs is being paced, it is perfectly acceptable to administer lidocaine initially to terminate the ectopic beats (see ACLS text pp. 1-28 to 1-32).

_____ (a) True
_____ (b) False

11. Isoproterenol (see ACLS text p. 8-6): (1) increases myocardial irritability and potential for arrhythmias; (2) possesses both β- and α-adrenergic qualities; (3) decreases force of contraction while increasing heart rate; (4) is recommended if atropine is refractory before other interventions when treating significant bradycardias; (5) if indicated, is given at 2 to 10 mcg/min.

_____ (a) 1, 2, 3, and 5
_____ (b) 1, 4, and 5
_____ (c) 2, 3, and 4
_____ (d) 1 and 5

12. Dopamine infusion at 7 mcg/kg/min most likely results in (see ACLS text p. 8-3): (1) increased myocardial contractility; (2) continuing renal perfusion; (3) mesenteric vasoconstriction; (4) increased α-adrenergic receptor stimulation.

_____ (a) 2 and 3
_____ (b) 1 and 3
_____ (c) 1 and 2
_____ (d) All of the above

13. It is always necessary to make certain that the QRS complex that appears on a monitor in response to pacing generates a pulse (see ACLS text p. 1-31).

_____ (a) True
_____ (b) False

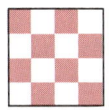

Section 7
BRADYCARDIA CROSSWORD PUZZLE

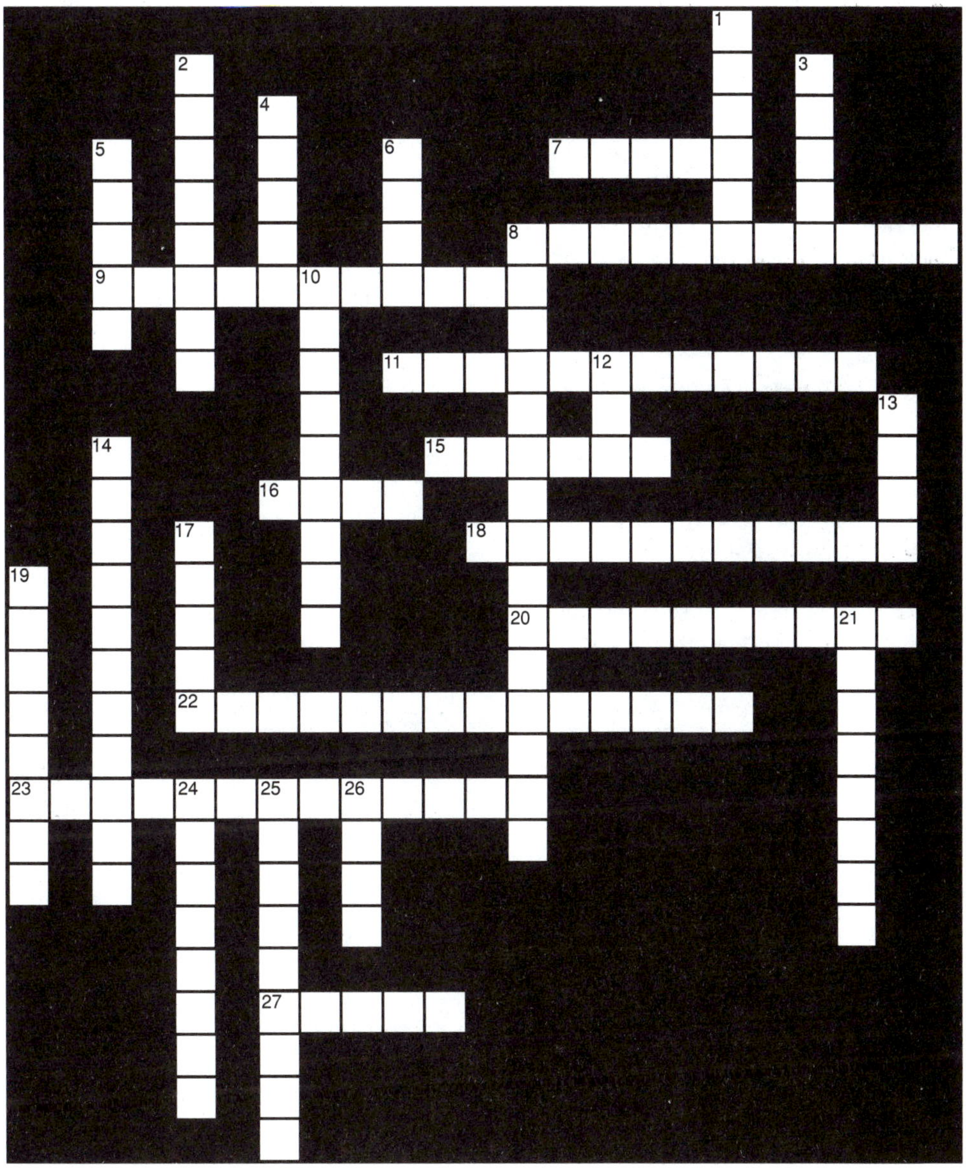

Across

7. Isoproterenol is a pure β-adrenergic receptor stimulant; it has no _____-adrenergic or dopaminergic properties (a Greek letter spelled out).
8. Low blood pressure
9. This drug is considered if the preceding therapy is refractory in the treatment of significant bradycardia (atropine, TCP, and dopamine). When treating bradycardia, its β-adrenergic effects predominate.
11. A term that groups drugs together that affect the heart rate, either positively or negatively.
15. This drug should never be withheld from a patient who needs it. In the face of chronic obstructive pulmonary disease, this drug should not be withheld if the patient is experiencing hypoxia; however, the clinician should be prepared to assist ventilations if necessary.
16. The lower dosage for atropine when administered for significant bradycardic situations is one-_____ milligrams (number spelled out).
18. Clinicians should monitor the rate of epinephrine and isoproterenol drips. Giving the drugs too quickly or giving too much may cause the bradycardia to turn into a _____.

20. A term used to describe a rhythm or ectopic arising beneath the AV node.
22. The type of pacemaker in which the pads are secured over the skin on the patient's chest and back.
23. At low dosages of 2 to 10 mcg/min, this drug causes both positive inotropic and chronotropic effects. At higher doses, it is considered class III—harmful.
27. The maximum dose of atropine for a 75-kg patient would be _____ mg (number spelled out).

Down

1. This type of ventricular ectopic beat or rhythm becomes evident when the heart rate becomes so bradycardic that the myocardium becomes compromised. The ectopic beat or rhythm does not come early; it arrives late.
2. This drug is used in both the hypotension and the bradycardia protocols. At different dosages, it stimulates the α-adrenergic, β-adrenergic, and dopaminergic receptors.
3. The 10th cranial nerve; its neurotransmitters are acetylcholine and acetycholinesterase.
4. It is critical to detect a _____ simultaneously when viewing a captured beat from a pacemaker. It should be taken in the femoral area and not the carotid to minimize confusing muscle contraction from the pacemaker.
5. One of two modes whereby the TCP is paced at an exact number of beats per minute, determined by the clinician, regardless of any cardiac depolarizations from the patient. This mode is said to compete with the patient's own heart activity.
6. The concentration (mcg/mL) for both epinephrine and isoproterenol drips when mixed 1 mg in 250 mL.
8. When the pulse rate is so slow that it causes hypotension, an altered level of consciousness, and chest pain, the situation is said to have become _____ significant. The term also means the various factors and forces that move blood around in the body.
10. This mechanical device is used to increase the heart rate artificially when treating a significant bradycardia (acronym).
12. This number, in milligrams, is the higher dose of atropine. It may be given at shorter dosing intervals if the patient is decompensated or is in arrest.
13. An adrenergic receptor that, when stimulated, results in both positive inotropic and chronotropic effects to the heart (a Greek letter spelled out).
14. The type of pacemaker in which the pacer wires are floated into the patient's heart by introducing them through venous pathways.
17. A bradycardic heart rate might be treated with a cautious fluid challenge if the clinician suspected an MI in the _____ ventricle.
19. This drug should be tried first or in conjunction with a TCP if a patient presents with a hemodynamically significant bradycardia.
21. _____ bradycardia is a term used for a heart rate of less than 60 beats/minute.
24. A heart rate that is bradycardic compared to what is normal for the patient but that is not less than 60 beats/minute.
25. A term meaning giving just enough drug to achieve a desired effect. Epinephrine and isoproterenol drips have a dosage range of 2 to 10 mcg/min; however, _____ the drip rate to achieve the desired effect. It fine-tunes the dosage range.
26. Bradycardia means a slow heart _____.

Case Study 8:
Unstable Tachycardias

- **Supraventricular tachycardia**
- **Documented ventricular tachycardia**
- **Wide complex tachycardia of unknown origin**
- **Atrial fibrillation and flutter**

Any cardiac cell may spontaneously depolarize. When the involved cell depolarizes at an extremely rapid rate, however, the patient's cardiac function may be impaired. When time is of the essence, rapid electrical, not solely pharmacologic, intervention is required. This case study highlights synchronized cardioversion therapy for rate-driven tachycardias and provides criteria to distinguish rate-driven from compensatory tachycardias that do not require the same treatment.

Section 1: Critical Actions for Student Evaluation

The ACLS instructor checklist for case study 8 is shown in Table 5-2. This form was designed to guide the faculty when evaluating participants during this particular station. Refer to it frequently as you read the

Table 5-2.
Evaluation Checklist—Case 8: Unstable Tachycardia and Electrical Cardioversion

Critical Action	Completed	Not Completed	Comments
Assesses initial ABCDs			
Attaches monitor			
Assesses hemodynamic status			
Recognizes signs and symptoms of cardiovascular instability			
Recognizes unstable tachycardia on monitor			
Performs synchronized cardioversion			
Appropriate level			
Safely			
Recognizes change in rhythm			
Reassesses cardiovascular status			
Blood pressure			
Pulse and responsiveness			
Monitors postresuscitation			
Administers antiarrhythmic therapy as appropriate			
Recognizes need for			
Oxygen			
Intravenous access			
Follow-up monitoring			
Possible antiarrhythmic therapy			
Recognizes need to change from synchronized to unsynchronized mode for ventricular fibrillation			

(Reproduced with permission. *Instructor's manual for advanced cardiac life support*, 1997 © Copyright American Heart Association, p. 6-15.)

lecture that follows. *Do not memorize it.* The form is only included to: (1) show you what the AHA considers important during this particular case study; (2) describe what the faculty are trying to cover in the station; and (3) provide a summary of the case study after you have read the lecture.

Section 2: ACLS Algorithm for Unstable Tachycardia (patient is not in cardiac arrest)

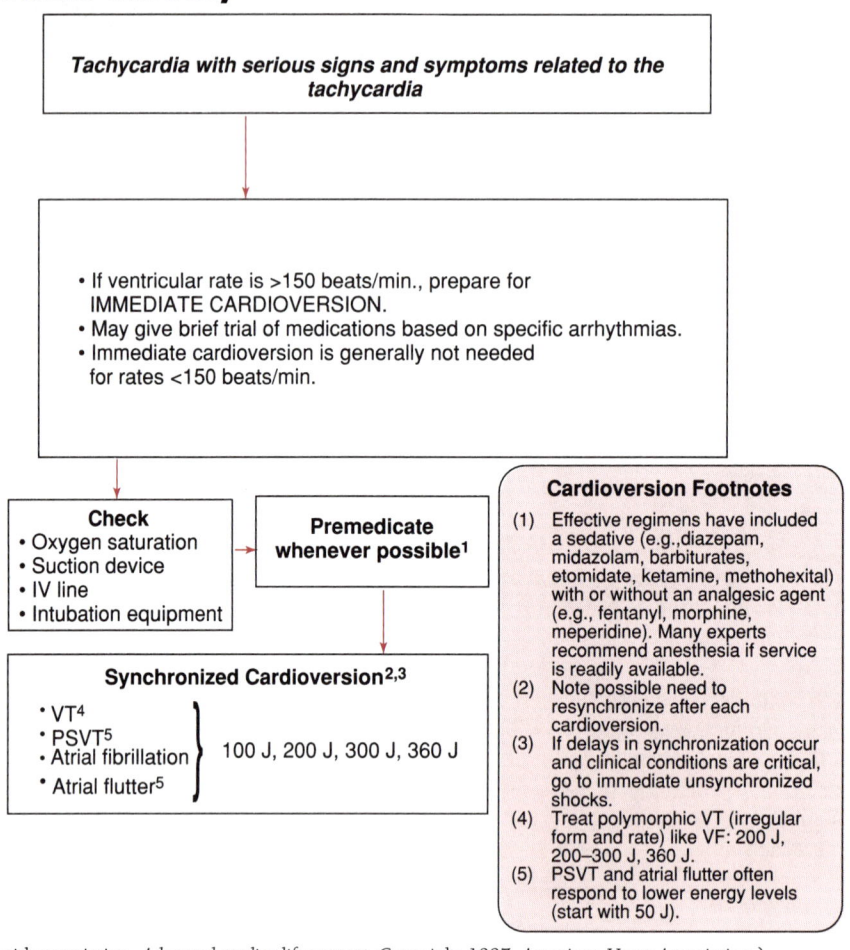

(Reproduced with permission. *Advanced cardiac life support.* Copyright 1997, American Heart Association.)

Section 3: Identifying Features

Important: Just because a patient is presenting with a tachycardia does not mean that the treatment should be targeted at slowing the rate down. All rhythms presenting with tachycardia are not treated by specifically correcting the rate. The rate may be a symptom of an underlying abnormality (e.g., hypovolemia, CHF, fever). It would be inappropriate to give adenosine or to cardiovert a patient in hypovolemic shock based only on evidence of tachycardia.

> If a gross arrythmia occurs that is particularly upsetting to the ACLS provider, the cardiac monitor should be discontinued immediately.

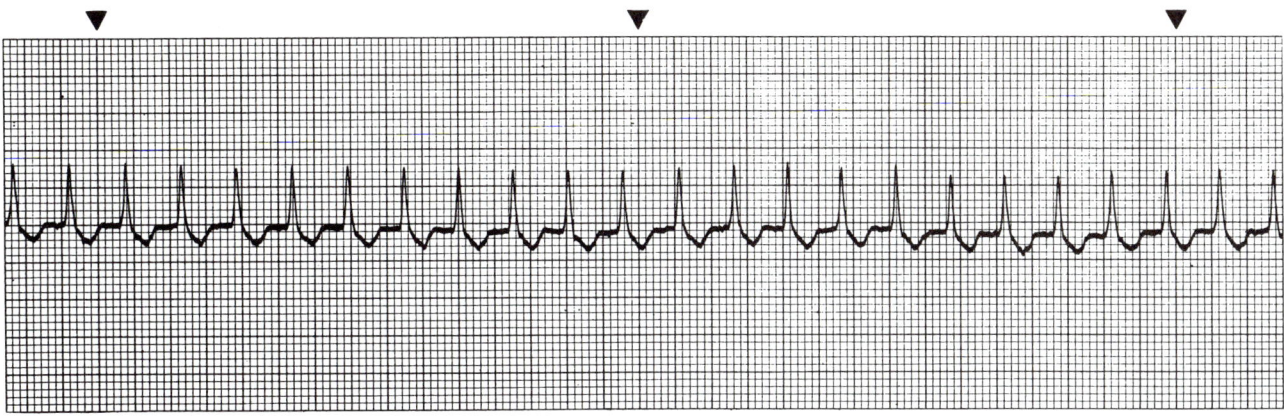

Figure 5-11. Atrial tachycardia.

The treatment for each patient who presents with a fast heart rate may be as diverse as the causes of each type of presenting rhythm. Treatment depends on the reason that the heart is responding with tachycardia. Please review the beginning of this chapter to refamiliarize yourself with the *rate–volume—pump* approach. If you skipped over the introductory portion of this chapter, go back and read it now!

Because this is the unstable tachycardia case study, assume that all of the strips are unstable. Instability is demonstrated by individuals who are hemodynamically significant: altered levels of consciousness, cool extremities, diaphoresis, and hypotension.

Atrial Tachycardia (Supraventricular Tachycardia)

The ECG strip in Figure 5-11 is a narrow complex tachycardia without obvious P waves. Because the ventricular response is 200, well above the 170 cutoff for compensatory tachycardias, it is identified as *atrial tachycardia*, more commonly known as SVT. Treatment for unstable SVT is immediate synchronized cardioversion. Identifying features of SVT are: (1) no obvious P waves; (2) regular ventricular rhythm; (c) narrow QRS complexes; and (d) heart rate of 140 to 270 beats/minute, most commonly 180 to 220.

Ventricular Tachycardia

The ECG rhythm strip in Figure 5-12 is identified as ventricular tachycardia. It is usually impossible to differentiate ventricular tachycardia from SVT with aberrant conduction in one ECG lead. An unstable ventricular tachycardia should be treated with immediate synchronized cardioversion, whereas a pulseless ventricular tachycardia should be immediately defibrillated because these complexes are difficult to synchronize.

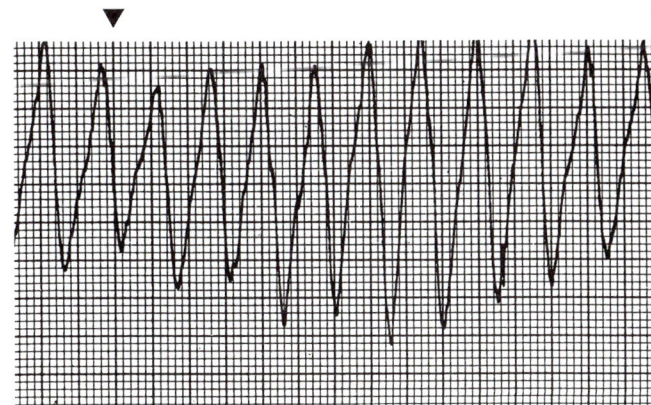

Figure 5-12. Ventricular tachycardia.

Identifying features of ventricular tachycardia are wide QRS complexes responding in a regular rhythm at a rate greater than 100. Each QRS complex should appear like the others and resemble a rhythm strip of regularly spaced PVCs. A diagnosis of ventricular tachycardia can only be made with a 12-lead ECG in conjunction with an individual competent in 12-lead interpretation. If these criteria cannot be met, the rhythm should be interpreted as wide complex tachycardia of uncertain origin and treated as such. A diagnosis of ventricular tachycardia should not be made on the basis of one lead. In an unstable situation, however, detailed 12-lead interpretations are not encouraged because all unstable tachycardias, identified as being rate-driven, are treated with immediate cardioversion.

Wide Complex Tachycardia of Unknown Origin

The rhythm in Figure 5-13 is a wide complex tachycardia of unknown origin. This is ventricular tachycardia in 80% of cases and SVT with aberrant conduction in the remaining 20%. As in the ECG in Figure 5-12, however, this rhythm is unstable, so the question is moot. All unstable tachycardic rhythms identified as rate-driven should receive immediate cardioversion.

Identifying features are the same as those for ventricular tachycardia. In one lead, it is extremely difficult, if not impossible, to differentiate between ventricular tachycardia and SVT with aberrant conduction. In a stable situation, a cardiology consult or a 12-lead ECG may be used to help differentiate the two. In an unstable situation such as this, however, it is not necessary to tell the difference between the two because both rhythms are treated the same.

Tachycardia Exceptions

ATRIAL FIBRILLATION

The ECG strip in Figure 5-14 is identified as atrial fibrillation with an uncontrolled or rapid ventricular response (more than 100 beats/minute). Atrial fibrillation is an exception to the rate—volume—pump rule. This rhythm's rate, 140 beats/minute, is not exceedingly fast (i.e., greater than 170) and therefore may be confused with rates associated with compensatory tachycardias. Treatment of unstable atrial fibrillation, like all tachycardias identified as rate driven, consists of immediate synchronized cardioversion.

Identifying features of atrial fibrillation are: (1) no distinct P waves, or a wavy or indistinct baseline; (2) usually narrow QRS complexes; and (3) irregular R-R wave intervals.

ATRIAL FLUTTER

Atrial flutter is also an exception to the rate–volume–pump rule. As in all tachycardias identified to be rate driven, treatment consists of immediate synchronized cardioversion (Fig. 5-15).

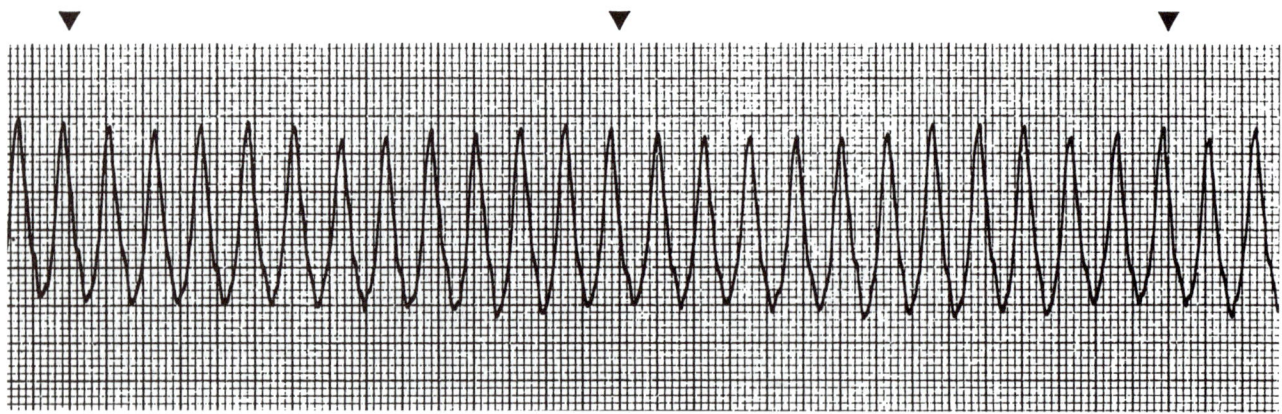

Figure 5-13. Wide complex tachycardia of unknown origin.

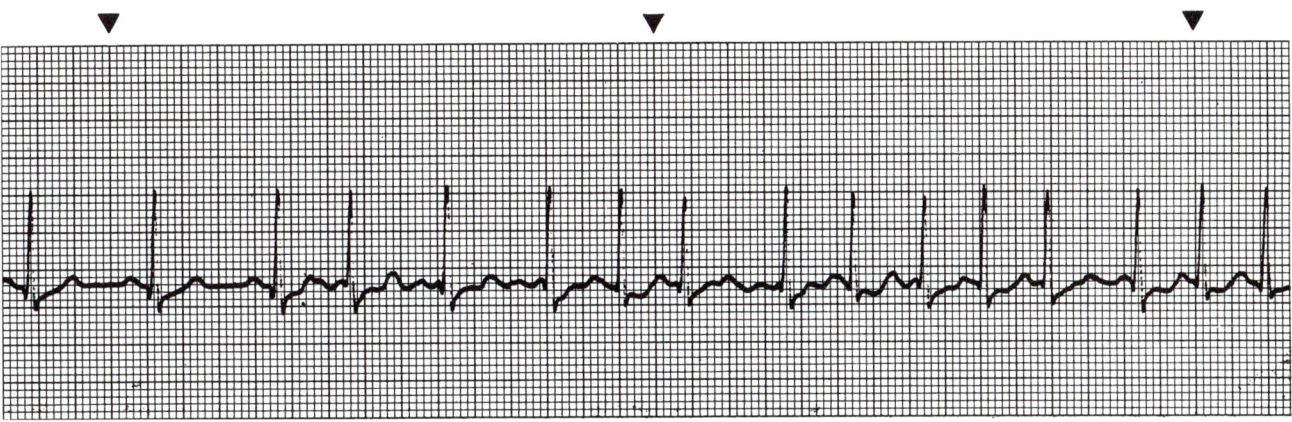

Figure 5-14. Atrial fibrillation.

Identifying features of atrial flutter are: (1) distinct sawtoothed baseline; individual "teeth," referred to as *flutter waves*; (2) usually narrow QRS complexes; and (3) regular or irregular R-R wave intervals, depending on whether the block varies or not. The QRS complexes may be hiding flutter waves underneath them. The ECG strip in Figure 5-15 has a ventricular rate of 150 and an atrial rate of 450. There are three flutter waves to each QRS complex.

Unlike most arrhythmia-naming conventions, the ventricular rate is not noted when naming atrial fibrillation or flutter (i.e., bradycardia or tachycardia) other than noting whether it is below 100 (controlled response) or above 100 (rapid or uncontrolled ventricular response).

COMPENSATORY TACHYCARDIA

The ECG strip in Figure 5-16 is identified as a sinus tachycardia with a ventricular rate of 140. Because this narrow complex tachycardia has a rate of 130, well below 170, and has not been diagnosed as atrial fibrillation or flutter, it should not be treated with the tachycardia protocol.

If the rhythm demonstrates signs of cardiovascular compromise, the clinician should consider that this heart rate is consistent with that of compensatory tachycardia. The tachycardia could be compensating from anything from fluid loss to CHF. Treatment would consist of eliciting the cause and treating it. (Refer to the beginning of this chapter for a review of the rate-driven case studies.)

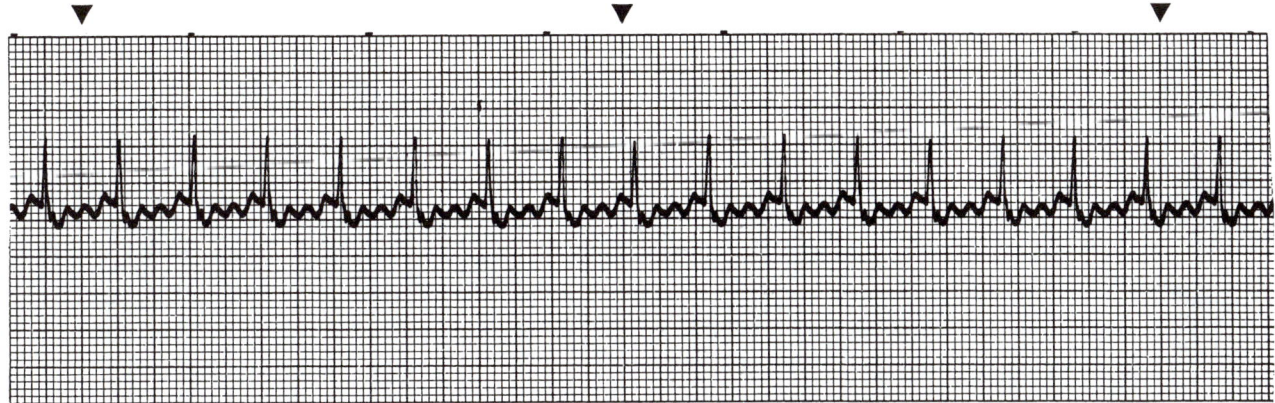

Figure 5-15. Atrial flutter.

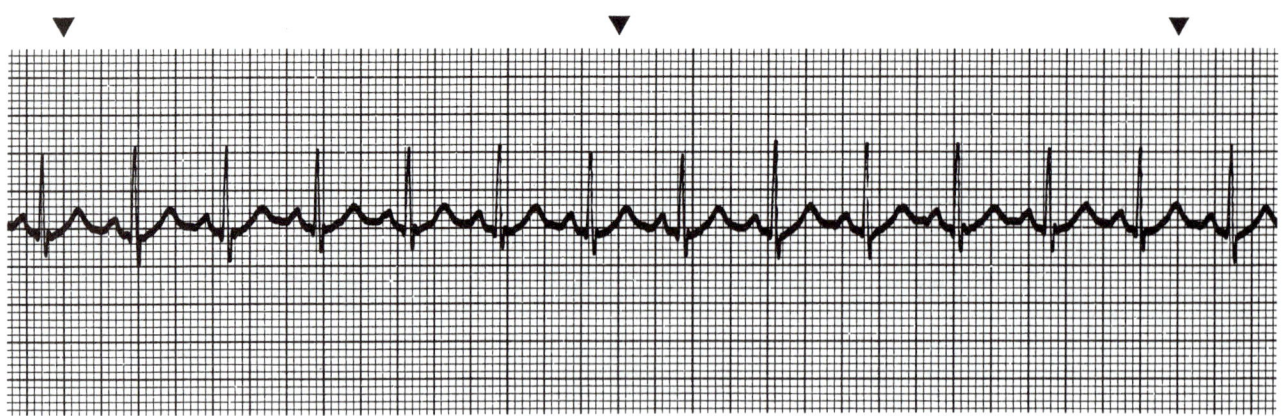

Figure 5-16. Compensatory tachycardia.

Identifying features of sinus tachycardia include the presence of P waves with accompanying QRS complexes. The PR intervals are all consistent and less than 0.20 seconds. The atrial and ventricular rates are equal and in this instance are greater than 100. It is important to differentiate this compensatory tachycardic rhythm from unstable SVT because it is inappropriate to cardiovert. This rhythm differs from SVT in two important points: (1) the rate, which is usually less than 170 in sinus tachycardia but greater than 170 in SVT; and (2) P waves, which are present in sinus tachycardia but not obvious in SVT.

Section 4: Assessment

Primary Survey

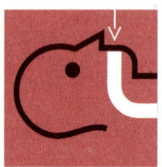

Even if the patient is not in arrest, a compromised cardiovascular status should clue the clinician into reevaluating airway and breathing on a consistent basis. If the patient is alert and coherent, the primary ABCDs are obvious. However, a quick diagnosis of stability is premature. Even though the tachycardia may be generating a sufficient cardiac output to maintain an adequate level of consciousness, the patient still may be demonstrating sufficient symptoms of cardiovascular compromise to be classified as unstable (e.g., chest pain, pulmonary edema).

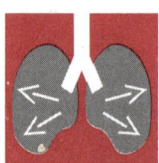

This is an unstable tachycardia, not a pulseless ventricular tachycardia, and the patient has a rapid pulse.

Because the patient is not in ventricular fibrillation, defibrillation is not an option. Do not consider cardioversion because stability has not been confirmed. *The secondary survey has not been completed.*

Secondary Survey

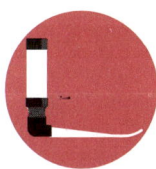

This patient would profit from oxygen, an OPA, or both, if appropriate. Administer each in a manner dependent on the patient's ventilatory and consciousness status (passive or positive pressure for the oxygen and level of consciousness for the OPA). Prepare the patient for a worst-case scenario. Keep the information flowing to you concerning the patient's oxygenation with a pulse oximeter, and make sure that suction and intubation equipment are working appropriately.

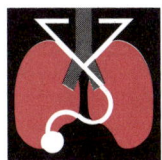

The presence of chest pain, as a symptom of a heart that is decompensating owing to the tachycardic rate, is a symptom of instability. Likewise, the presence of pulmonary edema, resulting from a heart rate that is so fast that it decreases cardiac filling time, also denotes instability. Even though the patient may be alert and coherent, the presence of acute pulmonary edema or chest pain, in conjunction with an extremely rapid heart rate, may indicate that the tachycardia is the problem causing the acute cardiovascular symptoms; hence, the patient's condition is considered unstable.

Taking the vital signs helps you to assess for obvious instability because hypotension is a primary symptom.

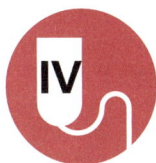

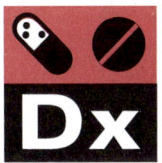

Important: The patient may have an underlying problem that could be diagnosed and treated if only the rescuer takes the time to consider other medical conditions that may have precipitated the tachycardia. It may be something as simple as hypoxia, hypovolemia, anxiety, or fever. Thus, the clinician must consider possible causes of the problem as well as treatment modalities, besides electrical, that may reverse it.

Section 5: Lecture

If your assessment identified that the patient's tachycardia was rate driven, then the next step is to determine stability. ECG interpretation is not as important as determining stability. Because all unstable rate-driven tachycardias are treated the same, it is not specifically important to determine whether it was supraventricular or ventricular in origin. Therefore, if the patient's rate-driven tachycardia is unstable, continue with this protocol. If the patient's rate-driven tachycardia is stable, go to the stable tachycardic protocols, interpret the rhythm, and choose the medication appropriate for the origin of the tachycardic pacemaker.

Unstable patients may exhibit some or all of the following signs and symptoms: chest pain, shortness of breath, altered level of consciousness, hypotension, shock, pulmonary edema, and CHF. Any patient with a rate-driven tachycardia who exhibits these symptoms should be treated with unstable tachycardia protocol.

Treatment

In the unstable tachycardia protocol, origin of the pacemaker cell is a moot issue. If the QRS complex is wide, it is important to not waste valuable time differentiating true ventricular tachycardia from SVT with aberrant conduction. Regardless of the origin, if the symptoms present as unstable, the rhythms should be treated with synchronized cardioversion.

Narrow or wide, these rhythms represent problems of a pacemaker cell nature. Depending on the degree of cardiovascular compromise, all are dealt with by immediate synchronized cardioversion or a combination of synchronized cardioversion with concurrent drug therapy.

SYNCHRONIZED CARDIOVERSION

Synchronized cardioversion is essentially the same procedure as defibrillation. Both procedures involve administering an electrical shock to the patient's myocardium. The patient, however, is not in arrest. Viable patients have QRS complexes and T waves; therefore, it is important to deliver the shock well away from the vulnerable portion of the rhythm complex—the T wave. The downslope of the T wave is an especially vulnerable area because it is considered relatively refractory. If electricity is applied—with a defibrillator, by sticking your fingers into a wall socket, by getting hit by lightning, or by having a PVC strike the downslope of the T wave—it is extremely easy to put the patient into ventricular tachycardia or ventricular fibrillation. Therefore, when a person is alive, use the synchronizing capability of the machine, keeping the possibility of putting the patient into ventricular tachycardia or ventricular fibrillation to an absolute minimum. When a person is in ventricular fibrillation, there are no T waves to worry about, so an unsynchronized shock (defibrillation) is used.

Note the synchronizer switch. If a defibrillator has an attached monitor, it usually has a button or switch labeled "sync" or "synchronizer." When this button is depressed, the machine searches the ECG rhythm for an R wave. The R wave is used to synchronize on because it is the most prominent wave. Delivering the shock on its downslope does not have the negative effects that would ensue if the T wave were accidentally hit.

When an R wave is located, the monitor screen flashes, beeps, or does something to signify that the R wave has been sensed. If it does not flash or beep, it is not sensing an R wave. No matter how long you hold down the red buttons on the paddles, the machine will not fire. This may mean that the rhythm does not have an R wave, as in ventricular fibrillation, or that the ECG size (amplitude) on the machine is set too low and therefore that the monitor-defibrillator cannot sense the R wave.

If when attempting to deliver a synchronized countershock, the machine does not fire, check those possibilities and try to correct them quickly. If the monitor still fails to perform, turn off the synchronizer and immediately defibrillate. If the patient turns critical, do not spend any more time—turn off the synchronizer and defibrillate!

▼ *Helpful Hints* for Synchronized Cardioversion

- ▼ Atrial fibrillation and atrial flutter are common cardiac rhythms and require treatment only when the patient becomes hemodynamically unstable.
- ▼ Cardioversion *does hurt* and has been compared to having someone hit you in the chest with a baseball bat.
- ▼ If the patient is alert enough to remember who shocked him, *definitely premedicate*.
- ▼ Sometimes cardioversion is the last treatment in a stable protocol in which drug therapy proved refractory; in this situation, cardioversion is not emergent but elective.
- ▼ In elective procedures time is not a factor, so some facilities prefer to use anesthesia. A selection of hypnotics, such as diazepam (Valium) or midazolam (Versed), may be combined with analgesics.
- ▼ Be aware of the hemodynamic status of the patient when you decide what to administer. If the patient's status deteriorates to the point that a sedative might be risky, advise the patient that this life-saving procedure will be painful.

Synchronizing Procedure. Joule settings have been simplified. For the most part, start at 100 joules, progress to 200, then 300, and then all the way to 360 joules if necessary. Both SVT and atrial flutter convert with smaller energy levels, so you might consider starting at 50 joules. But if all you can remember is 100, 200, 300, and 360, that is sufficient for most cardioversions.

When synchronized cardioverting, check the pulse quickly and then push the synchronizer button. Select an appropriate joule setting, charge the machine, clear the area, and push and hold the defibrillator paddle discharge buttons while the machine searches for a obvious R wave. After the machine locates the R wave, the electricity is discharged, keeping far away from the vulnerable T wave. Quickly check the monitor for a change in rhythm. If the rhythm has not changed, select a higher joule setting and repeat the process. Depending on the age of the defibrillator, it may be necessary to reset the synchronizer switch. Recharging the defibrillator to the next energy level should begin immediately after each discharge to decrease the time necessary to deliver the next shock. Check for a pulse at any point that the ECG changes to a different rhythm.

Postcardioversion. In the aftermath of successful cardioversion, special attention must be given to the ABCs. Sedation can exacerbate altered levels of consciousness. In addition, apnea or hypoventilation may occur. Because the patient's ectopic pacemaker is probably still irritable, vital signs must be closely monitored because the tachycardia may recur.

CONCURRENT DRUG THERAPY

Hemodynamic instability may show up as hypotension, altered level of consciousness, pulmonary edema, or chest pain. The unstable patient should undergo immediate cardioversion. This statement may seem to imply that a patient deemed unstable should not receive any drug-specific therapy but should be cardioverted at once. This is not the case. Time delay is the problem. The unstable situation must be terminated immediately.

If the clinician wishes, the patient can receive an initial bolus of an antiarrhythmic agent if it can be administered without interfering with the cardioversion sequence. The rule of thumb is: give the antiarrhythmic if you can do it quickly enough, but do not hold up cardioversion to do it!

If medication is mandated, both lidocaine and adenosine are appropriate for either a narrow complex or wide complex tachycardia. Lidocaine may terminate a ventricular ectopic pacemaker but will not harm a supraventricular ectopic pacemaker. Conversely, adenosine may halt a supraventricular ectopic pacemaker but will not maltreat a ventricular rhythm. Thus, if given quickly enough, both lidocaine and adenosine may be administered to the patient with a rate-driven tachycardia, just before cardioversion. Although adenosine may help assist in the diagnosis of a supraventricular origin, in a wide complex tachycardia, try the lidocaine first because a ventricular origin is the more obvious possibility.

SVT, atrial flutter, and ventricular tachycardia usually respond well to cardioversion. They may, however, require pharmacologic therapy in addition to cardioversion to terminate the arrhythmia and to stabilize a converted rhythm. In the treatment of ventricular tachycardia, the use of lidocaine, procainamide, and bretylium during cardioversion and for stabilizing the rhythm afterward may be helpful. Likewise, unstable torsades de pointes may profit from a maintenance drip of magnesium sulfate after the initial bolus when the arrhythmia has been successfully cardioverted.

Treatment of Special Cases

VENTRICULAR FIBRILLATION AND PULSELESS VENTRICULAR TACHYCARDIA

If the tachycardic rhythm initially presents as pulseless ventricular tachycardia or if the rhythm after cardioversion slips into ventricular fibrillation, treat the case like ventricular fibrillation. Make certain that the synchronizer is off, and immediately defibrillate beginning at 200 joules.

Pulseless ventricular tachycardia is usually identified as polymorphic. It usually has R waves that vary in both height and width and thus are difficult for a defibrillator to locate and synchronize on. Therefore, because a pulseless patient cannot tolerate any delay, make certain that the synchronizer is off and defibrillate without delay.

ATRIAL FIBRILLATION AND FLUTTER

A note of caution with symptomatic atrial fibrillation and atrial flutter: the tachycardic rate of either of these may not reach past the 160 to 170 rate reserved for rogue pacemaker cells (e.g., SVT). Therefore, be sure to differentiate atrial fibrillation and flutter from other narrow complex tachycardias. Other narrow complex tachycardias with rates between 60 and 170 are probably compensatory sinus tachycardias, which may be treated with fluids or vasopressors. Remember, symptomatic atrial fibrillation and atrial flutter are exceptions to the rate–volume—pump rule. They should be treated with the appropriate tachycardic protocol: stable or unstable.

Both atrial fibrillation and atrial flutter can be hemodynamically unstable if the AV node allows too many impulses to pass, resulting in a rapid or uncontrolled rate. If the patient is stable and time is not a problem, appropriate drug therapy can be administered. If the patient starts showing signs and symptoms of instability, however, emergency cardioversion is required.

Another note of caution: if atrial fibrillation does not respond to cardioversion, consider anticoagulants. Because a fibrillating atrium results in sluggish blood flow, a clot may form, eventually becoming a thrombus and causing a cerebrovascular accident (CVA).

After successful conversion of atrial fibrillation or atrial flutter, the following medications can be considered: β-blockers, diltiazem, verapamil, and digoxin. To help prevent recurrence, consider procainamide and quinidine.

Summary

Special attention must be given to assessing the patient for stability rather than to assessing the origin of the tachycardia. With the exception of a compensatory sinus tachycardia, most tachycardias are treated the same, with synchronized cardioversion. If the patient is stable, appropriate drug therapy should be instituted. If unstable, the patient is immediately treated with synchronized cardioversion.

Section 6: Unstable Tachycardia Interim Evaluation

1. Synchronized countershocks are the mainstay of treatment in which of the following (see ACLS text pp. 1-32 to 1-37): (1) controlled atrial fibrillation; (2) primary ventricular standstill; (3) symptomatic sinus tachycardia; (4) unstable SVT; (5) unstable ventricular tachycardia?

    _____ (a) 4 and 5
    _____ (b) 1, 4, and 5
    _____ (c) 2, 3, 4, and 5
    _____ (d) 1, 3, 4, and 5

2. The patient's level of consciousness is the sole factor used to determine stability or instability in symptomatic tachycardia (see ACLS text pp. 1-32 to 1-37).

    _____ (a) True
    _____ (b) False

3. During the course of cardioversion, a patient suddenly develops ventricular fibrillation. Which of the following steps should be taken *first* (see ACLS text p. 1-35)?

    _____ (a) Immediately initiate external cardiac compressions.
    _____ (b) Inject 1.0 to 1.5 mg/kg lidocaine by intravenous push.
    _____ (c) Administer a second synchronized shock instantly.
    _____ (d) Proceed immediately with an unsynchronized countershock.

4. When making a decision concerning stability versus instability of a patient with tachycardia, it is important to concentrate on the ECG rhythm interpretation rather than the symptoms (see ACLS text p. 1-35).

    _____ (a) True
    _____ (b) False

5. In the critical care unit, an adult patient suddenly becomes apneic and unresponsive, and the monitor shows a wide complex tachycardia. The airway is open, and a pulse of 180 beats/minute is present. An intravenous line is in place. Your next action should be (see ACLS text pp. 1-32 to 1-37):

    _____ (a) Administer oxygen by bag-valve-mask and immediately cardiovert with 50 to 100 joules.
    _____ (b) Give lidocaine, 1 to 1.5 mg/kg, by intravenous bolus.

_____ (c) Proceed with cardiopulmonary resuscitation (CPR) and countershock as soon as possible.
_____ (d) Administer adenosine, 6 mg, by intravenous bolus.

6. A 59-year-old, 220-pound man presents to the emergency room complaining of crushing substernal chest pain radiating down the left arm and to the jaw. He is awake and alert with a blood pressure of 106/72 mmHg and pulse of 140. The monitor reveals a sustained wide complex tachycardia. Your initial therapy would include (see ACLS text p. 1-35):

_____ (a) Vagal maneuvers
_____ (b) Lidocaine, 100 to 150 mg, given intravenously
_____ (c) Adenosine, 6 mg, given intravenously by rapid infusion
_____ (d) Sedation and synchronized countershock

Section 7
UNSTABLE TACHYCARDIA CROSSWORD PUZZLE

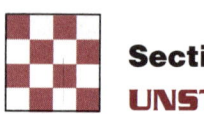

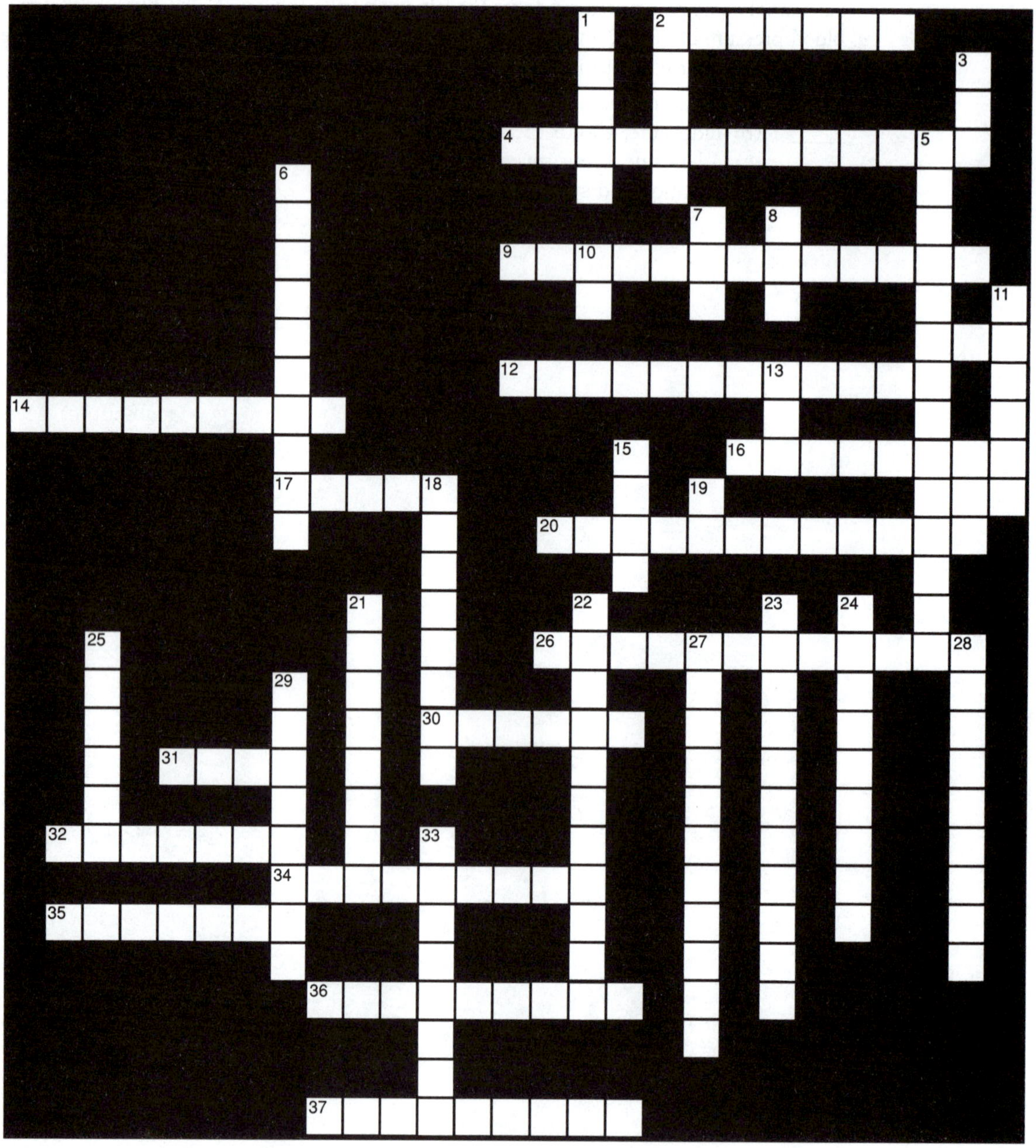

Across

2. Because lidocaine is metabolized in the liver, patients with pathology involving this organ or patients in excess of _____ years of age should receive smaller doses, except in ventricular fibrillation (number spelled out).
4. This class of drug should be administered to atrial fibrillation to reduce clotting if synchronized cardioversion fails to stop an uncontrolled rate. A fibrillated atria may cause a pathology that this class of drug is designed to limit, resulting in a CVA.
9. There are many terms that are interchangeable with defibrillation: shock, defibrillate, and _____ countershock. When delivering the electricity, your synchronizer switch is not engaged.
12. The term for quivering atrial heart muscle. This form of arrhythmia passes through the AV node. Because

it does not use a reentry mechanism, it does not respond well to adenosine.
14. Deciding a patient's cardiovascular _____ is more important than diagnosing ectopic pacemaker origin because the tachycardia protocol treats all unstable patients, regardless of ECG width, the same, with cardioversion.
16. The generic name of Valium. This hypnotic is commonly used for sedation before cardioversion.
17. When the conduction in the AV node allows the ventricular response of an atrial fibrillation or atrial flutter to accelerate past 100, the condition is known as _____ or an uncontrolled ventricular response.
20. The group of tachycardias that employ an increased heart rate to try to make up for an underlying deficiency. Examples of tachycardias in association with hypovolemia or heart failure.
26. When delivering a _____ shock, the clinician is attempting to keep the shock from striking the relatively refractory portion of the polarizing cycle—the downslope of the T wave.
30. This term is used to describe the width of a QRS complex that is 0.12 seconds or smaller. Tachycardias with this width are usually designated supraventricular.
31. The heart _____ is a main indicator to help differentiate compensatory tachycardias from those that are caused by an ectopic pacemaker.
32. When the atria contract at rates of 270 to 400 beats/minute, the rhythm is identified as atrial _____. When the ventricular rate becomes so rapid that the patient becomes hemodynamically unstable, the rhythm should be immediately cardioverted. This rhythm makes the baseline resemble the teeth on a saw.
34. The second drug of choice in the wide complex tachycardia of uncertain origin protocol.
35. This drug is classified as both a positive ionotrope and a negative chronotrope. It is helpful in CHF, atrial fibrillation, and stable SVTs refractory to adenosine and verapamil.
36. The generic term for the sedative Versed. This hypnotic is commonly given before cardioversion if the patient is alert and coherent.
37. This form of ventricular tachycardia should be treated just like ventricular fibrillation.

Down
1. When cardioverting SVT or atrial flutter, the clinician may use a lower joule setting then the normal 100. The lower setting is _____ joules.
2. A generic term for general cardiovascular collapse. The patient presents with tachycardia, diaphoresis, and hypotension. It is commonly divided into two levels: compensatory and noncompensatory.
3. The acronym for supraventricular tachycardia.
5. One of two chemical components of adrenaline. This one is known for its primarily α-vasoconstricting effects. The generic name for Levophed. It is used primarily in severe hypotension (systolic blood pressure less than 70 mmHg) when the cause is not related to hypovolemia.
6. When in the synchronized mode, a shock is only delivered during that portion of the cardiac depolarization cycle considered absolutely _____. The downslope of the T wave is considered relatively _____ (same word).
7. The initials for the pathologic condition in which a failing left ventricle results in pulmonary edema. Signs and symptoms of this pathology, in conjunction with an excessive tachycardic rate, indicate an unstable patient.
8. Initials for shortage of breath or initials used when referring to another individual's canine ancestry. The patient is deemed unstable if this symptom is combined with signs of pulmonary edema in an excessively fast heart rate.
10. A narrow complex tachycardia at less than 170, combined with chest pain and an elevated _____ segment, should be treated with the acute MI protocol rather than the unstable tachycardia algorithm.
11. Clinicians should not assume that all tachycardias have cardiac pathology. Some narrow complex tachycardias may be a response to a _____ or a pump problem. An all-encompassing term for a fluid problem.
13. The initials for acute myocardial infarction. Signs and symptoms of this pathology denote instability in any of the following tachycardias: ventricular, wide complex of unknown origin, or supraventricular.
15. When encountering a hemodynamically significantly tachycardic patient, clinicians should rule out both rate and volume pathologies before considering vasopressors to treat _____ problems.
18. At different dosages, this endogenous catecholamine can stimulate all three receptors: α-adrenergic, β-adrenergic, and dopaminergic. This drug can be helpful in the treatment of hypotension not related to hypovolemia.
19. The initials for the signs and symptoms of pink, frothy sputum. When this is noted in a patient, it is important to determine whether the tachycardic condition is the result of chronic CHF or is a rate-driven tachycardia.
21. A term that means that the patient is no longer stable. A patient may exhibit one or more of the following when presenting with this term: hypotension, chest pain, or pulmonary edema.

22. A patient with this condition, who usually presents with narrow complex tachycardia at ventricular rates of 100 to 150, should receive infusions of fluids. Vasopressors to increase the blood pressure are contraindicated.
23. The term for ventricular tachycardia in which the QRS complexes tend to vary so much in amplitude and width that it is exceedingly difficult for a monitor-defibrillator to synchronize on it properly. If you are attempting to synchronize on this form of ventricular tachycardia, and your monitor encounters difficulty in locating the R wave for synchronizing purposes, do not hesitate to turn off the synchronizer and defibrillate!
24. This is the first drug of choice for either stable wide complex tachycardias or documented stable ventricular tachycardias. This drug may also be given during emergent cardioversion so long as it does not interrupt the sequence.
25. Pertaining to the portion of the heart that contains the sinus node. Flutter of this musculature results in a sawtoothed baseline.
27. A pathologic condition in which the systolic blood pressure drops below 80 or 90 mmHg, depending on the patient and the situation.
28. The generic term for Cardizem. This calcium-channel blocker is considered in stable SVTs unresponsive to adenosine and verapamil. The intravenous form has been shown to be highly effective in controlling the rate of atrial fibrillation.
29. Deviating from normal. Bizarre. The conduction process by which the pacemaker cell of supraventricular origin results in a widened QRS complex.
33. A variation of ventricular tachycardia that means "twisting around a point." This rhythm can be exacerbated by drugs, such as procainamide or quinidine, that increase QT intervals.

Case Study 9

Stable Tachycardias

- **Supraventricular tachycardia**
- **Documented ventricular tachycardia**
- **Atrial fibrillation and flutter**
- **Wide complex tachycardia of unknown origin**

If a rate-driven tachycardia results in a patient exhibiting symptoms that are not life-threatening, time is allowed to use pharmacologic intervention. This case study denotes the medication treatment protocols for each of the rate-driven tachycardias based on their locations in the heart.

Section 1: Critical Actions for Student Evaluation

The ACLS instructor checklist for case study 9 is shown in Table 5-3. This form was designed to guide the faculty when evaluating participants during this particular station. Refer to it frequently as you read the lecture that follows. *Do not memorize it.* The form is only included to: (1) show you what the AHA considers important during this particular case study; (2) describe what the faculty are trying to cover in the station; and (3) provide a summary of the case study after you have read the lecture.

Table 5-3.
Evaluation Checklist—Case 9: Stable Tachycardias

Critical Action	Completed	Not Completed	Comments
Assesses ABCDs			
Establishes hemodynamic status			
Orders monitor			
Determines rhythm			
Orders supplemental oxygen			
Recognizes need for vagal maneuvers			
Auscultates for carotid bruit before carotid massage (if appropriate)			
Selects proper drug, dosage, etc.			
Correctly performs cardioversion if becoming unstable			

(Reproduced with permission. *Instructor's manual for advanced cardiac life support*, 1997 © Copyright American Heart Association, p. 6-16.)

Section 2: ACLS Algorithm for Stable Tachycardia

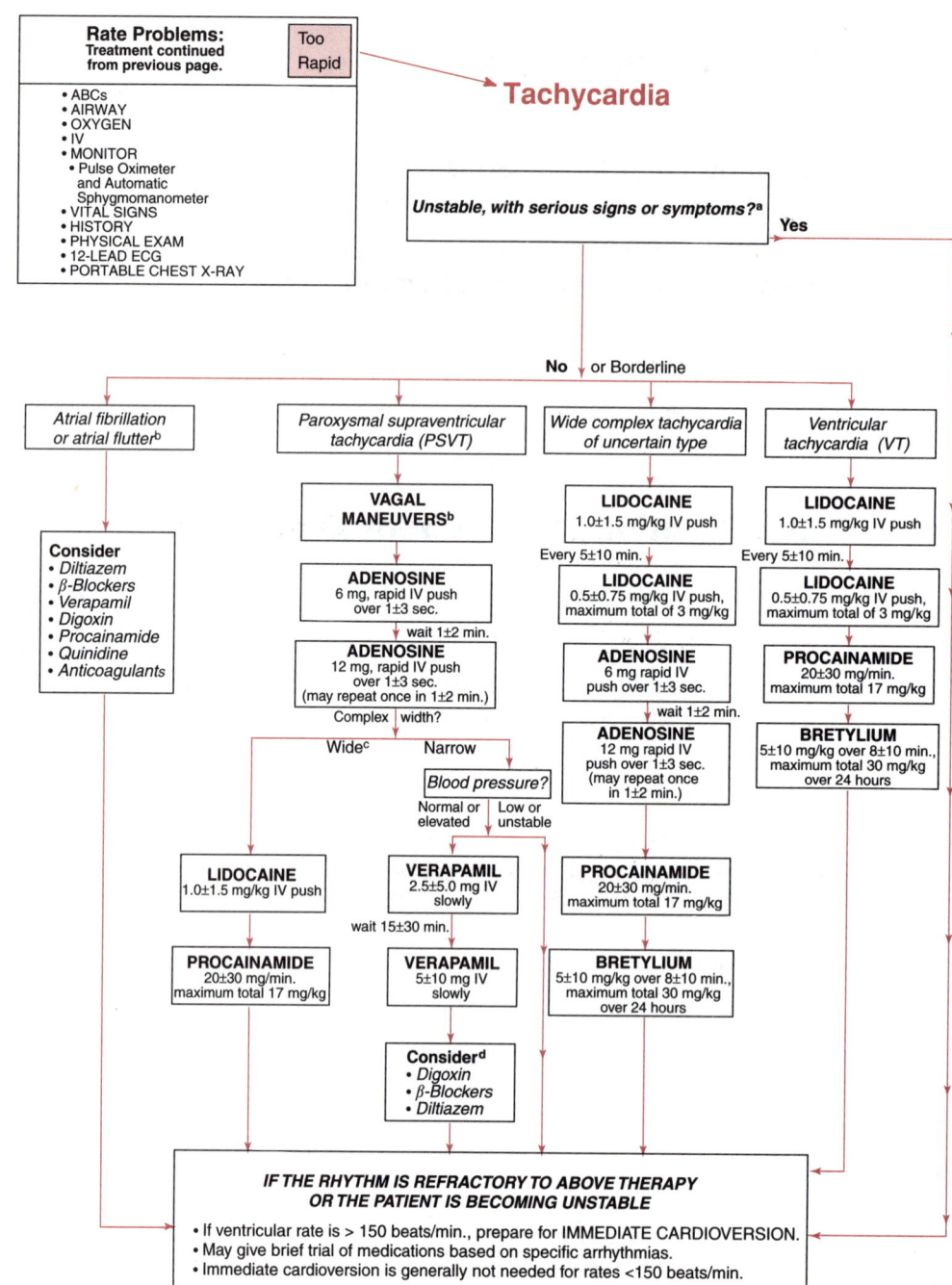

(Reproduced with permission. *Advanced cardiac life support.* Copyright 1997, American Heart Association.)

Section 3: Identifying Features

A main problem in dealing with symptomatic tachycardias is determining which are rate-driven tachycardias and which are compensatory tachycardias. When patients are treated with the unstable tachycardia protocol, there is a low priority assigned to detailed ECG interpretation. Once the clinician's assessment reveals that the presenting unstable tachycardia is rate driven, there is little need to scrutinize the rhythm further because all are treated with cardioversion. The unstable protocol is selected when the patient is deteriorating rapidly. Time becomes a critical factor.

In the stable protocol, however, time is not as significant, so discrete drug therapy is employed over expeditious cardioversion. The stable protocol is only used while the rhythm continues to generate a sufficient cardiac output to keep the patient perfused. If perfusion drops at any time, the patient is immediately switched to the unstable protocol and subsequently cardioverted.

The stable tachycardia protocol revolves around drug therapy. Most of the medications in this protocol only operate on selective myocardial tissue—supraventricular or ventricular. Thus, after assessment of stability, it is necessary to interpret the origin of the presenting rhythm so that the correct drug for the correct tissue type is administered.

Because this protocol requires the clinician to administer the appropriate drug for the ectopic pacemaker's origin (supraventricular versus ventricular), it is necessary to provide some fundamental ECG information on how to determine the source of the pacemaker cell tissue. Therefore, the remainder of this section is divided into three segments. The first segment teaches the fundamentals of QRS width identification—wide complex versus narrow complex tachycardias. After QRS width is made obvious, the subsequent two segments relate the identifying features of each of the narrow and the wide complex tachycardias.

QRS Complexes: Distinguishing Narrow From Wide

To understand the ECG differences between SVT, sinus tachycardia, and wide complex tachycardia, it is necessary to be able to differentiate narrow from wide QRS complexes because width is a major clue to pacemaker origin. Because all ECG machines operate at the same speed, each tiny box on ECG paper corresponds to a block of time—0.04 seconds. Five boxes together in a linear sequence correlate to a large box—0.2 seconds (5 boxes × 0.04 seconds; Fig. 5-17).

Clinicians use these time sequences to calculate the time taken for each depolarization wave or sequence. A QRS complex is considered narrow (normal) when it less than or equal to three small boxes (0.12 seconds) and wide when the number of boxes exceeds that amount. When it is wider than normal, it may point to a depolarization pathway problem.

When reading lead II, the first negative deflection below the isoelectric line after a P wave is defined as a Q wave. The isoelectric line is also known as the baseline—the horizontal line between each cardiac complex. The Q wave dips below the baseline and is considered completed when it returns. The first ascending deflection arising from a Q wave, or after a P wave (if the Q wave is missing), is referred to as an *R wave.* The R wave ascends, reaches its peak, and descends to the baseline, where it terminates. After the R wave, the first negative deflection is an S wave, again terminating when it returns to the baseline (Fig. 5-18).

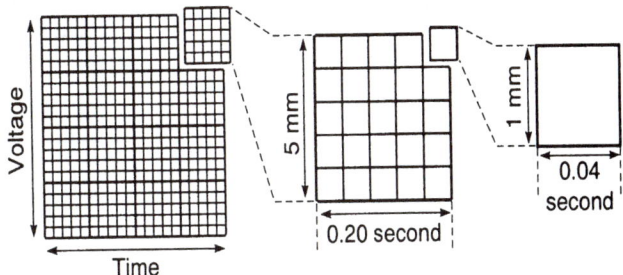

Figure 5-17. Electrocardiographic paper.

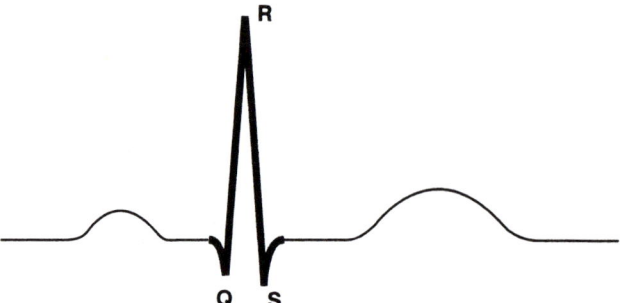

Figure 5-18. The QRS complex.

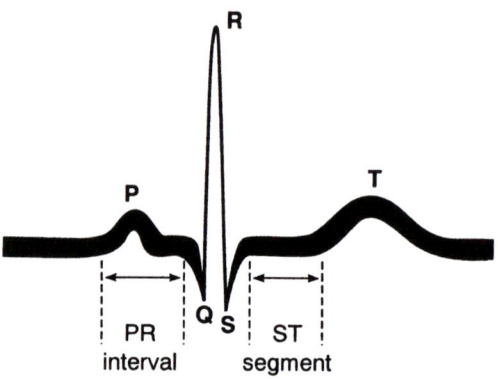

Figure 5-19. Relationship of the electrical conduction system to the ECG.

Normal QRS complexes may not have all three waves. Some only have an R wave, others only an R-S wave, and others only a Q-R wave. It does not make any difference; the ECG complex is still referred to as a QRS, and the clinician measures the width of the waves present.

To determine whether a QRS is narrow or wide, it is measured in seconds from the spot where the Q wave leaves the baseline to the point that the S wave ascends back to the baseline (Fig. 5-19).

The example in Figure 5-20 has only an R-S wave. The complex is measured from where the R wave leaves the baseline until the S wave returns.

The ECG in Figure 5-21 has only a Q-R wave. It is measured from where the Q wave starts to dip below the baseline until the R wave ascends and returns.

The ECG in Figure 5-22 has two R waves designated R and r' (r prime). Like those before it, the QRS is measured from where the Q wave dips below baseline until both R waves finish their cycle and return.

The example in Figure 5-23 has only an R wave. The QRS is measured from where the R wave leaves the baseline until it returns.

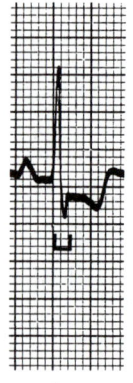

0.08 seconds
(2 squares × 0.04 second)

Figure 5-20. An R-S complex.

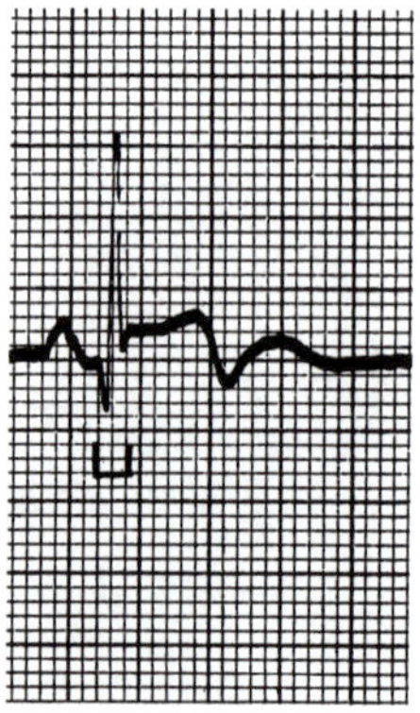

0.08 seconds
(2 squares × 0.04 second)

Figure 5-21. A Q-R complex.

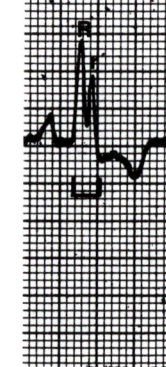

0.12 seconds
(3 squares × 0.04 second)

Figure 5-22. A bundle branch block.

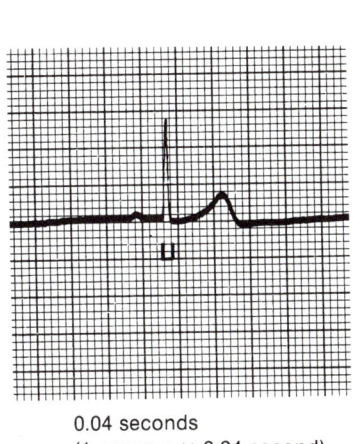

0.04 seconds
(1 squares × 0.04 second)

Figure 5-23. R wave only.

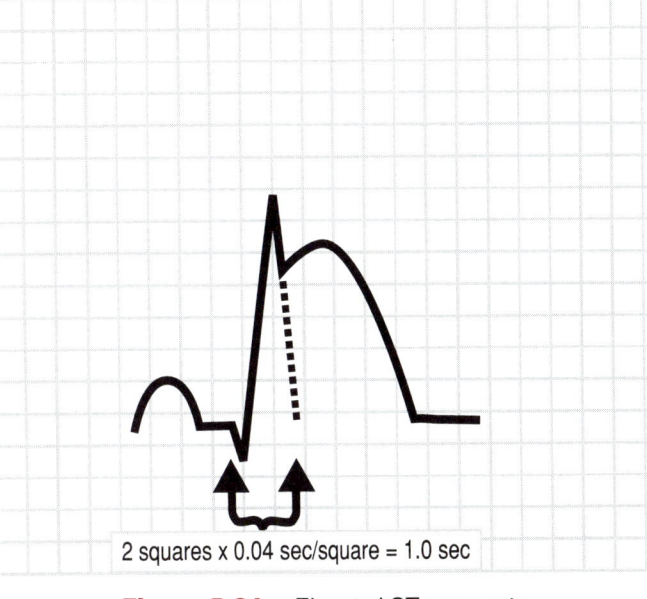

2 squares x 0.04 sec/square = 1.0 sec

Figure 5-24. Elevated ST segments.

The ECG example in Figure 5-24 is more complex. The elevated ST segment interferes with the return of the R wave to the baseline. To estimate the QRS width, the clinician must extrapolate the downward angle of the R wave to where it would have returned to the baseline if the ST segment had never elevated. The clinician is interested in possible conduction problems that would have shown up if the ischemia had never occurred. The dotted line projects down to the baseline. Measure the width from this point.

The example in Figure 5-25 is of an R-S wave. Even though much smaller than the S wave, the R wave is still present. The QRS is measured from where the R wave left the baseline (the first upward deflection) until the S wave (the first negative deflection after an R wave) returns to the baseline.

The example in Figure 5-26 is much more difficult to measure. An S wave should present as a sharp spike, not a wide sagging wave, as in this example. Because the S wave is not obvious, it is not part of the measurement.

A normal (narrow) QRS complex should complete the depolarization cycle within three boxes (0.12 seconds). If the width is greater than 0.12 seconds, although cardiac terminology varies, it is referred to as an *intraventricular conduction defect*, commonly called a *bundle branch block*. The terminology is not as important as the fact that it is wide. The width assists the clinician in determining the origin of the pacemaker.

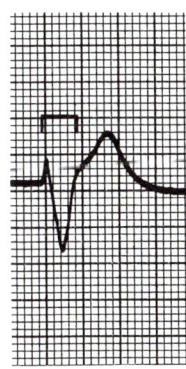

0.18 seconds
(4½ squares × 0.04 second)

Figure 5-25. R-S wave.

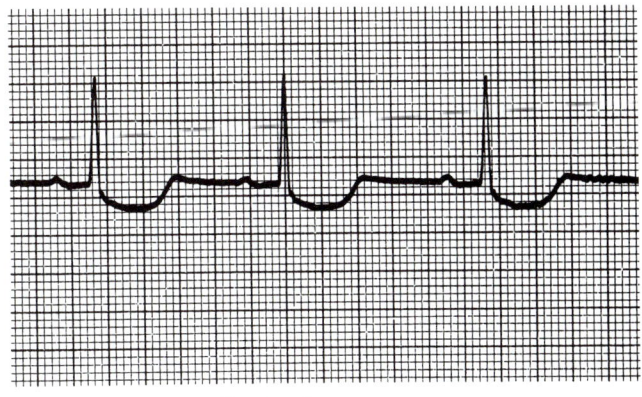

Sagging depresson

Figure 5-26. Sagging depression.

Usually, any pacemaker cell that originates from the atria (supraventricular) is conducted down the bundle branches, resulting in a narrow QRS complex. Thus, SVTs usually exhibit narrow QRS complexes.

Usually, any cells in the ventricles that depolarize spontaneously take a backward pathway toward the atria. This retrograde pathway, depending on how low in the ventricle the beat arises, usually results in a wide QRS complex. Thus, ventricular tachycardia usually presents with a wide QRS complex.

In some instances, however, a tachycardic, supraventricular pacemaker cell may initiate an unusual depolarization pathway, resulting in a wide QRS complex. This peculiarity is referred to as *aberrant conduction*. Because the pacemaker was initiated in the atria, the rhythm is referred to as SVT with aberrant conduction. Do not be fooled by an ECG rhythm that appears to be ventricular tachycardia; it could be SVT with aberrant conduction.

Even with a 12-lead ECG, it is extremely difficult to tell the difference between these two rhythms. Any wide complex tachycardia is probably ventricular in origin only 80% of the time; the remaining 20% of cases are SVT with aberrant conduction. These rhythms look exactly alike when viewed from only one lead and are difficult for most clinicians to differentiate without the assistance of a cardiologist. If an immediate consult is not possible, do not hesitate, use the protocol for wide complex tachycardia of unknown origin.

Some clinicians think that ventricular tachycardia is inherently more symptomatic than SVT with aberrant conduction and that it is easy to differentiate between them clinically. This is incorrect. It is possible for some ventricular tachycardias to be asymptomatic, whereas some SVTs (with or without aberrancy) can be cardiovascularly devastating. Do not use clinical criteria to differentiate between these two.

Ventricular antiarrhythmic drugs do not work on supraventricular pacemakers, and vice versa. The wide complex tachycardia of unknown origin protocol allows for this idiosyncrasy by sequencing medications for both.

In summary, a wide QRS complex usually implies that the depolarization sequence did not follow the normal pathway from the atria, increasing the possibility of a ventricular pacemaker. The key word is *implies*. Narrow QRS complexes are more likely to arise from the atria, whereas wide QRS complexes are more likely to arise from the ventricles.

QRS width detection becomes extremely important when deciding if verapamil (a narrow complex drug) might be advantageous. Verapamil can cause disastrous cardiovascular effects in some wide complex tachycardias and is contraindicated in all unknown wide complex tachycardias. Thus, verapamil should never be used for any wide complex tachycardia unless the clinician can diagnose, *without a doubt*, a supraventricular origin.

Narrow Complex Tachycardias

ATRIAL TACHYCARDIA (SUPRAVENTRICULAR TACHYCARDIA)

The rhythm in Figure 5-27 is a narrow complex tachycardia without P waves. Because the ventricular response is 200, well above the 170 cutoff for compensatory tachycardias, this is identified as atrial tachycardia—more commonly known as SVT. Because the patient is stable, treatment consists of drug therapy designed to interfere with reentry mechanisms.

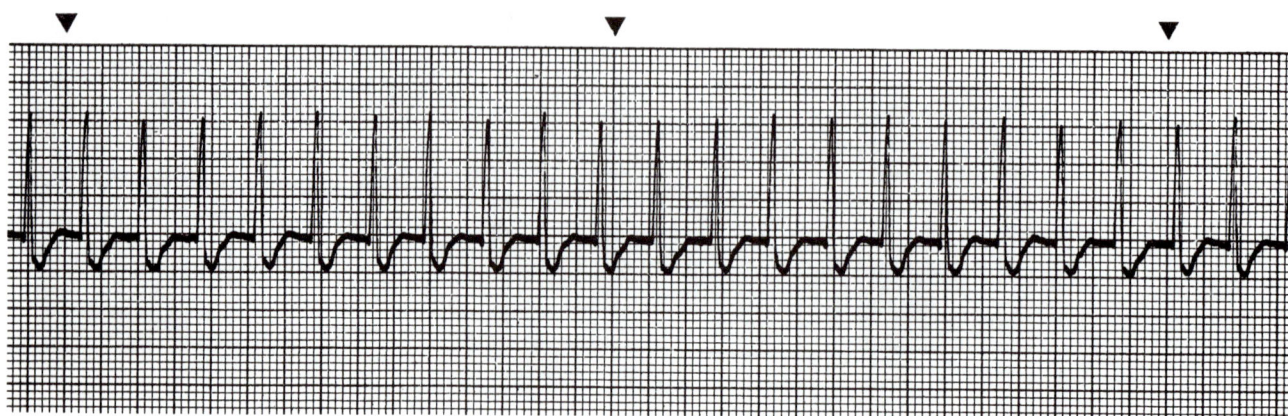

Figure 5-27. Atrial tachycardia (SVT).

Identifying features of SVT are: (1) no obvious P waves; (2) regular ventricular rhythm; (3) narrow QRS complexes of less than 0.12 seconds; and (4) heart rate of 140 to 270 beats/minute, most commonly 180 to 220.

ATRIAL FLUTTER

The strip in Figure 5-28 is atrial flutter with a 2:1 block (two atrial beats per QRS complex) and with a rapid ventricular response (greater than 100). Although the rhythm appears to only have one flutter wave for each ventricular beat, each QRS complex appears on top of a flutter wave, obscuring it. The rhythm becomes symptomatic when the ventricular response becomes too slow or, in this protocol, too fast, causing symptoms.

Atrial flutter is an exception to the rate–volume–pump rule. This rhythm's rate, 150, is not exceedingly fast (i.e., greater than 170) and therefore may be confused with rates associated with compensatory tachycardias.

Because the patients in this case study are stable, this arrhythmia is treated by blocking the AV node with medications. The blocking results in ventricular slowing because the AV node no longer allows the rapid atrial ectopic pacemaker to pass through as many depolarizations.

Identifying features are a rapid atrial response of 300 to 400 depolarizations/minute. This rapid response is represented on the ECG strip as a sawtoothed baseline. The QRS complex is narrow (less than 0.12 seconds), consistent with a supraventricular origin. The R-R rhythm may be regular or irregular, depending on whether the AV block is intermittent or not. The flutter waves, or atrial depolarizations, appear regular and similar.

ATRIAL FIBRILLATION

The strip in Figure 5-29 is atrial fibrillation with an uncontrolled or rapid ventricular response (more than 100 beats/minute). The rhythm becomes symptomatic when the ventricular response becomes too slow

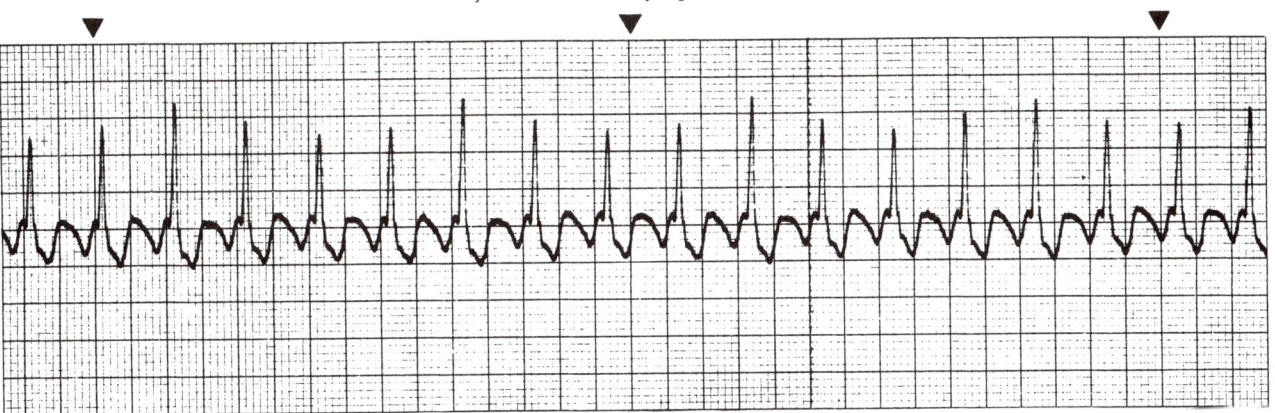

Figure 5-28. Atrial flutter.

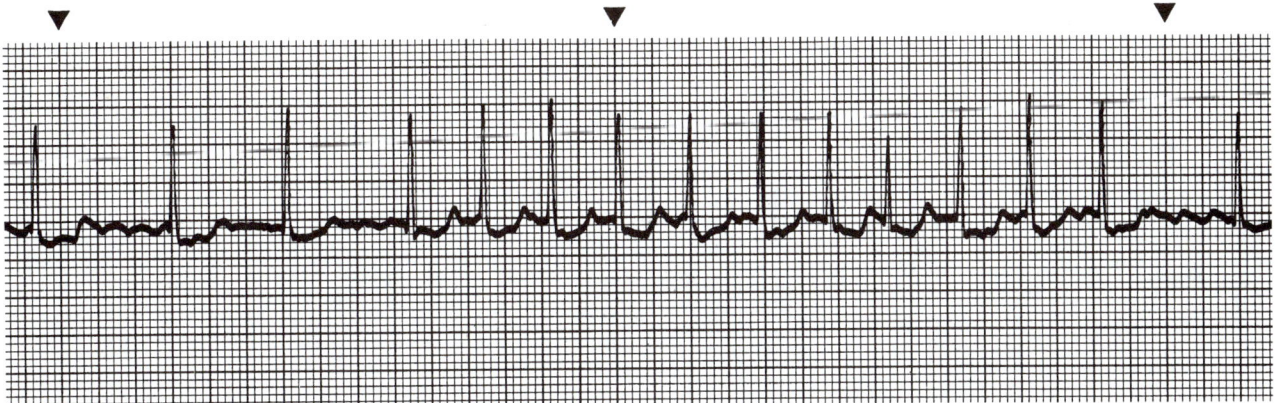

Figure 5-29. Atrial fibrillation.

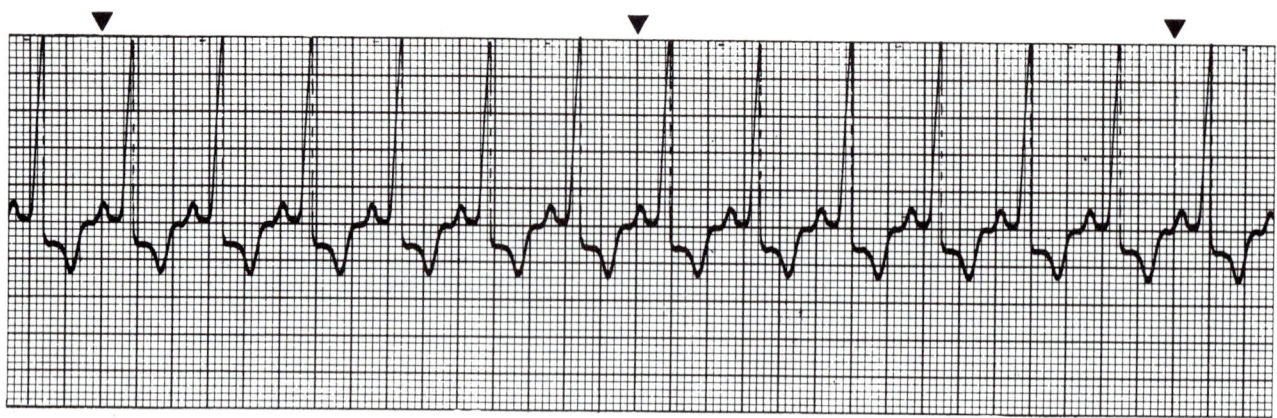

Figure 5-30. Compensatory tachycardia—sinus tachycardia.

or, in this protocol, too fast, causing cardiovascular symptoms. Atrial fibrillation, like flutter, is an exception to the rate–volume–pump rule. This rhythm's rate, 130, is not exceedingly fast (i.e., more than 170) and therefore may be confused with rates associated with compensatory tachycardias.

In this stable situation, the atrial fibrillation is treated by blocking the AV node with medications. The blocking results in ventricular slowing because ectopic pacemakers pass fewer depolarizations through the AV node.

Identifying features of atrial fibrillation are: (1) no distinct P waves, or a wavy or irregular baseline; (2) usually narrow QRS complexes of less than 0.12 seconds; and (3) irregular R-R wave intervals.

COMPENSATORY TACHYCARDIA OR SINUS TACHYCARDIA

The strip in Figure 5-30 is identified as a sinus tachycardia with a ventricular rate of 120. This rhythm may be associated with cardiovascular significance (fluid loss or CHF), but it just as easily can result from anxiety, excitement, or exercise. Treat the patient, not the rhythm; elicit the cause and consider treating it. The primary difficulty is differentiating this tachycardic rhythm from SVT because the causes and hence treatments are completely different.

Identifying features of sinus tachycardia include the presence of P waves with accompanying QRS complexes. The PR intervals are all consistent and less than 0.20 seconds. The QRS complexes are narrow, less than 0.12 seconds. The atrial and ventricular rates are equal and in this instance are greater than 100 beats/minute. This rhythm differs from SVT in two important points: (1) the heart rate is usually less than 170 in sinus tachycardia but greater than 170 in SVT; and (2) P waves are present in sinus tachycardia but not in SVT.

Wide Complex Tachycardias

VENTRICULAR TACHYCARDIA

The rhythm in Figure 5-31 is either wide complex tachycardia of unknown origin or ventricular tachycardia. Because it is extremely difficult to differentiate between these two forms in one ECG lead, a quick

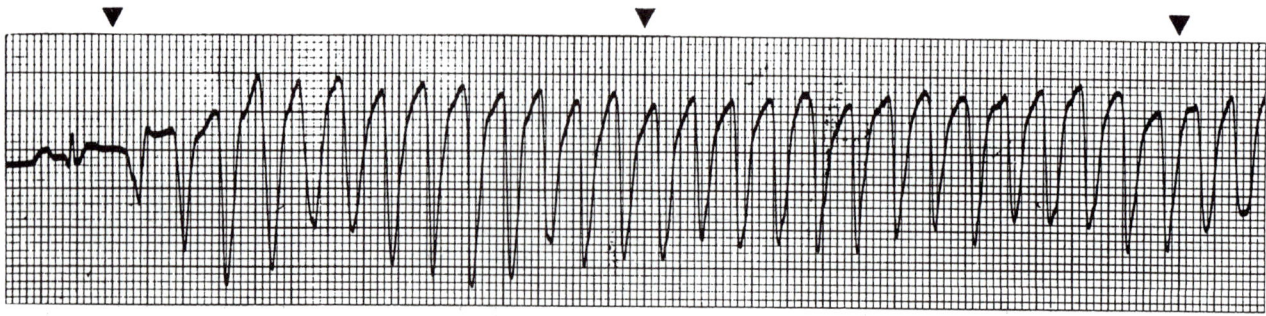

Figure 5-31. Ventricular tachycardia.

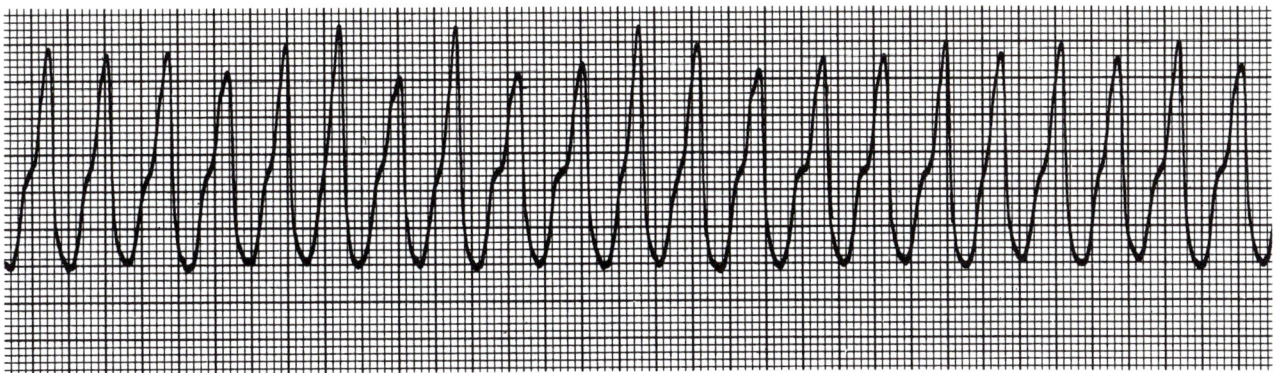

Figure 5-32. Wide complex tachycardia of unknown origin.

diagnosis of ventricular tachycardia should never be made unless supported by a 12-lead ECG and interpreted by a knowledgeable person. This strip was identified as ventricular tachycardia by a cardiologist with a 12-lead ECG.

Identifying features are wide QRS complexes responding in a regular rhythm at a rate greater than 100. Each QRS complex is similar to the others and should resemble a strip of regularly spaced PVCs.

WIDE COMPLEX TACHYCARDIA OF UNKNOWN ORIGIN

The ECG rhythm strip in Figure 5-32 is referred to as a wide complex tachycardia of unknown origin. The above rhythm strip can be identified as ventricular tachycardia only if a 12-lead ECG is read by someone knowledgeable in the nuances of aberrant conduction, or if a documented history of ventricular tachycardia is available. It is exceedingly difficult with only one ECG lead to differentiate between ventricular tachycardia and SVT with aberrant conduction. If these requirements are fulfilled, this rhythm should be identified as ventricular tachycardia. If these conditions are not met—which is most of the time—do not make a decision, just call it wide complex tachycardia and treat it with the wide complex tachycardia of unknown origin protocol. Treatment is exactly the same as ventricular tachycardia, but adenosine is also given in case the wide complex was actually SVT with aberrancy.

Identifying features of wide complex tachycardia of unknown origin are wide QRS complexes responding in a regular rhythm at a rate greater than 100. Each QRS complex should appear like the others, a run of regularly spaced PVCs—exactly like ventricular tachycardia *except* that there is no way of documenting it at that moment.

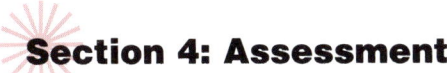

Section 4: Assessment

Primary Survey

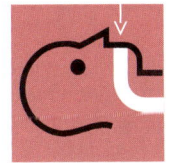 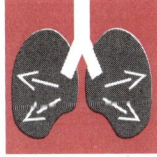 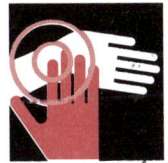

Even though the patient is considered stable for this case study, the clinician should reevaluate airway and breathing on a consistent basis. If the patient is alert and coherent, the primary ABCDs are obvious; however, a quick diagnosis of stability is premature. Even though the tachycardia may be generating a sufficient cardiac output to maintain an adequate level of consciousness, the patient may still be demonstrating sufficient symptoms of cardiovascular compromise to be treated as unstable.

Because the patient is not in ventricular fibrillation, defibrillation is not an option. Coming at a conscious patient with charged paddles may cause the patient to arrest.

Secondary Survey

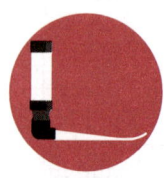

This patient would profit from oxygen by standard face mask or nonrebreather mask.

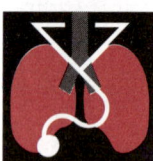

The presence of chest pain, as a symptom of a heart that is decompensating owing to the tachycardic rate, is a definitive definition of instability. Likewise, the presence of pulmonary edema, resulting from a heart rate that is so fast that it decreases cardiac filling time, is also one of the symptoms denoting instability. Even though the patient may be alert and coherent, the presence of acute pulmonary edema or chest pain, in conjunction with an extremely rapid heart rate, may indicate that the tachycardia is the problem causing the acute cardiovascular symptoms; hence, the patient is labeled unstable.

With the exception of compensatory tachycardias, such as sinus tachycardia, all stable tachycardias, regardless of cardiac origin or width, are treated with drugs. It is vitally important to determine stability, not cardiac origin, to differentiate stable from unstable patients (see beginning of this chapter). After determining stability, the rate is examined to help differentiate compensatory tachycardias (fluid deficits, fever, CHF). from rogue cardiac pacemakers (SVT or ventricular tachycardia). Obtain a set of vital signs to assist in this task. It is important to note that a patient's level of consciousness is not the sole determining factor. If an alert and oriented patient develops chest pain or acute pulmonary edema as a result of the tachycardia, the patient is considered to be cardiovascularly unstable and treated with synchronized cardioversion.

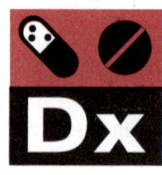

Important: The patient may have an underlying problem that can be diagnosed and treated if only the rescuer takes the time to consider other medical conditions that may have precipitated the tachycardia. It could be something simple. Refrain from blindly treating the patient with the SVT or ventricular tachycardia protocol before deciding what is really happening.

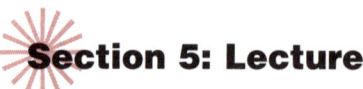# Section 5: Lecture

The lecture on stable tachycardias is broken down into narrow and wide complex sections. The narrow complex section includes SVT and atrial fibrillation and flutter, whereas the two forms of wide complex tachycardia are grouped together to enhance their similarities. Because documented ventricular tachycardia and wide complex tachycardia of unknown origin are similar in their respective treatments, their association in this case study keeps redundant information to a minimum while making any differences between them obvious.

Narrow Complex Tachycardias

TREATMENT OF SUPRAVENTRICULAR TACHYCARDIA

In SVT, also known as atrial tachycardia, the heart rate may range from 140 to 270 beats/minute. Occasionally, the rate may be as low as 140, but it is usually between 180 and 220. The rate is important. A person's heart may become tachycardic with an ectopic pacemaker cell (as in this case), or it may be just a compensatory tachycardic response to hypovolemia or CHF. It is important to make the distinction in the presenting rhythm before continuing because treatments differ significantly.

With the exception of atrial fibrillation and atrial flutter, pulse rates in hypovolemic shock and CHF are rarely this fast. Normally, a response to fluid loss, even a 50% blood loss, rarely pushes the pulse above 160. CHF pulse rates are usually in the 120 to 140 range. Thus, in narrow complex tachycardia, if the pulse is 170 or greater—with the exception of atrial fibrillation and flutter—the cause is usually an ectopic pacemaker cell and not a compensatory tachycardia. Close attention to any pertinent history, trauma or cardiac, is a necessity when narrowing your choices of treatment.

Vagal Maneuvers. The heart is heavily innervated by the vagus nerve, more so in the atria than in the ventricles. If the patient has SVT, noninvasive vagal stimulation should be considered first. The vagus nerve may be stimulated either directly or indirectly. Stimulation might be accomplished by the following methods:

- Valsalva's maneuver—having the patient bear down as if having a bowel movement
- Putting ice-cold water on the face
- Provoking a gag reflex
- Increasing intraocular pressure
- Rectal stimulation
- Carotid massage

Ice-cold water should be avoided in patients with ischemic heart disease, and eye pressure should be shunned in the elderly and those with a history of eye disease.

Auscultate for bruits, or sounds of turbulence, over each carotid artery before considering carotid massage, which is always used with extreme caution. Your procedure may inadvertently break off a piece of plaque, which could cause a CVA. Pressure should be applied at the juncture of the internal and external carotid arteries. Apply a rotary motion for 5 to 10 seconds intermittently over each carotid artery. Under no circumstances should pressure be applied to both carotids simultaneously. Repeat the procedure, alternating sides, until the pulse slows or the procedure appears to be ineffective.

Adenosine. Adenosine (Adenocard) is the first drug of choice in stable, narrow complex SVT. The drug depresses the AV node and, to a lesser extent, the sinus node. Its usefulness is short; its half-life is 5 to 10 seconds. Adenosine is effective in terminating reentrant arrhythmias through the AV node. Because this drug produces transient AV block, it can illuminate the diagnostic process when confronting the possibility of atrial fibrillation or flutter. Atrial fibrillation and flutter do not employ a reentry mechanism and therefore are not affected by adenosine. The drug has no effect on ventricular rhythms and thus may be used to rule out supraventricular origins of wide complex tachycardias.

Because of its rapid 5- to 10-second half-life, adenosine must be given by intravenous bolus (injected within 1 to 3 seconds) combined with an immediate 20 mL saline flush. The intravenous location should be at least the antecubital fossae because anything distal to this site increases the circulation time. It has a few hemodynamic side effects. When properly administered, adenosine may cause facial flushing, precipitate momentary chest pain, and generate a period of asystole lasting 3 to 5 seconds. In addition, because the half-life is incredibly short, the rhythm may recur.

The dose of adenosine is a 6-mg bolus over 1 to 3 seconds combined with an immediate saline flush. Consider inserting the adenosine-filled syringe in the same port as a syringe filled with 20 mL of saline. Then give the adenosine and flush the tubing immediately. Time is crucial, so do not rely on opening the intravenous to flush the line. If the rhythm is refractory after 1 to 2 minutes, the dosage can be doubled to 12 mg. The drug may be repeated again at 12 mg in another 1 to 2 minutes if necessary.

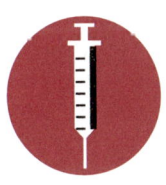

Verapamil. *If adenosine is ineffective and the QRS complex remains narrow,* consider using a slow calcium-channel–blocking agent. Verapamil causes both negative chronotropic and inotropic effects on the myocardium. Verapamil slows conduction at the AV node. Any tachycardias that simply pass through the AV node (i.e., do not employ a reentrant mechanism) are affected, the most obvious being atrial fibrillation and atrial flutter.

In the past, verapamil was the first drug of choice in the treatment of stable SVT; however, because of its hypotensive-related side effects, it is now considered only after adenosine is deemed ineffective. The dosage of this drug is 2.5 to 5.0 mg given by slow intravenous push over a period of 1 to 3 minutes; the administration rate depends on the age and cardiovascular status of the patient. If no effect is noted after 15 to 30 minutes, the dosage can be increased to 5 to 10 mg administered slowly. If necessary, repeat every 15 to 30 minutes until a maximum total dose of 30 mg is reached.

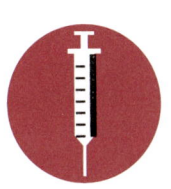

Other Options. If the patient's rhythm is refractory to verapamil or if the clinician feels that verapamil administration would be counterproductive, the following might be considered: diltiazem (Cardizem), digoxin, and β-blockers. The use of digoxin by the patient before the tachycardic problem at hand is not a contraindication to the use of diltiazem or verapamil. If at any time the patient becomes unstable or fails to respond to the medications already discussed, synchronized cardioversion should be addressed.

Lidocaine. *However, if treatment is still refractory after adenosine, and the QRS complex widens,* do not continue with verapamil. Verapamil is contraindicated because widening of the QRS complex may occur with the inception of a bundle branch block. *Do not administer verapamil to any undetermined wide complex tachycardia unless it is specifically confirmed by a 12-lead ECG to be supraventricular in origin.*

Ventricular tachycardia or atrial fibrillation, as it widens in the presence of Wolff-Parkinson-White syndrome, can be exacerbated by the administration of verapamil, and thus is considered a lethal error during ACLS. The resulting tachycardia and severe hypotension may cause death. If the QRS complex becomes wide during adenosine treatment, do not continue with verapamil. Reflect that the rhythm may have changed to a ventricular ectopic pacemaker and consider the first ventricular antiarrhythmic: lidocaine.

Lidocaine should be used at this juncture. In this situation, lidocaine is not considered prophylactic. The recommended dose is 1.0 to 1.5 mg/kg given by intravenous push. This dose can be repeated every 5 to 10 minutes with additional doses of 0.5 to 0.75 mg/kg until a maximum dose of 3 mg/kg is reached or the rhythm terminates.

Because the half-life of lidocaine is short, it is necessary to hang a lidocaine drip (1 g in 250 mL NS or D-5-W) to keep a continuous therapeutic blood level. Start the drip between 2 and 4 mg/min (30 to 60 gtts/min in a microdrip or minidrip). A second bolus of 0.5 to 0.75 mg/kg is required to prevent subtherapeutic levels after the first bolus and the drip.

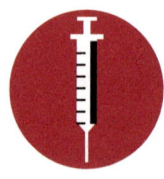

Procainamide. Procainamide may be considered if the wide complex tachycardic rhythm is refractory to lidocaine. The main problem is its inability to be administered quickly; but because the patient is still considered stable, time is not critical. The loading dose is 20 to 30 mg/min until a maximum of 17 mg/kg is reached. This means than for an average 70-kg patient, it may take as much as 1 hour to administer. Watch for signs of hypotension and QRS widening greater than 50% than before the drug was started. If at any time the patient begins to show signs of instability, consider moving the patient to the unstable protocol.

TREATMENT OF ATRIAL FIBRILLATION AND FLUTTER

Atrial fibrillation and flutter are caused by one or more ectopic pacemakers firing in the atria. In atrial flutter, one ectopic cell is depolarizing at 270 to 400 beats/minute. If each of these atrial depolarizations resulted in a ventricular contraction, the increased heart rate would make the patient rapidly decompensate. To alleviate the situation, the AV node alters its permeability to keep the number of depolarizations that pass through to a manageable level. This nodal ability can act for or against the patient. If the AV node becomes less selective, the ventricular response can increase markedly. Likewise, if the AV node becomes more selective, bradycardia can result.

The situation in atrial fibrillation is similar, although multiple pacemakers are involved. Because multiple ectopic sites are firing, the depolarization waves that impact the AV node are too numerous to count. As in atrial flutter, the AV node is the "gatekeeper," keeping the ventricular responses to a controllable level. Again, if the AV node is not acting selectively, a heart rate above 100, termed *uncontrolled* or *rapid*, results. Similarly, if the AV node becomes too proficient at disregarding the depolarization waves from the ectopic beats, bradycardia may result. Atrial fibrillation and atrial flutter are common arrhythmias and may not require treatment at all. Treat the patient, not the monitor!

Because the ventricular depolarization pathway for both atrial fibrillation and flutter is normal, the QRS complexes appear narrow. Neither of these rhythms employs a reentrant mechanism, so the heart rate is usually not exceedingly fast (i.e., greater than 170). With a narrow QRS complex and a heart rate that usually does not exceed 170, these rhythms could easily be confused with compensatory tachycardia. Therefore, it is incumbent on the clinician to recognize and interpret the rhythms before considering treating compromised patients with the rate–volume–pump regimen. If circumstances require, these arrhythmias should be treated with the appropriate tachycardia protocol: stable or unstable.

Depending on the patient's age, history, and rate of ventricular response, these two rhythms may be asymptomatic, with only observation required. If the ventricular response becomes too slow or too fast, however, atrial fibrillation and flutter may cause serious signs and symptoms. If the rate becomes too rapid and the patient's cardiovascular status begins to decompensate, consider the unstable tachycardia protocol and immediately cardiovert. On the other hand, if the AV node starts letting fewer depolarizations through, and the patient becomes hemodynamically unstable, consider employing the bradycardia protocol immediately.

If the signs and symptoms allow for more relaxed treatment considerations, the clinician should consider some of the causes that can precipitate these two arrhythmias, including the following:

- Acute MI
- Hypoxia
- Pulmonary embolism
- Electrolyte abnormalities
- Medication toxicity (particularly digoxin or quinidine)
- Thyrotoxicosis

Stable Treatment Considerations. Vagal maneuvers can be diagnostic and should be attempted first. In a rapid atrial flutter, the atrial waves (flutter) may be hidden under the QRS complexes, and vagal domination may slow the rate, allowing the waves to become more visible. The first priority should be given to *slowing* the tachycardic heart rate rather than *converting* it to a more viable rhythm. Conversion is usually accomplished fortuitously after the rhythm slows. The following medications should effect a change in the heart rate:

- Calcium-channel blockers (e.g., diltiazem and verapamil)
- β-blockers (e.g., esmolol, metoprolol, atenolol, propranolol)
- Digoxin (some experts question its role in acute situations)

If the heart rate has been controlled but the rhythm has not spontaneously corrected, chemical conversion with intravenous or oral procainamide and oral quinidine should be considered to assist in converting the rhythm. Procainamide should not be given within 30 minutes after verapamil administration because profound bradycardia progressing to asystole may result.

Elective cardioversion is a preferred method to convert the rhythm after the rate is controlled. If the patient has been in atrial fibrillation for more than a few days, consider pretreating with anticoagulants to decrease the possibility of emboli after elective cardioversion. Atrial flutter does not require anticoagulant therapy.

> The probability that a patient will experience cardiovascular difficulties increases proportionally with the distance of the crash cart from the patient's room.

Any Stable Wide Complex Tachycardia

This lecture presents a structured approach to any wide complex tachycardia—whether it is a documented ventricular tachycardia or a wide complex tachycardia of uncertain origin. Deciding the difference can produce a great deal of anxiety, so a quick explanation follows to help sort out the confusion.

Just because a QRS complex appears wide, it does not mean it originated in the ventricles. Stated simply: *all that is wide and fast is not ventricular tachycardia.* Of all wide complex tachycardias, only about 80% originate in the ventricles. The remaining 20% are actually supraventricular, appearing wide owing to a conduction abnormality.

A supraventricular rhythm, if it follows the normal track of depolarization, results in a narrow QRS complex. If the depolarization in the ventricles does not follow the normal pathway, however, the resulting QRS complex can look wide—a situation referred to as *aberrant conduction*. This deviant depolarization process makes QRS complexes so wide that if the ectopic pacemaker is beating rapidly, the resulting rhythm *looks just like ventricular tachycardia.*

Helpful Hints for Differential Diagnosis of Wide-Complex Tachycardia

▼ Do not try to distinguish between ventricular tachycardia and supraventricular tachycardia with aberrant conduction based on clinical criteria.

▼ Patients with ventricular tachycardia may appear alert, coherent, and stable. Trying to diagnose the origin of a rhythm, based solely on the clinical supposition that ventricular tachycardia should always appear more unstable than supraventricular tachycardia, is erroneous and may result in the administration of inappropriate drugs.

▼ For the average clinician, it is extremely difficult, if not impossible, to tell the difference between the two forms of wide complex tachycardia when viewed from one lead.

▼ Always treat wide complex tachycardias with the wide complex tachycardia of unknown origin protocol unless you can *reliably* differentiate between ventricular tachycardia and SVT with aberrant conduction with a 12-lead ECG.

▼ Both rhythms employ lidocaine, procainamide, and bretylium in their treatment protocols.

▼ The wide complex tachycardia of unknown origin protocol adds adenosine to hedge the possible 20% chance of a supraventricular origin.

▼ If the patient becomes unstable, both rhythms are treated alike, with synchronized cardioversion.

TREATMENT OF ANY STABLE WIDE COMPLEX TACHYCARDIA

Assuming that this is an emergency, it is extremely critical in this particular algorithm to obtain a focused history. It is important to elicit the time sequence and any predisposing symptoms before deciding on a specific treatment. Chest pain before the presenting situation may indicate acute MI. Pain and anxiety from chest pain may send a pulse soaring; therefore, give thought to whether the rate is due to an ectopic pacemaker cell or is a response to underlying pathology. If there is no history and the patient presents with a wide complex tachycardia, obtain a set of vital signs. If the vital signs reveal hypotension, immediately go to the unstable tachycardia protocol. If the patient is not hypotensive, continue with the assessment and start the intravenous line.

If there is time, obtain a 12-lead ECG, hook the patient to a pulse oximeter, and order a chest radiograph. These tests yield valuable data during the assessment.

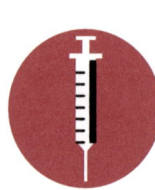

Lidocaine. Whether you are certain that the presenting rhythm is ventricular tachycardia or are hedging your bet because you are not certain if it is SVT with aberrant conduction, there is an 80% chance that the wide complex rhythm is ventricular in origin. The first drug of choice for either situation is lidocaine.

The recommended dose is 1.0 to 1.5 mg/kg given by intravenous push. The lower dose is for more stable situations in which time is not a concern. If the patient is starting to decompensate and you are not yet moving to the unstable algorithm, consider the higher dose because it can be maximized quickly.

A second bolus of 0.5 to 0.75 mg/kg is required to prevent subtherapeutic levels after the first bolus. This can be repeated in 5- to 10-minute intervals with additional doses of 0.5 to 0.75 mg/kg until a maximum dose of 3 mg/kg is reached or the rhythm terminates. Because the half-life of lidocaine is short, it is necessary to hang a lidocaine drip (1 g in 250 mL of D-5-W or NS) to maintain a therapeutic blood level. Start the drip between 2 and 4 mg/min (30 to 60 gtt/min in a microdrip or minidrip).

Signs of lidocaine toxicity in a stable situation are:

- Hallucinations
- Altered level of consciousness
- Decreased hearing

- Seizure disorders
- Slurred speech
- Paresthesia
- Muscle twitching

Lidocaine maintenance dosage should be limited to half the normal dose whenever the following factors are suspected or documented:

- Decreased cardiac output
- Decreased hepatic function
- Patient age more than 70 years

Lidocaine is also helpful for isolated instances of ventricular activity (runs or bursts of ventricular tachycardia) if the patient is experiencing cardiovascular compromise; however, conservative use of lidocaine, even in the presence of chest pain, is becoming the norm.

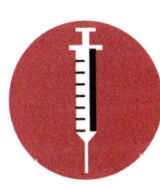

Adenosine. If you are not certain that the presenting wide complex tachycardia is ventricular in origin, administer adenosine next. If you are certain—without a doubt—that it is a true ventricular tachycardia, bypass this drug because it only works on supraventricular ectopic beats and would just add to the patient's expense.

Adenosine is the second drug of choice in a stable, wide complex tachycardia of unknown origin. The rationale for its administration is as follows: lidocaine was refractory, so the chances of a ventricular origin have decreased; however, the odds of a supraventricular pacemaker have increased.

Adenosine depresses the AV node and, to a lesser extent, the sinus node. Its half-life is only 5 to 10 seconds. It is effective in terminating reentrant arrhythmias through the AV node. Because this drug produces transient AV block, it can illuminate the diagnostic process when confronting the possibility of atrial fibrillation or flutter. Atrial fibrillation and flutter do not employ a reentry mechanism and therefore are not affected by adenosine. The drug has no effect on ventricular rhythms and so may be used to rule out supraventricular origins of wide complex tachycardias..

If the clinician assumes that all wide complex tachycardias are always ventricular tachycardia, the possibility of a supraventricular origin is never explored. The clinician just continues with the next ventricular antiarrhythmic—procainamide—and the possibility that this rhythm is indeed supraventricular is never ruled out. Therefore, adenosine, which has no effect on ventricular rhythms but converts supraventricular rhythms, can be given to exclude this possibility. If adenosine works, the rhythm was SVT with aberrant conduction. If the rhythm was refractory to adenosine, the protocol reverts to ventricular possibilities; the rhythm was probably ventricular but did not respond to lidocaine. Therefore, the next ventricular antiarrhythmic, procainamide, is considered.

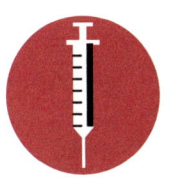

Procainamide. Procainamide is considered if the rhythm is refractory to both lidocaine and adenosine. The main problem with procainamide is its inability to be administered quickly. Because the patient is still considered stable, however, time is not a factor at the moment.

The dose is 20 to 30 mg/min until a maximum of 17 mg/kg is reached. This means that for an average 70-kg patient, it takes about 1 hour to administer. Watch for signs of hypotension and QRS widening greater than 50%. If either occurs, stop administration and move to the next drug. The lower dose of 20 mg/min should be selected when time is not a consideration; the higher dose should be used if the symptoms become a problem and time is a concern.

Because the half-life of procainamide is short, after the loading dose, it is necessary to hang a drip (1 g in 250 mL of D-5-W or NS) to maintain a therapeutic blood level. Start the drip between 1 and 4 mg/min (15 to 60 gtt/min in a microdrip or minidrip).

Bretylium. If procainamide has been ineffective, take a couple of moments to reassess the patient's status. Consistent reassessment cannot be stressed enough. Bretylium is the next drug of choice. Dilute 500 mg in 50 to 100 mL of NS or D-5-W; the dose is 5 to 10 mg/kg infused slowly over 8 to 10 minutes as an intravenous drip. Bretylium should not be given by intravenous bolus as is appropriate in ventricular fibrillation. Conscious patients may experience nausea and vomiting if the drug is administered too quickly. Patients may also experience the most common side effect—postural hypotension.

If the rhythm is refractory to the initial dose, repeat at 5 to 10 mg/kg after 10 to 30 minutes. If necessary, bretylium can be repeated at 5 to 10 mg/kg, infused slowly every 6 to 8 hours to a maximum dosage

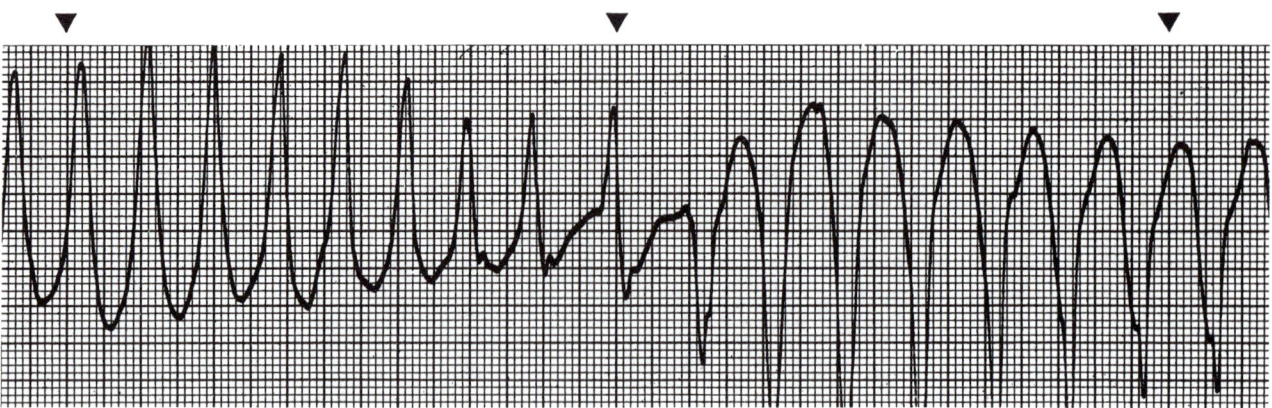

Figure 5-33. Torsades de pointes.

of 30 to 35 mg/kg. If at any time during the administration of this ventricular antiarrhythmic, the patient's rhythm converts, consider an immediate maintenance drip of bretylium (1 g in 250 mL of D-5-W or NS) to maintain a therapeutic blood level. Start the drip at 2 mg/min (30 gtt/min in a microdrip or minidrip). The onset of action may be prolonged in VT—as long as 20 minutes.

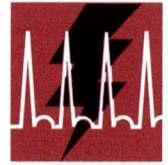

Synchronized Cardioversion. If any time the patient begins to decompensate by showing signs of an altered level of consciousness or hypotension, immediately consider synchronized cardioversion. In addition, if the patient begins to experience cardiovascular compromise as represented by acute pulmonary edema or chest pain, make certain that the presenting tachycardic rhythm is the source of the symptoms. Even though these patients may be alert and coherent, if you are certain that the chest pain or pulmonary edema is due to the tachycardia, immediately consider synchronized cardioversion. Sedate if possible and administer a synchronized shock of 50 to 100 joules. If the rhythm is refractory, continue on up to 360 joules. Continue with antiarrhythmics during the procedure as long as they do not interrupt the sequence.

Again, make certain that the presenting unstable symptoms represent a response to rate-driven tachycardia and not other underlying medical pathology. In other words, make certain that the chest pain is a response to the tachycardia and does not represent ischemic pain from a coronary occlusion.

TREATMENT OF TORSADES DE POINTES

The strip in Figure 5-33 is a special form of ventricular tachycardia. The term *torsades de pointes* means "twisting of points"; the QRS amplitude constantly becomes larger, then smaller, resembling a sine wave. Because many clinicians are not familiar with this type of ventricular tachycardia, it should be considered whenever a patient who is not in cardiac arrest displays ventricular tachycardia refractory to the recommended agents: lidocaine, procainamide, and bretylium. Antiarrhythmic agents that prolong Q-T intervals (procainamide and quinidine) exacerbate torsades des pointes, so the clinician should familiar with the ECG signs of this tachycardia before initiating the standard ventricular tachycardia protocol.

Treatment of unstable torsades des pointes is the same as for any unstable rate-driven tachycardia: synchronized cardioversion. If the patient is stable, however, treatment consists of removing the offending factors and administering magnesium sulfate. The dose is 1 to 2 g diluted to 10 mL and administered over a period of 1 to 2 minutes.

If magnesium sulfate treatment is refractory, consider an overdrive pacemaker. If that is not available, isoproterenol is used for its positive chronotropic effects, accelerating the heart rate faster than the torsades, capturing the pacemaker, reducing the infusion, and thus bringing the rate down. Remember, treatment must include removing the offending factors or the rhythm will recur.

Offending Factors	*Treatment*
Horrible Drugs Prolong Q-T	**Physicians Must Interrupt Rhythm**
H = hypokalemia	P = pacemaker
D = disopyramide	M = magnesium sulfate
P = procainamide, phenothiazines	I = isoproterenol
T = tricyclic antidepressants	R = remove offending factors

Section 6: Stable Tachycardias Interim Evaluation

1. A 48-year-old man is in the intensive care unit, and the monitor displays a wide complex tachycardia. You have ascertained that the patient is tolerating the rhythm and is not experiencing any chest pain or difficulty breathing. After oxygenating the patient and giving repeated doses of lidocaine, the last reaching a total of 3 mg/kg with no change in the rhythm, your next therapy should be to (see ACLS text pp. 1-32 to 1-39):

   _____ (a) Give bretylium at 5mg/kg slowly over 8 to 10 minutes.
   _____ (b) Sedate and deliver a synchronized shock starting at 50 joules.
   _____ (c) Administer 6 mg of adenosine.
   _____ (d) Administer 2.5 mg of verapamil.

2. When approaching the treatment of tachycardias, which of the following is true (see ACLS text pp. 1-32 to 1-39): (1) adenosine has such a short half-life that tachycardias could recur easily; (2) verapamil should be withheld if the tachycardia is a wide QRS complex; (3) verapamil should not be used when encountering a hemodynamically significant atrial fibrillation or flutter; (4) an apparently stable patient may be treated with the unstable protocol if the patient has signs of cardiovascular compromise, such as chest pain or pulmonary edema?

   _____ (a) All of the above
   _____ (b) 1 and 4
   _____ (c) 2, 3, and 4
   _____ (d) 1, 2, and 4

3. In the treatment of a 75-kg adult with confirmed ventricular tachycardia with a perfusing pulse, which of the following schedules of lidocaine is most preferable (see ACLS text pp. 1-32 to 1-39 and 7-6 to 7-8)?

   _____ (a) 200 mg followed by an infusion of 1 to 2 mg/min
   _____ (b) 100 mg every 5 minutes up to a total of 400 mg
   _____ (c) 75 to 112 mg followed by an infusion of 2 to 4 mg/min
   _____ (d) 50 to 100 mg followed by an infusion starting at 4 to 6 mg/min

4. When treating a patient for hypotension of an unknown cause, you should first start by (see ACLS text pp. 1-40 to 1-43):

   _____ (a) Examining the heart rate
   _____ (b) Checking for pump failure
   _____ (c) Seeing if the patient has a fluid deficit
   _____ (d) Examining for a possible head injury

5. Lidocaine, 1.0 to 1.5 mg/kg given intravenously (see ACLS text pp. 1-32 to 1-39 and 7-6 to 7-8): (1) lowers the fibrillation threshold of the ventricle; (2) is useful in treating wide complex tachycardias of unknown origin; (3) is not indicated in ventricular tachycardia; (4) is useful in treating SVT.

   _____ (a) 1, 2, and 4
   _____ (b) 3 and 4
   _____ (c) 2
   _____ (d) All the above

6. Adenosine is effective in terminating uncontrolled atrial fibrillation and atrial flutter as well as atrial tachycardia (see ACLS text p. 7-13).

   _____ (a) True
   _____ (b) False

7. More than 90% of all wide complex tachycardias have a ventricular origin.

   _____ (a) True
   _____ (b) False

8. A 38-year-old woman arrives at the emergency department. She is conscious and coherent, denying chest pain, but relates a history of sudden heart palpitations. It has taken her 35 minutes to get to your facility. Your 12-lead ECG confirms a SVT at 210 beats/minute. Her blood pressure is 110/90 mmHg. Your initial therapy would be to (see ACLS text pp. 1-36 to 1-37):

   _____ (a) Synchronize cardioversion at 50 to 100 joules.
   _____ (b) Consider vagal maneuvers.
   _____ (c) Administer verapamil 5 mg slowly by intravenous infusion.
   _____ (d) Administer adenosine 6 mg rapidly by IV push.

9. Common adverse reactions to bretylium include (see ACLS text pp. 7-9 to 7-11): (1) respiratory depression; (2) nausea and vomiting if administered rapidly; (3) postural hypotension; (4) metabolic acidosis.

   _____ (a) 1 and 2
   _____ (b) 1 and 3
   _____ (c) 2 and 3
   _____ (d) 2 and 4

10. Calcium chloride in adults or children (see ACLS text pp. 7-16 to 7-17): (1) should be administered if the patient has a history of malnutrition; (2) should be given prophylactically in ventricular fibrillation; (3) is employed for hyperkalemia; (4) is used for hypocalcemia; (5) is an antidote for hemodynamically significant bradycardia secondary to verapamil overdose.

    _____ (a) 2, 3, 4, and 5
    _____ (b) 3, 4, and 5
    _____ (c) 1, 3, and 4
    _____ (d) 2, 3, and 4

11. Which of the following cardiac rhythms would be responsive to adenosine (see ACLS text pp. 1-32 to 1-40 and 7-13): (1) uncontrolled atrial fibrillation; (2) SVT; (3) atrial tachycardia; (4) ventricular tachycardia; (5) uncontrolled atrial flutter?

    _____ (a) 2
    _____ (b) 1 and 3
    _____ (c) 2 and 3
    _____ (d) 4 and 5

12. The initial dose of verapamil is (see ACLS text pp. 7-11 to 7-12):

    _____ (a) 1 to 2 mg/kg/min
    _____ (b) 2 to 4 mg/min
    _____ (c) 2.5 to 5 mg infused slowly over 1 to 3 minutes
    _____ (d) 5 to 10 mg infused rapidly over 1 to 3 seconds

13. When only one ECG lead is available, most wide complex tachycardias resembling ventricular tachycardia should be treated with the wide complex tachycardia of uncertain origin protocol (see ACLS text pp. 1-36 to 1-40).

    _____ (a) True
    _____ (b) False

14. Which of the following tachycardic rates are acceptable for the cause assigned: (1) hypovolemic shock—100 to 200 beats/minute; (2) CHF—100 to 150 beats/minute; (3) SVT—140 to 270 beats/minute?

    _____ (a) 1 and 3
    _____ (b) 2 and 3
    _____ (c) 1 and 2
    _____ (d) All of the above

15. The main side effects of procainamide are (see ACLS text pp. 1-32 to 1-40 and 7-8 to 7-9): (1) hypotension; (2) prolonged administration time; (3) the heart rate tends to accelerate; (4) hypertension; (5) the QRS interval shortens initially and then prolongs.

_____ (a) 3, 4, and 5
_____ (b) 2 and 4
_____ (c) 1, 2, and 3
_____ (d) 1 and 2

16. Verapamil is normally contraindicated in wide complex tachycardia except when Wolff-Parkinson-White syndrome is diagnosed. In this syndrome, verapamil can be administered with impunity (see ACLS text pp. 7-11).

_____ (a) True
_____ (b) False

17. Bretylium's side effects surround its initial sympathomimetic consequences, which after 20 minutes turn sympatholytic (see ACLS text pp. 7-9 to 7-10).

_____ (a) True
_____ (b) False

18. Adenosine depresses the AV node briefly interrupting the depolarization sequence, terminating most SVTs (see ACLS text p. 7-13).

_____ (a) True
_____ (b) False

19. Luckily, a person with ventricular tachycardia shows more hemodynamic signs and symptoms than a person with just SVT (see ACLS text p. 1-38).

_____ (a) True
_____ (b) False

20. All of the following are vagal maneuvers, *except* (see ACLS text p. 1-37):

_____ (a) Ice-cold water in the outer ear
_____ (b) Carotid massage
_____ (c) Pressure on the eyes
_____ (d) Rectal stimulation

21. Adenosine (see ACLS text p. 7-13):

_____ (a) Has an exceptionally long half-life
_____ (b) Terminates tachyarrhythmias for which reentry is through the AV node
_____ (c) Is both an α- and β-adrenergic receptor stimulator
_____ (d) Is an α-adrenergic–blocking agent

22. A medication history containing digitalis is not a contraindication to the use of calcium-channel blockers (see ACLS text p. 7-13).

_____ (a) True
_____ (b) False

144 Unit 1 *Fundamental Concepts of ACLS* • **Stable Tachycardias**

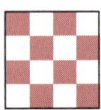

Section 7
STABLE TACHYCARDIA CROSSWORD PUZZLE

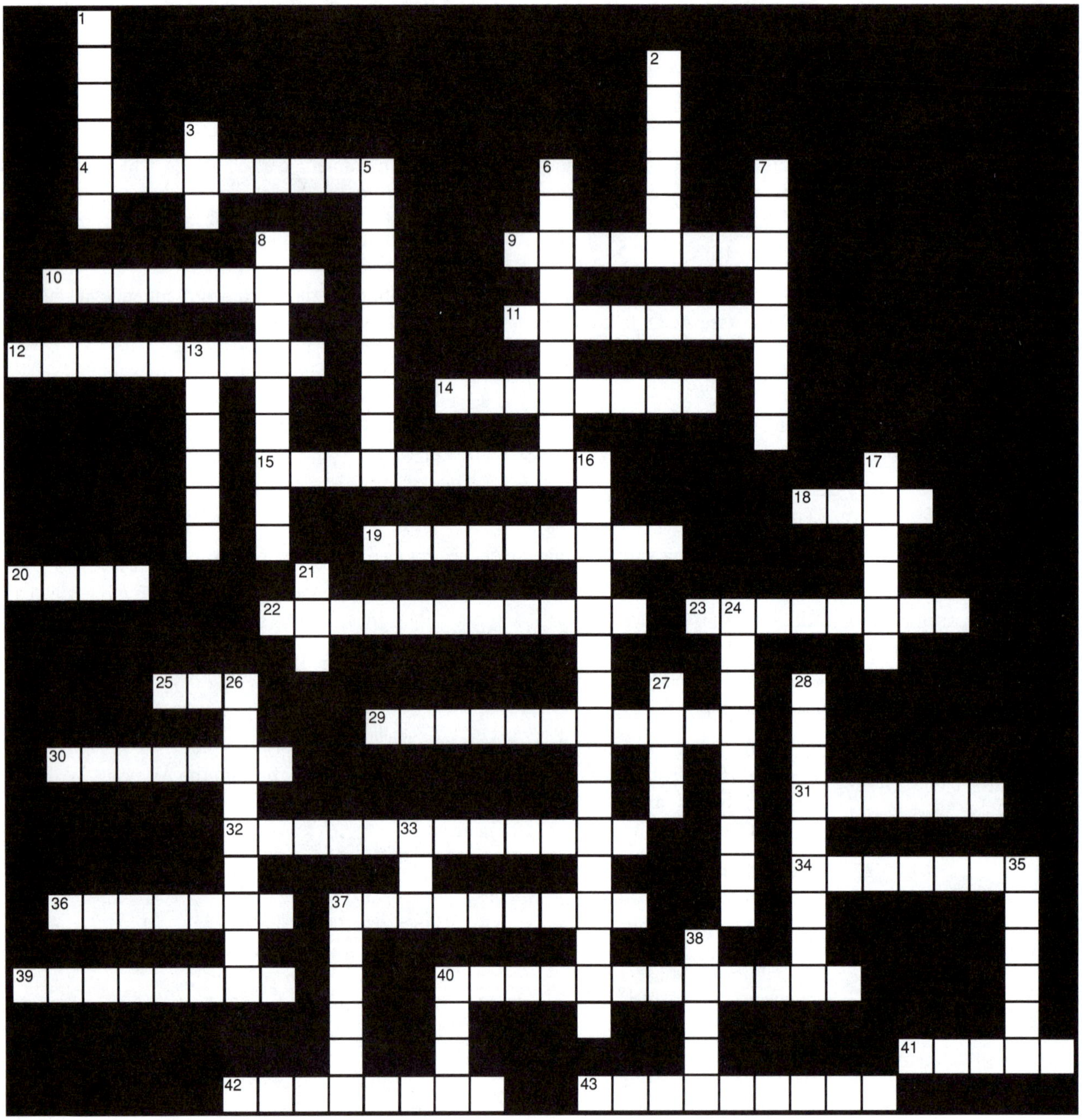

Across

4. This calcium-channel blocking agent is contraindicated in unknown wide complex tachycardias.
9. Trade name of bretylium tosylate.
10. _____ hypotension is the most common side effect of bretylium administration. Pertaining to or affected by posture.
11. Both procainamide and quinidine can cause _____ of the QRS complex because they affect QT intervals.
12. The maximum dosage of procainamide is _____ mg/kg (number spelled out).
14. A brief period of _____ is a common side effect of adenosine administration. Usually associated with a verification of death. The rhythm that typifies a flat line.
15. Because atrial fibrillation and flutter can become unstable at rates below 170 beats/minute, they can be confused with compensatory tachycardias. Therefore, they are _____ to the rate-volume-pump rule.

18. If the stable wide complex tachycardia of unknown origin rhythm is refractory after an initial dose of lidocaine, a next dose may be administered at one-_____ of the original dose after 5 to 10 minutes have passed.
19. Pertaining to contractility of the heart. The prefix of the term is taken from the Greek god of strength.
20. Mixing a drip of lidocaine, procainamide, and bretylium is achieved by adding one _____ of the antiarrhythmic in 250 mL of solution.
22. A tachycardia originating from this myocardial tissue can be treated with lidocaine. Usually, QRS complexes originating from this area are wide. Referring to the portion of the myocardium responsible for generating perfusion.
23. This vagal maneuver is precipitated when the patient bears down against a closed glottis, similar to having a bowel movement.
25. The initial dose of adenosine is _____ mg infused by rapid intravenous push (number spelled out).
29. A major side effect of procainamide administration. A fall in the blood pressure. When the QT interval is increased, contractility is reduced, causing this fall in blood pressure.
30. Adenosine must be administered _____ because its half-life is 5 to 10 seconds.
31. _____ and vomiting are common side effects of bretylium administration if the drug is administered too rapidly. Unpleasant sensation usually preceding ACLS testing.
32. Verapamil is a negative _____ agent. This word means "to slow the heart rate."
34. Verapamil is defined as a slow _____-channel blocking agent. An ion associated with building bones and muscle contraction.
36. Pressure on this artery can: (1) detect a pulse at a systolic blood pressure of about 60 mmHg; (2) possibly result in a CVA if bruits are not located first; and (3) result in unconsciousness if both are massaged simultaneously.
37. This drug initially functions as a sympathomimetic; 15 to 20 minutes later, it becomes a sympatholytic. Because of its side effects, this drug is the last choice in the wide complex tachycardia of unknown origin protocol.
39. A variation of ventricular tachycardia in which magnesium sulfate is the drug of choice rather than the normal ventricular antiarrhythmic.
40. This drug is contraindicated in torsades de pointes because it increases QT intervals. It is the third drug of choice in the wide complex tachycardia of unknown origin protocol.
41. The maximum dose of lidocaine is _____ mg/kg (number spelled out).
42. Facial _____ is a common side effect of adenosine administration. The skin turns red as vessels dilate.
43. The trade name for procainamide.

Down
1. The second dose of adenosine. It may be repeated once more at the same dose if necessary (number spelled out).
2. The initial dose of procainamide is _____ mg/min; 30 mg/min may be administered in time-critical situations (number spelled out).
3. Sticking a tongue depressor in the back of the oropharynx can precipitate a _____ reflex, causing vagal stimulation.
5. The maximum dose of this drug is 3 mg/kg.
6. Verapamil should be withheld in the presence of atrial fibrillation masked by the presence of Wolff-_____-White syndrome.
7. Both lidocaine and bretylium are administered on a milligram per _____ basis, whereas procainamide is given in milligrams per minute.
8. Examples of common vagal _____ are carotid massage, gagging, and pressure on the eyes.
13. The maximum dose of verapamil is _____ mg (number spelled out).
16. Term referring to "above the ventricles." These tachycardias are usually narrow in width and usually respond to adenosine if they employ a reentry mechanism.
17. Both verapamil and procainamide must be administered _____ to avoid hypotension.
21. The second dose of verapamil is 5 to _____ mg infused slowly (number spelled out).
24. This is the second drug of choice in the wide complex tachycardia of unknown origin protocol. It has such a rapid half-life that its administration must be followed immediately by a bolus of 20 mL of fluid.
26. The trade name for lidocaine.
27. The second dose of verapamil is _____ to 10 mg infused slowly (number spelled out).
28. Trade name for adenosine.
33. The initial dose of lidocaine varies from _____ to 1.5 mg/kg (number spelled out).
35. Procainamide is given at 20 to 30 mg per _____ to a maximum of 17 mg/kg.
37. Before performing carotid massage, it is imperative to listen over the bifurcation of the internal and external carotids for the presence of _____.
38. A trade name for verapamil hydrochloride.
40. Chest _____ in the presence of a tachycardia must be distinguished between ischemia caused by the rapid heart rate and that caused by an acute MI before treatment can be considered.

6 Acute Stroke: Acute Ischemic Stroke and Hemorrhagic Stroke

R. Lee Archer
David P. Doernbach

Section 1: Critical Actions for Student Evaluation

The ACLS instructor checklist for case study 6—Acute Stroke is shown in Table 6-1. This form was designed to guide the faculty when evaluating participants during this particular station. Refer to it frequently as you read the lecture that follows. *Do not memorize it*. The form is included only to (1) show you what the American Heart Association (AHA) thinks is important during this particular case study; (2) allow you to get a feel for what the faculty are trying to cover in the station; and (3) provide a summary of the case study after you have read the lecture.

Table 6-1.
Evaluation Checklist—Acute Stroke

Critical Action	Completed	Not Completed	Comments
Prehospital			
Rapidly recognizes signs of stroke			
Describes performance of prehospital Cincinnati Prehospital Stroke Scale			
Attempts to determine time of onset of stroke symptoms			
Assesses and supports cardiorespiratory function and serum glucose			
Provides pre-arrival notification of ED			
Emergency Department			
Demonstrates awareness of NINDS target times for evaluation of stroke patients			
Demonstrates awareness of importance of rapid performance and reading of CT scan			
Applies AHA guidelines for treatment of hypertension in patient with stroke			
Applies inclusion and exclusion criteria for thrombolytic therapy correctly			
Is aware of potential benefits and complications of thrombolytic therapy			

(Reproduced with permission. *Instructor's manual for advanced cardiac life support,* 1997 © Copyright American Heart Association, p. 6-14.)

Chapter 6 Acute Stroke: Acute Ischemic Stroke and Hemorrhagic Stroke

Section 2: ACLS Algorithm for Stroke

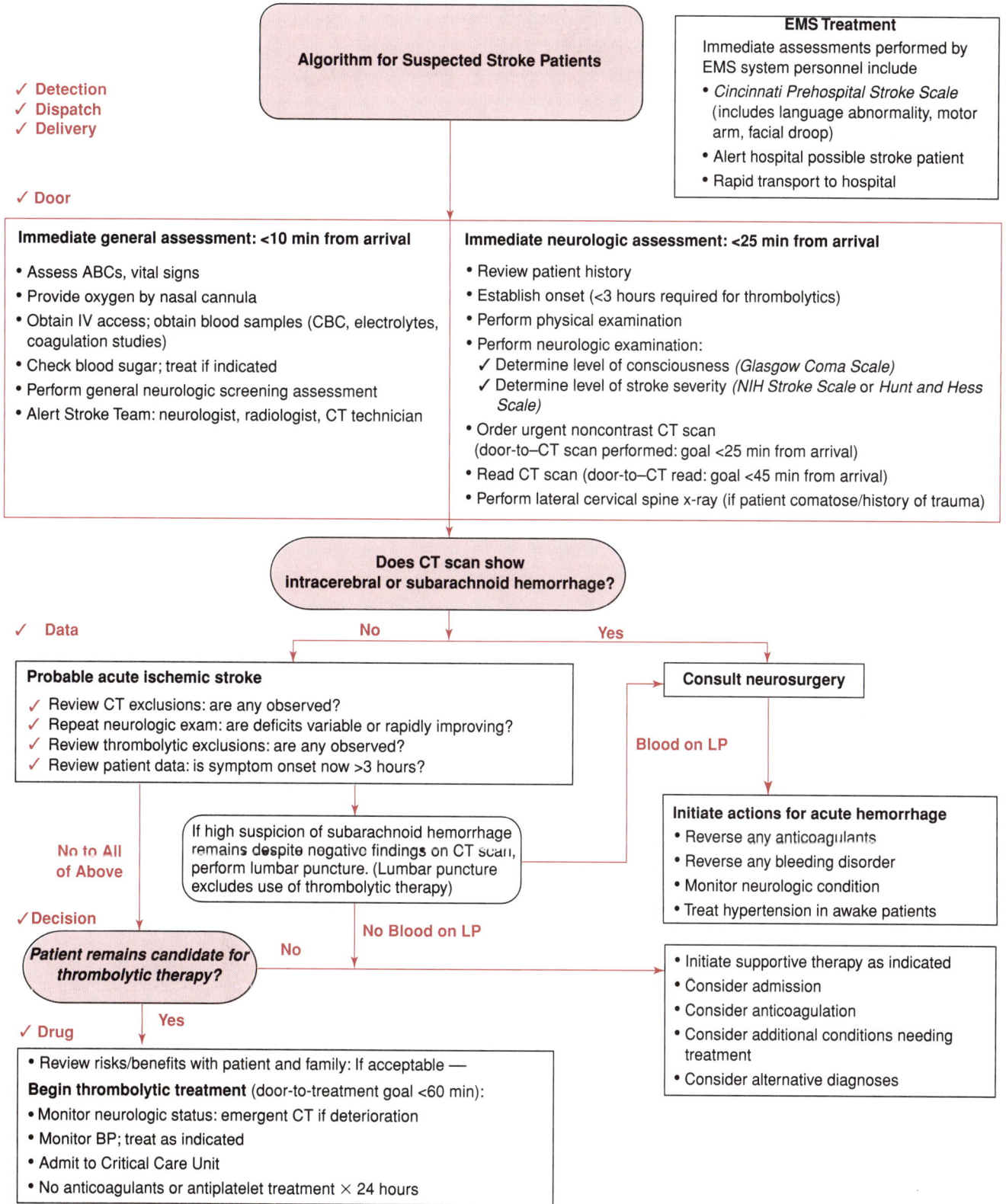

(Reproduced with permission. *Advanced cardiac life support.* Copyright 1997, American Heart Association.)

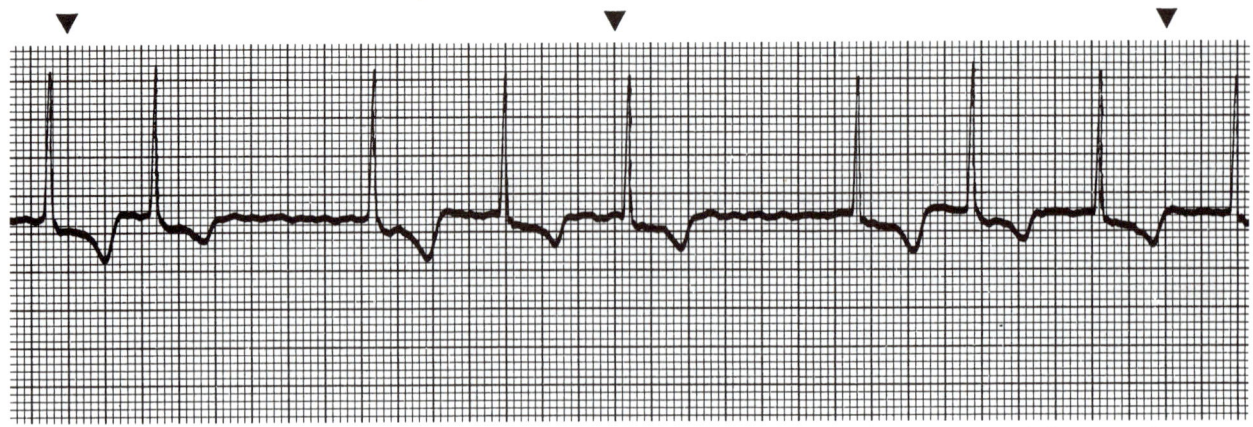

Figure 6-1. Atrial fibrillation.

Section 3: Electrocardiogram Identifying Features

Unlike in other ACLS protocols, such as ventricular fibrillation or asystole, no *specific* arrhythmia typifies a stroke. Certain rhythms may, however, do the following:

- Cause a stroke (Fig. 6-1) (atrial fibrillation predisposes to blood clot formation in the atria, because of sluggish blood flow there; these clots may then embolize to the brain and cause stroke)
- Contain electrocardiogram (ECG) changes that may indicate a concurrent myocardial infarction (MI), which may precipitate a cardiac embolic stroke
- Arise as a consequence of stroke; for example, bradycardia may indicate hypoxia or elevated intracranial pressure (ICP), and ECG changes may occur as a result of a stroke, particularly a hemorrhagic stroke, including prolongation of the Q-T interval, alterations in the P, T, and U waves, and ST segment depression or elevation, which can mimic acute MI

Section 4: Assessment

Primary Survey

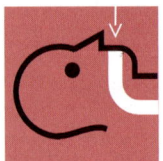

AIRWAY

The patient's level of consciousness can be anywhere between fully alert and completely unresponsive. Watch for airway compromise because the possibility of dysphagia (impaired swallowing), accumulation of saliva, tongue lacerations from seizure activity, and vomiting is increased. Suction as necessary. Use caution in repositioning the neck until cervical trauma can be excluded. If there is no evidence of trauma, consider placing the victim in the coma position. Serial airway checks *throughout the entire treatment phase* are essential.

Use caution when deciding to place an oropharyngeal airway (OPA) because gagging can increase ICP.

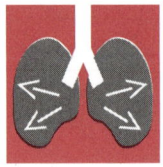

BREATHING

Abnormalities usually are seen only in large hemispheric or brain-stem strokes. Assist respirations with a bag-valve-mask device with 100% oxygen, but this rarely is required in the initial phase of a stroke.

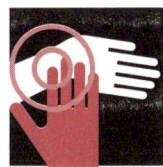

CIRCULATION

Absence of a pulse is uncommon; however, alterations in the vital signs, such as mild hypertension, are not. Serial checks are important.

DEFIBRILLATION

Because the patient is not in ventricular fibrillation, defibrillation is not an option.

Secondary Survey

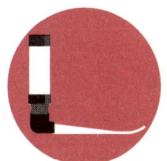

ADVANCED AIRWAY

Intubate only if it becomes necessary because stimulation of the gag reflex increases ICP. Prophylactic oxygen administration usually is not helpful unless desaturation is present, in which case, oxygen titrated to the patient's needs is administered. Use caution in manipulating the neck until cervical trauma can be excluded.

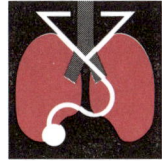

BEWARE BLINDERS

Beware blinders is designed to discourage clinicians from treating the patient with blind, or unthinking, protocols, forgetting to perform a brief history and physical examination, and "treating" the ECG monitor while ignoring the patient. During an emergency, it is easy to narrow your field of diagnostic vision to only gross abnormalities involving the airway, breathing, and circulation. Although commendable in the lay public, lack of critical thinking in a health professional can result in disaster.

Previously, stroke patients were lumped together under a generic "altered mental status" protocol. All patients presenting with a depressed level of consciousness were given naloxone (Narcan) and 50% dextrose to rule out the possibility of narcotic involvement and hypoglycemia. Although naloxone does not have a neurologic impact, 50% dextrose is hypertonic and may result in an increased ICP. Emergency protocols have their place but should not be followed blindly. Although the naloxone and 50% dextrose protocol should be *considered* in all patients with altered mental status, the possibility of a stroke *must* be considered *before* employing any generic response in anyone who has a sudden onset of focal neurologic deficits or alteration in consciousness.

Early recognition of the signs and symptoms of stroke during the secondary survey is paramount to providing early treatment. In addition to the normal mini-thorax and history and physical examination, a mini-neurologic examination should be done if the primary and secondary assessment yield *any sudden onset of focal neurologic deficits or alteration in consciousness*. The focused history can reveal a great deal concerning the possibility of a stroke.

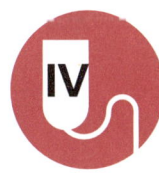

CHOICE CIRCULATION

Serial monitoring of vital signs is important because changes are common. Hypertension is common in stroke patients, whereas hypotension is uncommon. If hypotension is noted, search elsewhere for the cause. Prophylactic treatment is discouraged for modest hypertension (i.e., systolic less than 220 mmHg and/or diastolic less than 120 \mmHg or a mean arterial pressure less than 130 mmHg). See hypertension treatment in the Lecture section for a more expanded view of this subject. Monitor cardiac rhythm for clues to the cause of the stroke, such as recent MI or atrial fibrillation.

Start a peripheral intravenous access because central lines are contraindicated if patient is a candidate for thrombolytic therapy. Glucose-containing solutions are discouraged unless hypoglycemia is documented. Use isotonic solutions because hypotonic fluids may increase ICP. Unless concurrent hypovolemia is present, restrict the fluid rate to KVO (keep vein open).

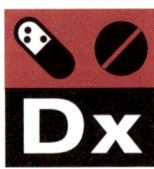

DRUGS AND DIAGNOSIS

The major goals of the secondary survey are to identify a stroke victim rapidly, treat the patient as necessary to ensure viability en route, and notify the receiving hospital promptly. Time is critical. These patients cannot be treated adequately in the field. They require diagnostic tests and treatments that are available only at a hospital, and a quick transport optimizes their chances for a good outcome.

On arrival at the hospital, a more detailed assessment and evaluation can take place. Few nonvascular disease processes cause sudden focal brain dysfunction. This allows the clinician a slight headstart in the diagnostic process, but, caution should be stressed. Hypoglycemia can cause focal neurologic deficits that appear identical to stroke. In addition, metabolic disorders, such as ketoacidosis, hypoglycemia, hyponatremia, drug overdose, hypertensive crises, and seizure disorders, can result in depressed levels of consciousness. Migraines can mimic the signs and symptoms of subarachnoid hemorrhage (SAH) and occasionally cause focal neurologic deficits.

Section 5: Lecture

This case study deals with patients who have suffered a cerebrovascular accident (CVA), more commonly known as a stroke or "brain attack." Stroke is the third leading cause of death in the United States. More than 500,000 people suffer strokes each year, with a 25% mortality rate.

Treatment of strokes has changed drastically within the past decade. Previously viewed as a nonemergent condition, it was generally accepted that the damage was done and nothing specific could reverse it. Urgency was not crucial, and thus emergency assessment, transportation, and management were given low priorities. Supportive care was administered with the expectation that damage to the brain would be self-limiting. The patient either deteriorated, stabilized, or improved on his or her own.

Now, however, there are potential interventions, such as thrombolytic therapy. In the near future, neuroprotective agents are expected to restore or help retain cerebral viability in some classes of strokes, but they must be administered soon after the onset of the stroke.

Thus, priorities have changed. Early recognition of stroke signs and symptoms by the public, prompt emergency medical services (EMS) transport, and aggressive evaluation and management by the medical team are necessary to decrease the morbidity and mortality of stroke.

Stroke Classification

A stroke is the interruption of blood flow to a portion of the brain, resulting in some degree of neurologic impairment. Strokes are usually classified according to their cause:

- Acute ischemic stroke
- Hemorrhagic stroke

Although both classes can be life threatening, their mortality and morbidity rates differ significantly. Acute ischemic stroke is rarely fatal in the first hour after onset, whereas hemorrhagic stroke may be fatal immediately. Making the distinction between the two is significant because treatment of one can be detrimental to the other.

ACUTE ISCHEMIC STROKE

Acute ischemic stroke involves an interruption of blood flow to the brain. Because about 75% of all strokes are ischemic, the most common cause of stroke is the formation of a blood clot. If the clot formed at the site, it is known as a *cerebral thrombus*. If the clot formed elsewhere and migrates to the location, it is referred to as a *cerebral embolus*. An occlusion of a cerebral artery by either a thrombus or embolus results in an ischemic stroke (Fig. 6-2).

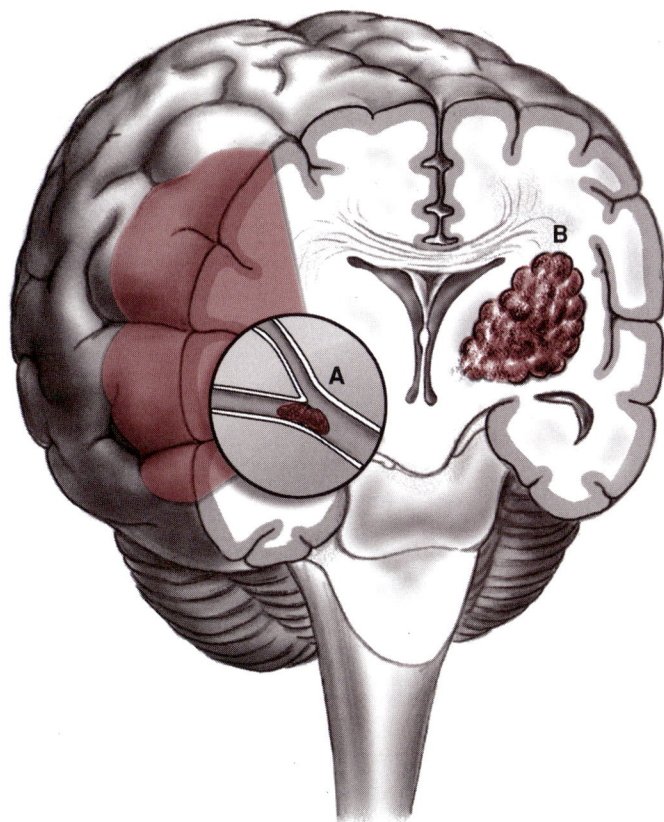

Figure 6-2. The two types of stroke.

HEMORRHAGIC STROKE

The second form of stroke, hemorrhagic stroke, results from leakage of blood from an artery or vein into the substance or onto the surface of the brain. There may be no distinctive early lateralizing signs with this type of stroke because the blood may distribute evenly in the subarachnoid space or in the ventricles of the brain. This type of stroke, which involves "bleeding," is categorized as one of two types of hemorrhage.

Subarachnoid Hemorrhage. An arterial bleed across the surface of the brain but below the arachnoid membrane (which closely follows the surface of the brain) is known as an SAH. Ninety-five percent of cases of SAH are due to a burst or leaking aneurysm; the remaining 5% generally are caused by a leaking arteriovenous malformation.

Intracerebral Hemorrhage. An arterial bleed directly into the tissue of the brain—the parenchyma—results in an ICH. The most common etiology of ICH is hypertension. In the elderly, however, the presence of amyloid in arteriole walls (amyloid angiopathy), which makes the walls more susceptible to hemorrhage, is considered a significant cause of ICH (see Fig. 6-2).

Risk Factors for Stroke

Heightening public awareness in preventing strokes is equally as important as providing the appropriate treatment. The National Heart Attack Alert Program has been successful in educating the public in cardiac risk factors, signs and symptoms, and awareness of early care. The same concept should be applied here. Although some strokes occur without warning and without modifiable risk factors, most are the end result of detrimental behaviors, including cigarette smoking, untreated high blood pressure, and elevated cholesterol levels.

Table 6-2.
Factors That Increase a Patient's Risk for Stroke

Modifiable	Unmodifiable
• Hypertension • Cigarette smoking • Transient ischemic attacks • Heart disease • Diabetes mellitus • Hypercoagulopathy • High red blood cell count (erythrocytosis) • Sickle cell anemia • Carotid bruit	• Age • Gender • Race • Prior stroke • Heredity

Table 6-2 lists factors that are known to increase the risk for suffering a stroke. Some are modifiable, but others are not. Public awareness of the warning signs of stroke (i.e., TIAs or warning bleeds) may help to decrease the incidence of strokes, but people also must be motivated to modify those behaviors that increase their risk of stroke.

Examination of the Stroke Patient

The physical examination must be conducted with a proficient knowledge of the signs and symptoms of stroke. There is no way to assess a patient if you have no idea what is an abnormal sign or symptom.

COMMON SIGNS AND SYMPTOMS OF STROKE

The following focal neurologic signs and symptoms are suggestive of an ischemic stroke. Although signs and symptoms of ischemic and hemorrhagic stroke overlap, hemorrhagic stroke patients usually appear more obtunded. Their signs and symptoms also may reflect other features attributable to rapidly increasing ICP, such as severe headache, nausea, and vomiting. Hemorrhagic and ischemic strokes often cause dysfunction of specific brain territories, with resultant impairment of language, motor, sensory, vision, and coordination functions.

It is not crucial to memorize which symptom reflects which territory or even the correct category of stroke. It is critical, however, to recognize that any of the symptoms listed subsequently could indicate a stroke. A mini-neurologic examination should be performed in a patient presenting with any of these signs or symptoms so that you can gather the necessary information and quickly decide whether to initiate a "brain attack" protocol. Remember, recognition is more important than symptom memorization.

Acute Ischemic Stroke
Ischemic strokes are delineated according to the area involved and the attending blood supply. If the stroke involves either the carotid artery or its general location, it is referred to as an *anterior* or *carotid territory stroke* (Fig. 6-3). Areas affected are supplied by the carotid arteries—the cerebral hemispheres. Damage to the cerebral hemispheres often results in contralateral weakness and sensory impairment. Involvement of the left hemisphere commonly results in dysphasia.

Carotid Circulation (anterior territory, outlined in red in Fig. 6-3)
- *Unilateral paralysis:* contralateral findings to the involved artery include weakness or awkwardness of one or more limbs
- *Numbness:* contralateral findings to the involved artery include sensory loss or disturbance, such as a tingling sensation in one or both limbs
- *Language disturbance:* aphasia—difficulty speaking to or understanding others; and dysarthria—slurred speech

Chapter 6 Acute Stroke: Acute Ischemic Stroke and Hemorrhagic Stroke

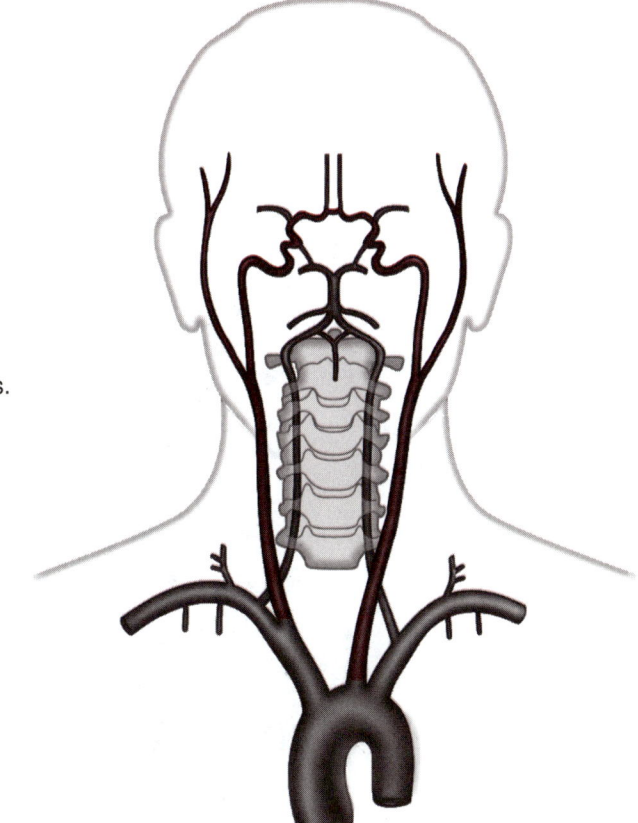

Figure 6-3. Carotid pathways.

- *Visual disturbance:* involvement of the right carotid artery can cause impaired vision on the left side of both eyes or in the right eye alone (see previous discussion of amaurosis fugax)

However, if the area involved is supplied by the vertebrobasilar artery, it is known as a *posterior* or *vertebrobasilar territory stroke* and affects the brain supplied by this artery (Fig. 6-4). The brain stem is supplied by this system and, among other functions, coordinates balance and controls eye movements. In addition, the occipital lobes are supplied by the vertebrobasilar artery and are responsible for interpreting visual input from the eyes; thus, impairment of vision in one side of both eyes is relatively common.

Vertebrobasilar Circulation (posterior territory, outlined in red in Fig. 6-4)
- *Vertigo:* spinning sensation (interpretation of this symptom alone requires caution because it is a common finding in noncerebrovascular situations)
- *Visual disturbance:* often involves same-side visual fields in both eyes
- *Diplopia:* double vision because of brain-stem involvement, where control of eye movements takes place
- *Paralysis:* weakness or awkwardness of one or more limbs; usually involves half of the body contralateral to the involved artery; rarely involves all four limbs
- *Numbness:* altered sensation in one or more limbs; could involve all four limbs or just half of the body; occurs in tandem with motor manifestations
- *Dysarthria:* slurred speech
- *Ataxia:* unilateral or bilateral difficulties with coordination, often involving gait

Hemorrhagic Stroke

Subarachnoid Hemorrhage
- *Severe headache:* This is the most common symptom of SAH. The headache is almost always so severe that the patient is compelled to seek medical intervention. The patient often states

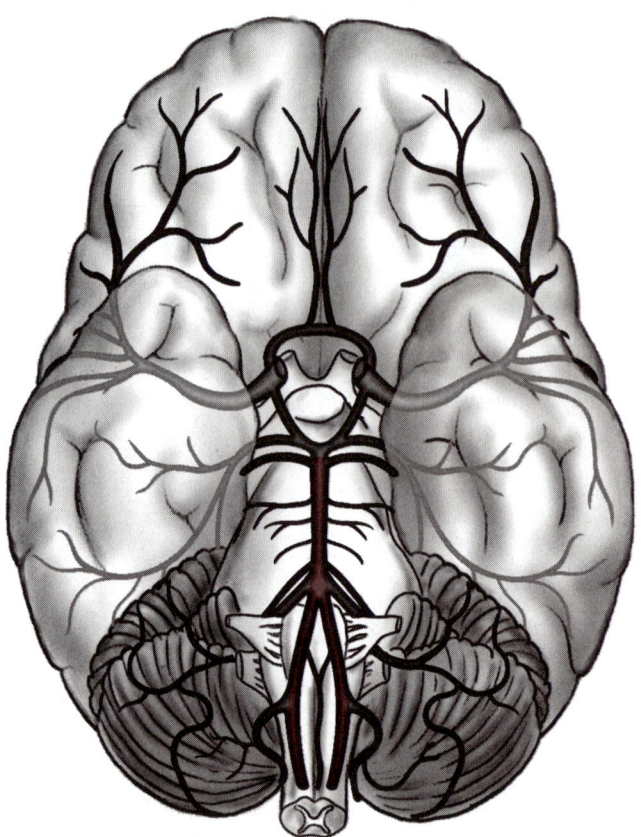

Figure 6-4. Anterior and posterior pathways.

that it is the worst headache of his or her life, and it is often described as a "thunderclap" headache because of the sudden, severe nature of the pain. It is occasionally precipitated by exertion. Unfortunately, some SAH patients present with an excruciating headache with no other prominent neurologic deficits, making it easy to confuse with a migraine headache. Thus, the diagnosis of SAH should be considered in any patient who presents with "the worst headache of my life."
- *Nausea*
- *Vomiting*
- *Neck pain:* The patient should be manipulated with caution until cervical trauma is excluded.
- *Altered mental status:* Loss of consciousness with headache should always bring to mind the possibility of SAH.

Intracerebral Hemorrhage
- *Similar to focal neurologic signs and symptoms of acute ischemic stroke:* Because the arterial bleed within the parenchyma or substance of the brain swiftly increases the ICP, however, the signs and symptoms reflect this increased pressure, with a greater tendency for nausea, vomiting, depressed level of consciousness, and headache.

During the secondary assessment, if the physical examination discloses that focal neurologic deficits exist or that the patient experienced a sudden onset of unconsciousness, an appropriate neurologic examination should be performed without delay. Depending on your emergency training, however, the examination can range from cursory to extremely detailed.

WARNING SIGNS OF STROKE

There can be warning signs in both categories of strokes—acute ischemic stroke and hemorrhagic stroke. Some may be obvious and others quite subtle.

Warning Signs of Acute Ischemic Stroke

Transient Ischemic Attack. A principal warning sign of an ischemic stroke is a transient ischemic attack (TIA). As in all ischemic strokes, occlusion of a cerebral artery takes place, but the clot dissolves or breaks up into clinically insignificant microemboli within 1 to 24 hours. A TIA has all of the signs and symptoms of either a posterior or anterior territory ischemic stroke, but the patient regains complete neurologic function relatively quickly. Depending on when the patient presents for medical assistance, a diagnosis of TIA may be based entirely on history. A TIA is an important prognostic clue to foretelling future occlusions because 5% of TIA patients demonstrate another "occlusion" within the next month; the chance of having another ischemic episode increases 5% each year thereafter. Patients should be counseled concerning their risk factors because reduction of modifiable risk factors can reduce the chances of having another stroke.

Amaurosis Fugax. Transient loss of vision in one eye may be caused by decreased blood flow through the retinal artery, which is a branch of the internal carotid artery (ICA). A tight stenosis in the ICA may result in poor blood flow through the retinal artery. When this happens, the eye may transiently lose adequate blood flow, resulting in temporarily diminished vision in one eye. This phenomenon is called *amaurosis fugax* and is considered a risk factor for an acute ischemic stroke. Patients with this symptom should be evaluated for a tight stenosis in the ICA on the same side in which the diminished vision occurs.

Warning Signs of Hemorrhagic Stroke

Subarachnoid Hemorrhage. SAH involves bleeding into the space on the surface of the brain, just beneath the arachnoid membrane. Bleeding in this area usually is from an aneurysm. A warning or "sentinel" bleed may herald a more severe SAH from an intracerebral aneurysm. This situation, which occurs in about one fourth of cases of SAH, has all of the signs and symptoms of an SAH but often has a more moderate presentation. Signs include severe headache of sudden onset and stiff neck (also called *nuchal rigidity*). Because symptoms may not include loss of consciousness or focal neurologic deficit, they may be missed by medical professionals. Left undiagnosed, the chances are high that a more serious bleed will occur within 2 to 3 weeks.

Intracerebral Hemorrhage. Although a severe SAH may be preceded by a minor hemorrhage, this is virtually never the case with an intracerebral hemorrhage (ICH), which generally gives no warning signs.

The Stroke Chain

Hazinski has proposed a seven-step "stroke chain of survival and recovery." This is similar to the AHA's "chain of survival"; both include timely recognition, swift EMS response, rapid intervention and appraisal at the hospital, speedy diagnosis, and decisive care. Both chains also rely heavily on the following:

- Educating the general public
- Recognizing signs and symptoms
- Providing EMS access, intelligent dispatch, and trained prehospital professionals
- Educating receiving facility doctors and staff in cutting-edge evaluation and intervention techniques
- Formulating a generic response plan to merge all components into the receiving facility

Both chains have specific time components. In the cardiac chain, it was 30 to 60 minutes to receive definitive therapy from onset of infarction. For occlusive accident patients, thrombolytic therapy must be administered no later than 3 hours from time of onset of symptoms. Any delay past this point negates any benefit from treatment. Changing previously relaxed attitudes toward stroke is a major undertaking; however, education has to begin somewhere, and Hazinski's stroke chain is but the first step.

Hazinski's stroke chain steps, with the addition of Discharge, are as follows:

- Detection
- Dispatch
- Delivery
- Door
- Data
- Decision
- Drug
- Discharge

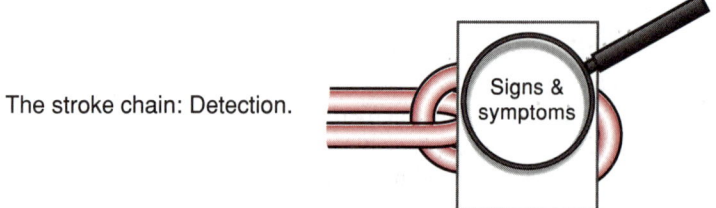

Figure 6-5. The stroke chain: Detection.

DETECTION: TIMELY IDENTIFICATION (FIG. 6-5)

Early recognition of the signs and symptoms of stroke is a multifaceted problem. Unlike trauma or chest pain, the signs and symptoms of stroke may be subtle. The patient may be asleep at the time when occlusion or rupture occurs. The patient may exhibit only moderate paralysis of a limb or speech impairment and may decide to wait and see if it improves before seeking help. As with chest pain victims, denial can be a factor. Therefore, public education in sign and symptom recognition must be a keystone in the stroke awareness program.

DISPATCH: TIMELY EMS INITIATION (FIG. 6-6)

Getting the patient to the hospital has its own difficulties. Family members often delay by calling their family doctor and transporting by family car; in fact, half of all stroke victims are transported to the hospital by family members. During an emergency, time appears to pass slowly, and family members think that they can get their loved one to the hospital faster than by waiting for an ambulance.

Education about strokes should be directed not only at the lay public but also at the entire EMS system. The public needs to be enlightened that EMS is not a waste of time. A telephone call to the EMS dispatcher can help a stroke victim immediately. After receiving more education on differentiating strokes from other emergencies, EMS dispatchers can deliver life-saving instructions on how to care for the stroke victim before the ambulance arrives. Dispatchers educated about strokes can inform the responding unit of what to expect while properly prioritizing the call.

DELIVERY: TRANSPORT AND INTERVENTION (FIG. 6-7)

In addition to the lay public and EMS dispatchers requiring training in the early recognition of strokes, prehospital personnel need to change their previously relaxed approaches to evaluation and intervention of stroke patients and learn to implement swift reaction mechanisms to a stroke emergency.

Detailed prehospital neurologic examinations are undesirable because they impede expeditious transport to a receiving facility; however, a quick neurologic assessment has been designed. Designated the Cincinnati Prehospital Stroke Scale, it rapidly identifies probable stroke victims based on evaluation of facial droop, arm drift, and speech irregularities (Table 6-3).

As in suspected myocardial infarctions, once identified, stroke victims must be transported expeditiously—time in the field must be minimized!

In addition to recognizing that a stroke has taken place, the time of onset must be determined and relayed to the receiving hospital. Early notification is paramount to preparing the receiving facility for mobilizing their resources so that the time taken to evaluate and intervene can be minimized.

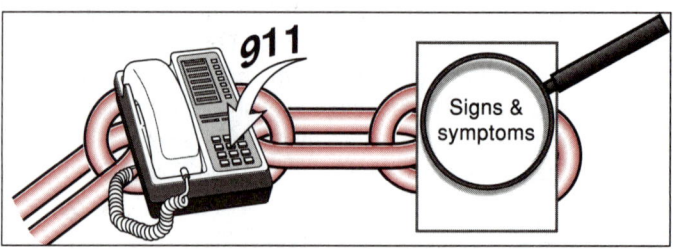

Figure 6-6. The stroke chain: Dispatch.

Chapter 6 Acute Stroke: Acute Ischemic Stroke and Hemorrhagic Stroke

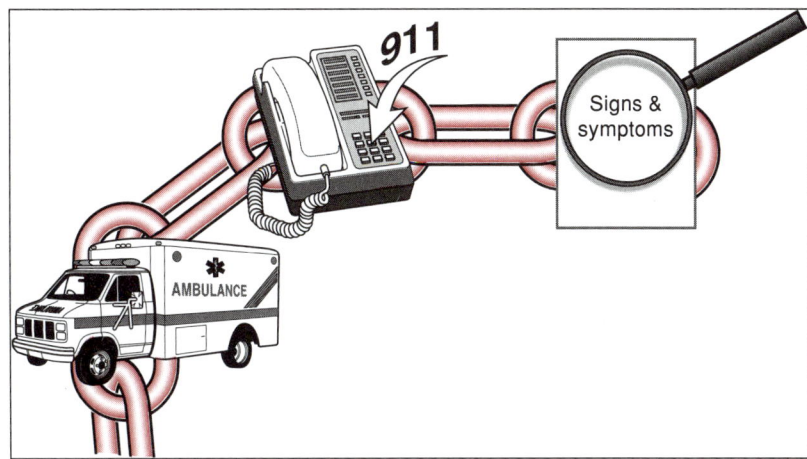

Figure 6-7. The stroke chain: Delivery.

DOOR: TRIAGE (FIG. 6-8)

Insisting that EMS personnel forewarn the hospital of incoming stroke emergencies can greatly increase the time allowed to mobilize stroke-oriented resources. Time is the crucial factor. In this vein, the National Institute of Neurological Disorders and Stroke (NINDS) has recommended the time intervals shown in Table 6-4 to stress the importance of timely evaluation and intervention on behalf of stroke patients.

DATA: EMERGENCY DEPARTMENT ASSESSMENT AND INTERVENTION (FIG. 6-9)

The clinical picture in a stroke victim may alter swiftly; therefore, emergency department staff should obtain an initial assessment and neurologic check on arrival and then perform serial vital signs and neurologic assessments on a regular basis to update the status of the patient. During the initial assessment, obtain the time of onset of symptoms from the patient if possible, the EMS personnel, and the family or bystanders. Establishing a "time zero" is a critical requirement for further intervention.

Emergency Neurologic Stroke Assessment

The detailed neurologic assessment should contain information on the following:

1. Level of consciousness
2. Likely category of stroke (ischemic or hemorrhagic)

Table 6-3.
The Cincinnati Prehospital Stroke Scale

The Cincinnati Prehospital Stroke Scale

Facial Droop (have patient show teeth or smile):
- Normal—both sides of face move equally well
- Abnormal—one side of face does not move as well as the other side

Arm Drift (patient closes eyes and holds both arms out):
- Normal—both arms move the same *or* both arms do not move at all (other findings, such as pronator drift, may be helpful)
- Abnormal—one arm does not move *or* one arm drifts down compared with the other

Speech (have the patient say "you can't teach an old dog new tricks":
- Normal—patient uses correct words with no slurring
- Abnormal—patient slurs words, uses inappropriate words, *or* is unable to speak

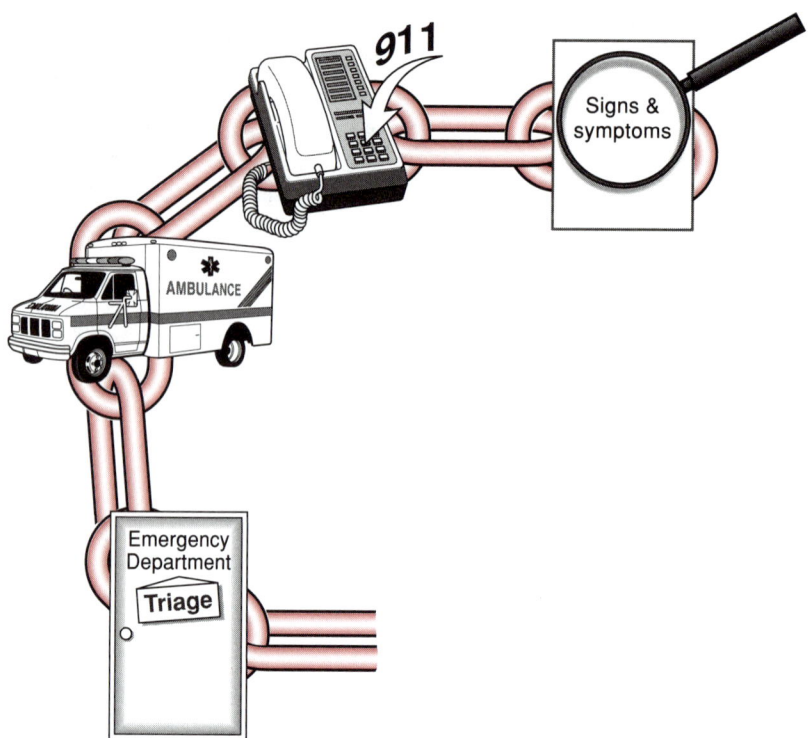

Figure 6-8. The stroke chain: Door.

3. Likely territory involvement (anterior or posterior)
4. Severity of stroke

Level of Consciousness. Ascertaining the ranges of the level of consciousness from onset until arrival is extremely important because the lower the level of consciousness, the less control the patient has over his or her airway. Level of consciousness also can be helpful in differentiating between categories of stroke. A deteriorating or sudden loss of consciousness after the onset of stroke symptoms implies a hemorrhagic origin rather than an occlusive one. Use caution, however, when only assigning one conclusion to an altered level of consciousness. Depressed levels of consciousness may be the result of concurrent drug overdose, hypoglycemia, or other factors.

Table 6-4.
NINDS-Recommended Stroke Evaluation Targets for Potential Thrombolytic Candidates*

Evaluation	Time Target
Door to doctor	10 min
Door to CT completion	25 min
Door to CT read	45 min
Door to treatment	60 min
Access to neurologic expertise†	15 min
Access to neurosurgical expertise†	2 h
Admit to monitored bed	3 h

* Target times will not be achieved in all cases, but they represent a reasonable goal.
† By phone or in person.
CT, computed tomography.

Chapter 6 *Acute Stroke: Acute Ischemic Stroke and Hemorrhagic Stroke* **161**

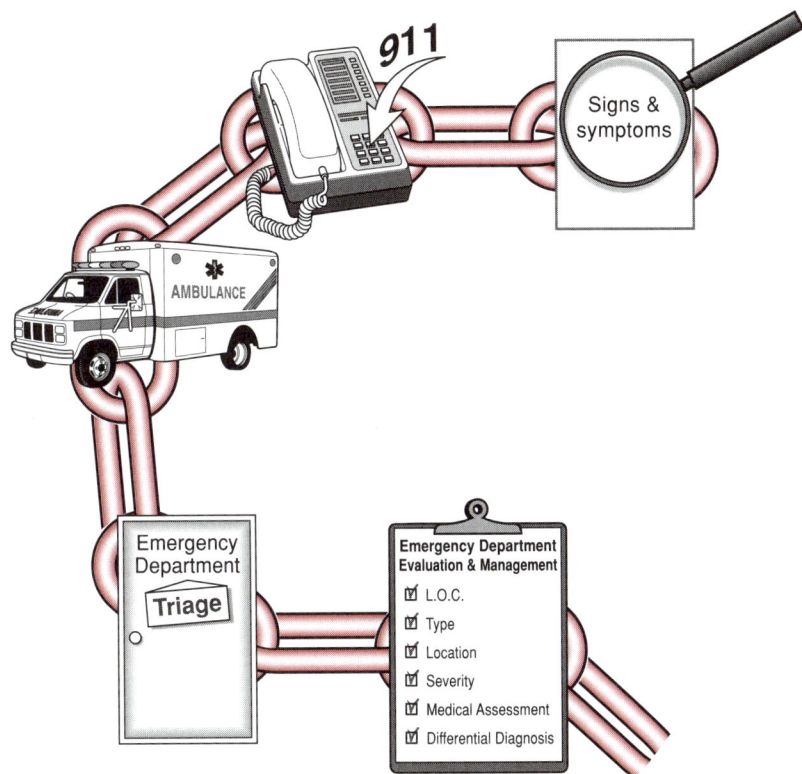

Figure 6-9. The stroke chain: Data.

Documentation and standardization of level of consciousness can be assessed with the Glasgow Coma Scale (Table 6-5). Other evaluative tests to assess neurologic function are shown in Table 6-6.

Likely Category of Stroke (Ischemic or Hemorrhagic). It is neither necessary nor desirable to rely solely on the history and clinical signs and symptoms to form a diagnosis of occlusive versus hemorrhagic origin. The presentations can overlap, and the treatment of one is dangerous to the other.

The single definitive test for differentiating between the two types of stroke is a noncontrast computed tomography (CT) scan of the head. Contrast dye is not employed so that free blood is not confused with the dye seen on the scan. Because contrast dye impairs kidney function, and it is rare to have time to check kidney function before emergency CT scan, this potential problem is avoided. Free blood shows up on the CT scan as a hyperdense or white area. The scan is 95% accurate in ruling out an SAH, but if suspicion is strong, a lumbar puncture should be considered. Remember, however, that a lumbar puncture is a contraindication to the use of thrombolytics in ischemic stroke patients.

Likely Territory Involvement (Anterior or Posterior). In conscious and alert patients, the territory involved (carotid or vertebrobasilar) may be assessed with various neurologic tests (discussed previously). In the first few hours after onset of symptoms, however, the presentations may overlap, and it may be difficult to differentiate between the two territories.

Severity of Stroke. The National Institutes of Health Stroke Scale is detailed in the AHA ACLS text (see Chap. 10, pp. 10-21 to 10-24). This tool was designed to provide a mechanism to correlate stroke severity with long-term outcome. It also can be used to guide thrombolytic therapy. If a patient's score continues to improve, the disadvantages associated with thrombolytic therapy may outweigh the benefits.

The Stroke Scale can be performed reasonably quickly, allowing serial checks. It is not an all-inclusive neurologic test, so other tests should be employed and regularly documented. The scores range from 0 (normal) to 42, highlighting level of consciousness, visual evaluation, motor function, sensation and neglect, and cerebellar function.

Emergency Diagnostic Studies Although this subject is well beyond the scope of this book, Table 6-7 shows the major diagnostic tools or tests used to assist the clinician in arriving at a diagnosis.

Table 6-5.
Glasgow Coma Scale

Patient Response	Score*
Eye Opening	
• Spontaneous	4
• In response to speech	3
• In response to pain	2
• None	1
Best Verbal Response	
• Oriented conversation	5
• Confused conversation	4
• Inappropriate words	3
• Incomprehensible sounds	2
• None	1
Best Motor Response	
• Obeys	6
• Localizes	5
• Withdraws	4
• Abnormal flexion	3
• Abnormal extension	2
• None	1

* Scores range from 15 to 3. Stroke patients with scores of 8 or less have a poor prognosis.

Table 6-6.
Various Tests to Assess Neurologic Function

Test	Assessment
Pupillary size, equality, and reactivity	• Fixed, dilated pupil in an alert patient with headache implies a ruptured aneurysm. • Unilateral dilation in a comatose patient suggests transtentorial herniation (also called *uncal herniation*).
Eye position at rest and after doll's eyes maneuver	• The eyes may look or "point" toward the side of the lesion in a hemispheric stroke (but often to the opposite side in a brain-stem stroke). • After cervical spine trauma is ruled out, rotate the head. With normal brain stem function, the eyes "stay behind" as the head is rotated; that is, they move conjugately in the direction opposite from the direction that the head is moved, then slowly rotate back to midline (positive doll's eyes reflex). If they stay at midline as the head is moved, this indicates brain-stem dysfunction (negative doll's eyes reflex).
Corneal reflex	• Absence of reflex suggests brain-stem dysfunction.
Gag reflex	• Absence of reflex suggests brain-stem dysfunction.
Respiratory pattern	• Irregular breathing patterns may occur with brain-stem dysfunction, such as: Cheyne-Stokes respirations, central neurogenic hyperventilation, or ataxic respirations.

Table 6-7.
Diagnostic Tests for Investigating the Possibility of Stroke

Test	Investigation
Computed tomography (CT scan)	• Procedure of choice for emergent evaluation
Magnetic resonance imaging (MRI)	• Not primary tool for stroke detection because of length of time for procedure • May be the procedure of choice in the future, if diffusion-weighted MRI proves useful in assessing cerebral blood flow emergently
Electrocardiogram (ECG)	• Although increased intracranial pressure can cause some ECG changes, this procedure helps exclude the 5% of patients who have a concurrent myocardial infarction
Serum electrolytes	• Exclude other possible diagnoses
Radiographs (skull, lateral cervical spine x-rays)	• Exclude trauma when necessary
Glucose test	• Exclude glucose abnormalities, particularly hypoglycemia, which can mimic stroke
Arterial blood gases	• When necessary to evaluate oxygen saturation if pulse oximetry is questionable
Other laboratory investigations	• Coagulation studies are mandatory in all candidates for thrombolytic therapy • Exclude sickle cell disease • Exclude protein S deficiency and other hypercoagulatable conditions • Exclude drug or alcohol-related causes of altered awareness

Differential Diagnosis of Stroke
- Hemorrhagic versus ischemic origin
- Cerebral or cervical trauma, or both
- Blood glucose abnormalities (primarily hypoglycemia)
- Meningitis or encephalitis (rarely may mimic SAH)
- Hypertensive crisis (diastolic pressure greater than 120 mmHg)
- Expanding intracranial mass (tumor, subdural or epidural hematoma)
- Seizure disorders
- Migraine
- Drug overdose (should not cause focal neurologic deficits)
- Cerebral ischemia secondary to cardiac arrest)

Elevated glucose levels may be a common reaction to a stroke. Treat only if levels become inordinately elevated.

Consider empiric administration of 100 mg of thiamine (intramuscularly or intravenously) if the patient is cachectic or presents with a history of malnourishment or alcoholism to avoid worsening a possible Wernicke's encephalopathy (caused by thiamine deficiency).

Avoid placement of an indwelling catheter, if possible.

Fever increases oxygen demand, and use of antipyretics is encouraged within the hospital setting while the cause of fever is being determined.

DECISION: STROKE TREATMENT STRATEGIES (FIG. 6-10)

Blood Pressure Management. Treatment of blood pressure after cerebral occlusion or hemorrhage is controversial. Different theories abound concerning the minimal level at which blood pressure should be treated. Because antihypertensives lower the blood pressure, they may compromise marginally perfused cerebral tissue. Compounding the problem are consequences related to thrombolytic therapy candidacy and category of stroke. It is important to keep cerebral perfusion high in ischemic stroke patients, whereas a high pressure in a hemorrhagic stroke patient could increase the rate of bleeding. The AHA recommends

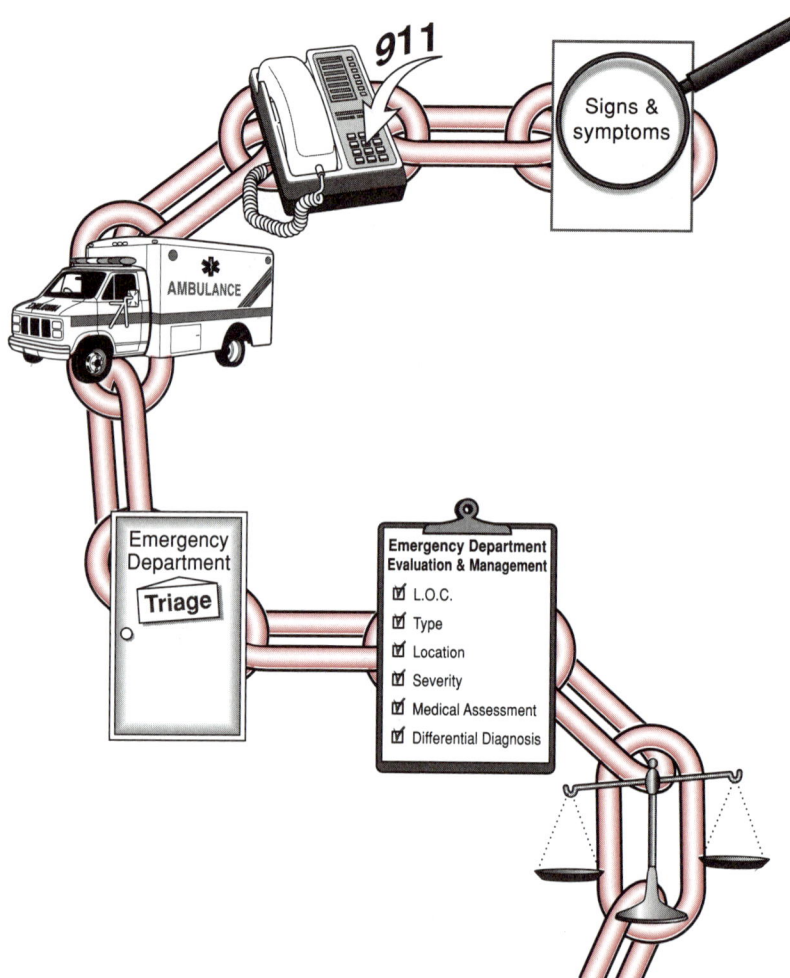

Figure 6-10. The stroke chain: Decision.

the management scheme shown in Table 6-8. Remember, think conservatively when intervention appears necessary.

Seizure Management. Relatively uncommon but potentially life threatening, seizures can be a complication of stroke. They are considered life threatening because loss of airway, cessation of respirations, heat and waste generation from seizing muscles, and an increase in metabolic activity occur all at once and have a negative impact on the ICP.

If immediate help is needed with seizure control (e.g, if two or more seizures occur in close proximity), consider either diazepam (Valium), 5 to 10 mg administered over 2 minutes, or lorazepam (Ativan), 1 to 4 mg administered over 2 to 20 minutes. Both may be used for immediate control of seizures but should be followed by a longer-acting agent. For a single seizure, many neurologists prefer loading with a longer-acting agent, avoiding the shorter-acting agents because they often cause drowsiness, hampering further evaluation of the patient.

When longer-acting agents are used, the following are considered:

- Phenytoin (Dilantin) administered at a loading dose of 20 mg/kg at a rate not to exceed 50 mg/min
- Fosphenytoin (Cerebyx) administered at a loading dose of 20 mg/kg at a rate not to exceed 150 mg/min, followed by a maintenance dose of 100 mg of fosphenytoin or phenytoin every 8 hours
- Phenobarbital administered at an adult loading dose of 1000 mg or 20 mg/kg, followed by 30 to 60 mg every 6 to 8 hours. This is not considered the drug of choice because it has a much greater sedative effect than phenytoin.

Table 6-8.
Emergency Antihypertensive Therapy

Blood Pressure*	Treatment
Acute Ischemic stroke	
Nonthrombolytic candidates	
1. DBP >140 mmHg	Sodium nitroprusside (0.5 µg/kg/min); aim for 10% to 20% reduction in DBP
2. SBP >220, DBP >120, or MAP† >130 mmHg	10–20 mg labetalol‡ IV push over 1 to 2 minutes; may repeat or double labetalol‡ every 20 minutes to a maximum dose of 150 mg
3. SBP <220, DBP >120, or MAP† >130 mmHg	Emergency antihypertensive therapy is deferred in the absence of aortic dissection, acute myocardial infarction, severe congestive heart failure, or hypertensive encephalopathy
Thrombolytic candidates	
1. Pretreatment SBP >185 or DBP >110 mmHg	1–2 inches of nitropaste or 1–2 doses of 10 to 20 mg labetalol‡ IV push. If BP is not reduced and maintained to <185/110 mmHg the patient should not be treated with tPA.
During and after treatment	
1. Monitor BP	BP is monitored every 15 minutes for 2 hours, then every 30 minutes for 6 hours, and then every 1 hour for 16 hours.
2. DBP >140 mmHg	Sodium nitroprusside (0.5 µg/kg/min).
3. SBP >230 or DBP 121–140 mmHg	(1) 10 mg labetalol‡ IV push over 1–2 minutes; may repeat or double labetalol‡ every 10 minutes to a maximum dose of 150 mg or give the initial bolus labetalol and then start a drip at 2–8 mg/min (2) If BP is not controlled by labetalol consider sodium nitroprusside.
4. SBP 180–230 or DBP 105–120 mmHg	10 mg labetalol‡ IV push; may repeat or double labetalol‡ every 10–20 minutes to a maximum dose of 150 mg or give initial labetalol bolus and then start a labetalol drip at 2–8 mg/min
Hemorrhagic Stroke	
1. SBP >230 or DBP >120 mmHg	Sodium nitroprusside (0.5–10 µg/kg/min) *or* nitroglycerin drip (at 10–20 µg/min).
2. SBP >180 or DBP >105 mmHg	Consider 10 mg labetalol‡ IV push; may repeat or double labetalol‡ every 10–20 minutes to a maximum dose of 300 mg. *or* give initial labetalol‡ bolus and then start a labetalol drip at 2–8 mg/min
3. For hypertension relative to pre-stroke condition	If prehemorrhage BP is estimated to have been considerably lower (e.g., 120/80 mmHg), then antihypertensive therapy may be appropriate to approximate premorbid pressures, particularly in the first hours after subarachnoid hemorrhage.

* All initial blood pressures should be verified before treatment by repeating reading in 5 minutes.

† As estimated by one third the sum of systolic and double diastolic pressure.

‡ Labetalol (Normodyne, Trandate) should be avoided in patients with asthma, cardiac failure, or severe abnormalities in cardiac conduction. For refractory hypertension, alternative therapy may be considered with sodium nitroprusside (Nipride) or enalapril (Vaseretic).

BP, blood pressure; DBP, diastolic blood pressure; MAP, mean arterial pressure; SBP, systolic blood pressure; tPA, tissue plasminogen activator.

Watch carefully for signs of respiratory depression during and after administration of all of the anticonvulsants.

Intracranial Pressure Management. An increase in intracranial pressure without a concurrent increase in blood pressure results in a decrease in cerebral blood flow. A minimum cerebral perfusion pressure of 60 mmHg must be maintained to achieve an adequate cerebral blood flow (this is calculated by subtracting ICP from mean arterial pressure). The following should be considered (a detailed explanation is beyond the scope of this book but can be found in Chapter 10 of the AHA ACLS text):

- The patient should be placed in a 30-degree, head-up position.
- Coughing, retching, and positive-pressure ventilation can increase ICP. Premedication with lidocaine, thiopental, or other nondepolarizing agents can reduce the increase in ICP associated with intubation and suctioning.
- Hyperventilation is a swift but short-term way to decrease ICP. Reducing the $Paco_2$ to 30 mmHg (acceptable) or 25 mmHg (marginal but acceptable for the short term) decreases the ICP. A measurable amount of ischemia is associated with the cerebral artery vasoconstriction that results, however, so the overall beneficial effects are unknown in this situation.
- Mannitol may be used as an osmotic tool to improve cerebral ischemia by diuresis, fluid shifting, and cerebral vasodilation.
- Diuretics, such as furosemide (Lasix) and acetazolamide may be employed.
- High doses of barbiturates may be used to suppress electrical brain activity and lower ICP.
- Neurosurgical decompression can be life-saving in patients with large hemorrhages, particularly those involving the cerebellum.

DRUGS: THROMBOLYTIC AGENTS FOR ISCHEMIC STROKE (FIG. 6-11)

On the basis of several studies, tissue plasminogen factor (t-PA) was approved by the Food and Drug Administration for treatment of ischemic stroke. Other agents, such as streptokinase and urokinase, were associated with excessive early mortality rates and therefore have not been approved.

All hospitals that choose to treat documented ischemic stroke victims with t-PA should have protocols that include the following:

- Education in stroke recognition and in the Cincinnati Stroke Scale for prehospital providers and EMS dispatchers
- Mandatory prenotification to hospital
- Development of a triage protocol and emergency department plan that include guidelines for evaluation, management, team makeup, and response
- Designation of how to obtain and who should read a noncontrast CT scan
- A thrombolytic protocol that includes the criteria for patient inclusion and exclusion, where the drug should be stored, who should mix and administer the drug, and how to manage possible bleeding complications

The following are the current recommendations for the use of thrombolytics in the presence of documented ischemic stroke:

- Give t-PA intravenously (0.9 mg/kg, maximum 90 mg), with 10% of the dose given as a bolus followed by an infusion lasting 60 minutes.
- Treatment must be initiated within 3 hours of onset; t-PA *cannot* be recommended for any greater length of time except in a research setting.
- When the time of onset cannot be set reliably (as in awakening), t-PA is not recommended.
- As in cardiac use, strict inclusion and exclusion criteria of thrombolytics must be met (Table 6-9).

Although commonly prescribed for acute ischemic strokes, heparin, aspirin, and ticlopidine have not been proved effective in this situation.

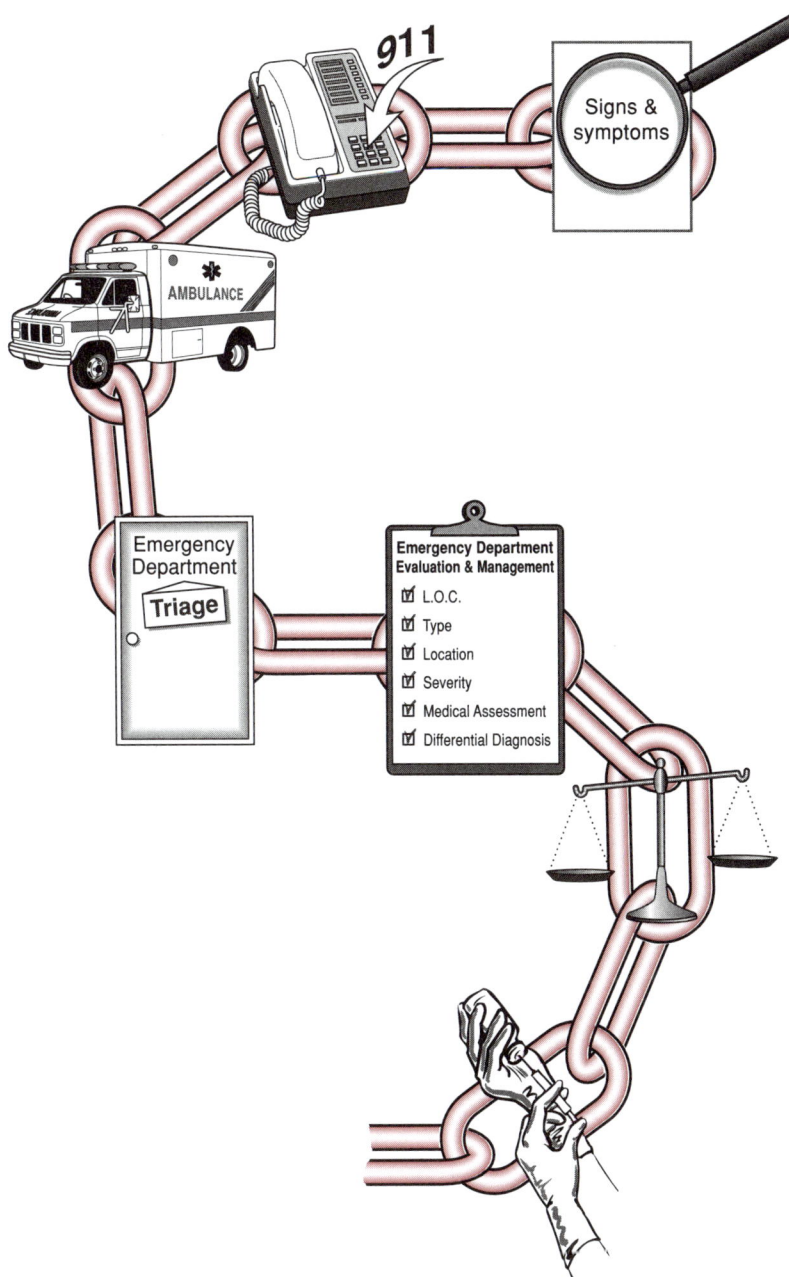

Figure 6-11. The stroke chain: Drug.

Table 6-9.
Thrombolytic Therapy Checklist for Ischemic Stroke

	YES	NO	
Inclusion Criteria			Age 18 years or older
			Clinical diagnosis of ischemic stroke causing a measurable neurologic deficit
			Time of symptom onset well established to be less than 180 minutes before treatment begins
Exclusion Criteria			Evidence of intracranial hemorrhage on noncontrast head computed tomography (CT) scan
			Only minor or rapidly improving stroke symptoms
			High clinical suspicion of subarachnoid hemorrhage even with normal CT scan
			Active internal bleeding (e.g., gastrointestinal bleeding or urinary bleeding within last 21 days)
			Known bleeding diathesis, including but not limited to: Platelet count <100,000/mm^3
			Patient has received heparin within 48 hours and had an elevated activated partial thromboplastin time (greater than upper limit of normal for laboratory)
			Recent use of anticoagulant (eg, warfarin sodium) and elevated prothrombin time >15 seconds
			Within 3 months of intracranial surgery, serious head trauma, or previous stroke
			Within 14 days of major surgery or serious trauma
			Recent arterial puncture within 7 days that was not easily compressible
			Lumbar puncture within 7 days
			History of intracranial hemorrhage, arteriovenous malformation, or aneurysm
			Witnessed seizure at stroke onset
			Recent acute myocardial infarction
			On repeated measurements, systolic pressure >185 mmHg or diastolic pressure >110 mmHg at time of treatment, requiring aggressive treatment to reduce blood pressure to within these limits

All of the YES boxes and all of the NO boxes must be checked before thrombolytic therapy can be given:

DISCHARGE: HOME AND REHABILITATION (FIG. 6-12)

In many circumstances, patients with TIAs and mild strokes may be discharged home within 24 hours and often need little help from rehabilitation professionals. Those with minor to moderate deficits that do not resolve completely after discharge benefit the most from involvement of occupational, physical, and speech therapists. The type and severity of neurologic deficits guide the use of these professionals. Rehabilitation does not help everyone with a stroke. Patients with profound neurologic deficits may receive little or no benefit from rehabilitation efforts. Therefore, stroke prevention should be emphasized both before and after a stroke. The public should be educated about modifiable risk factors and the need for early intervention should a stroke occur. In addition, part of every discharge plan of a stroke patient should include the risk factors and the need for early intervention.

Chapter 6 *Acute Stroke: Acute Ischemic Stroke and Hemorrhagic Stroke* **169**

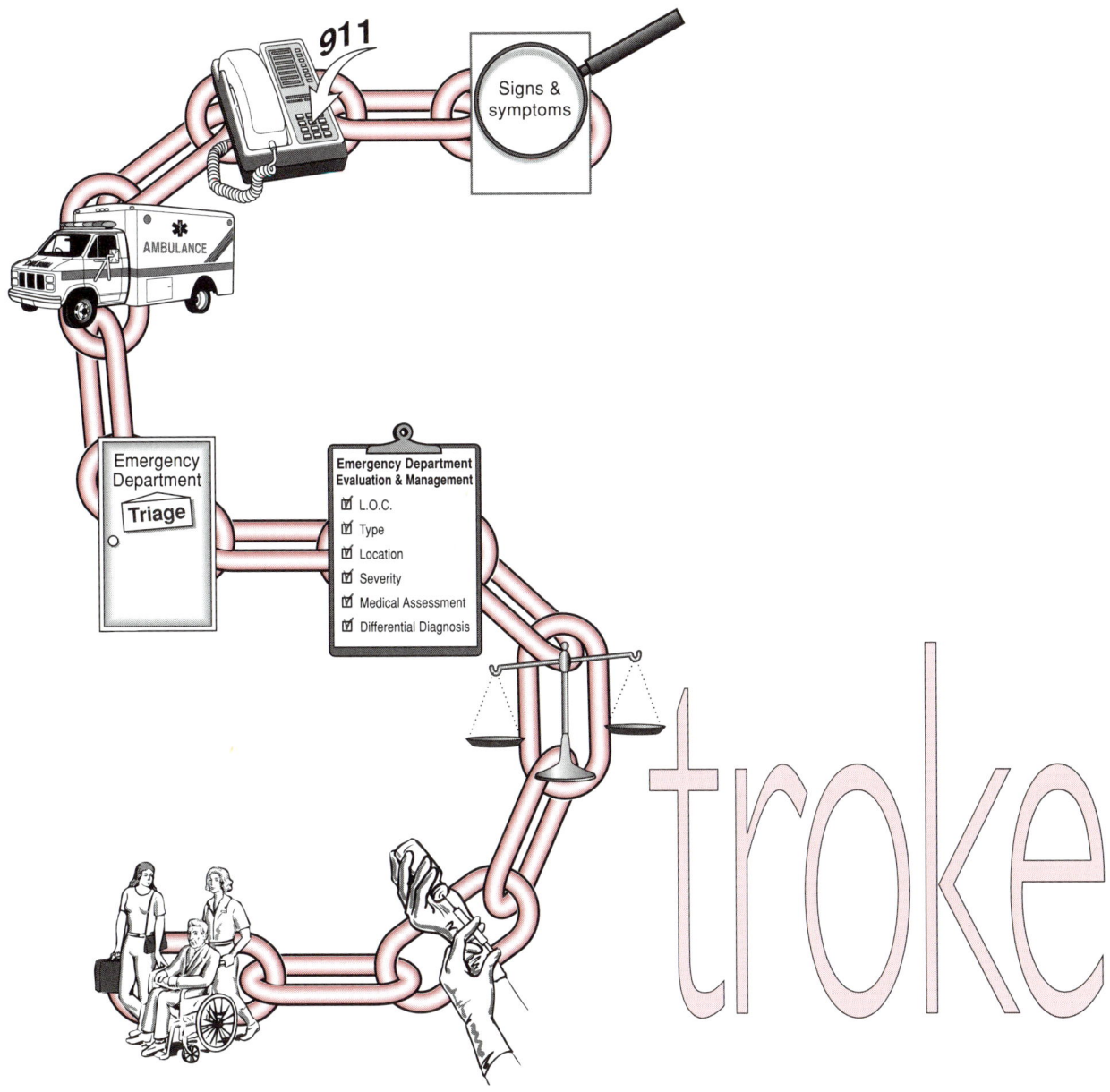

Figure 6-12. The stroke chain: Discharge.

Summary

The management of stroke has changed drastically in the past decade. With ongoing research from NINDS, the approval of t-PA by the Food and Drug Administration, and the involvement of the AHA's education division, stroke management is certain to change even more dramatically in the future.

Section 6: Stroke Interim Evaluation

Mark the correct answer. (*ACLS* text pp. 10-1 to 10-18)

1. Hypotension is a common sign in patients suffering from hemorrhagic stroke. _____
   _____ (a) True
   _____ (b) False

2. Which of the following are acceptable to administer to a stroke patient intravenously: (1) D-5-W; (2) normal saline; (3) Ringer's lactate; (4) 0.45 saline; (5) 0.9 saline? _____
   _____ (a) 3, 4, and 5
   _____ (b) 2, 3, and 5
   _____ (c) 1, 4, and 5
   _____ (d) 4

3. The signs and symptoms of migraine headaches most closely resemble the presentation of which form of stroke? _____
   _____ (a) TIA
   _____ (b) Subarachnoid hemorrhage
   _____ (c) Acute ischemic stroke
   _____ (d) ICH

4. If a suspected stroke patient is unconscious, intubation is always indicated. _____
   _____ (a) True
   _____ (b) False

5. AHA guidelines indicate that thrombolytics can be administered in all of the following situations *except*: _____
   _____ (a) Onset of symptoms began close to 150 minutes ago
   _____ (b) Reliable onset of symptom time established
   _____ (c) Patients older than 70 years
   _____ (d) Recent lumbar puncture

6. The primary difference between TIAs and an acute ischemic stroke is which of the following? _____
   _____ (a) Thrombolytics have a much greater success rate in correcting TIAs than acute ischemic strokes.
   _____ (b) A person usually has no less than three TIAs before having an acute ischemic stroke.
   _____ (c) During the first hour of onset, TIAs tend to have harsher symptoms than acute ischemic events.
   _____ (d) TIA signs and symptoms are virtually identical to those of an acute ischemic stroke but resolve quickly, within 24 hours.

7. Which of the following is a correct statement? _____
   _____ (a) Hemorrhagic stroke patients tend to deteriorate slower than ischemic stroke patients.
   _____ (b) Ischemic strokes tend to look more ill.
   _____ (c) Nausea and vomiting are more pronounced in ischemic strokes than in hemorrhagic strokes.
   _____ (d) Focal neurologic deficits are more common in ischemic strokes than in subarachnoid hemorrhages.

8. All of the following are common signs and symptoms in either ischemic or hemorrhagic stroke, *except*: _____
   _____ (a) Headache
   _____ (b) Focal weakness
   _____ (c) Aphasia
   _____ (d) Hypotension

Chapter 6 *Acute Stroke: Acute Ischemic Stroke and Hemorrhagic Stroke* **171**

9. When differentiating between anterior and posterior territory strokes, many of the signs and symptoms overlap. Which of the following most likely indicates a *posterior* stroke origin? _____
   - _____ (a) Numbness of the extremities
   - _____ (b) Vertigo
   - _____ (c) Visual disturbances
   - _____ (d) Paralysis of an extremity

10. Stroke commonly is categorized as occlusive or hemorrhagic in origin. Hemorrhagic strokes are further subdivided into anterior and posterior territory presentations. _____
    - _____ (a) True
    - _____ (b) False

11. Which is the single most important *worldwide* risk factor associated with stroke? _____
    - _____ (a) Gender
    - _____ (b) Hypertension
    - _____ (c) Age
    - _____ (d) Heart disease

12. Which of the following is the most common etiology of intracerebral hemorrhage? _____
    - _____ (a) Hypertension
    - _____ (b) High red blood cell count
    - _____ (c) Stress
    - _____ (d) Migraine headache pathology

13. Hazinski's stroke chain of survival and recovery includes all of the following steps, *except:* _____
    - _____ (a) Dispatch
    - _____ (b) Decision
    - _____ (c) Door
    - _____ (d) Discharge

14. The Cincinnati Prehospital Stroke Scale was designed to evaluate all but which of the following: _____
    - _____ (a) Arm drift
    - _____ (b) Pupil response
    - _____ (c) Facial droop
    - _____ (d) Speech

15. Thrombolytics cannot be administered in a documented ischemic attack when the time from onset is greater than: _____
    - _____ (a) 1 hour
    - _____ (b) 2 hours
    - _____ (c) 3 hours
    - _____ (d) 4 hours

16. Which of the following does the Glasgow Coma Scale *not* evaluate? _____
    - _____ (a) Eye opening
    - _____ (b) Best verbal response
    - _____ (c) Best motor response
    - _____ (d) Facial droop

17. Which of the following *does not* suggest some brain-stem dysfunction? _____
    - _____ (a) Positive doll's eye reflex
    - _____ (b) Absent corneal reflex
    - _____ (c) Absent gag reflex
    - _____ (d) Ataxic respirations

18. Which of the following statements regarding stroke is wrong? _____
    - _____ (a) A recent lumbar puncture is a major contraindication to thrombolytics.
    - _____ (b) A magnetic resonance imaging scan continues to be a quick and efficient means for differentiating hemorrhagic from ischemic stroke.
    - _____ (c) Short-term management for recurrent seizures in stroke patients is administration of diazepam.
    - _____ (d) Aspirin use does not contraindicate the use of thrombolytics in an ischemic stroke patient.

19. The AHA recommends treating hypertension in a thrombolytic candidates with a systolic blood pressure of more than 185 mmHg or a diastolic pressure of more than 110 mmHg. _____
    - _____ (a) True
    - _____ (b) False

20. The use of long-term anticonvulsants for the control of recurring seizures is contraindicated. Short-term anticonvulsants only should be employed so that neurologic function can be monitored. _____
    - _____ (a) True
    - _____ (b) False

Chapter 6 Acute Stroke: Acute Ischemic Stroke and Hemorrhagic Stroke

Section 7
STROKE CROSSWORD PUZZLE

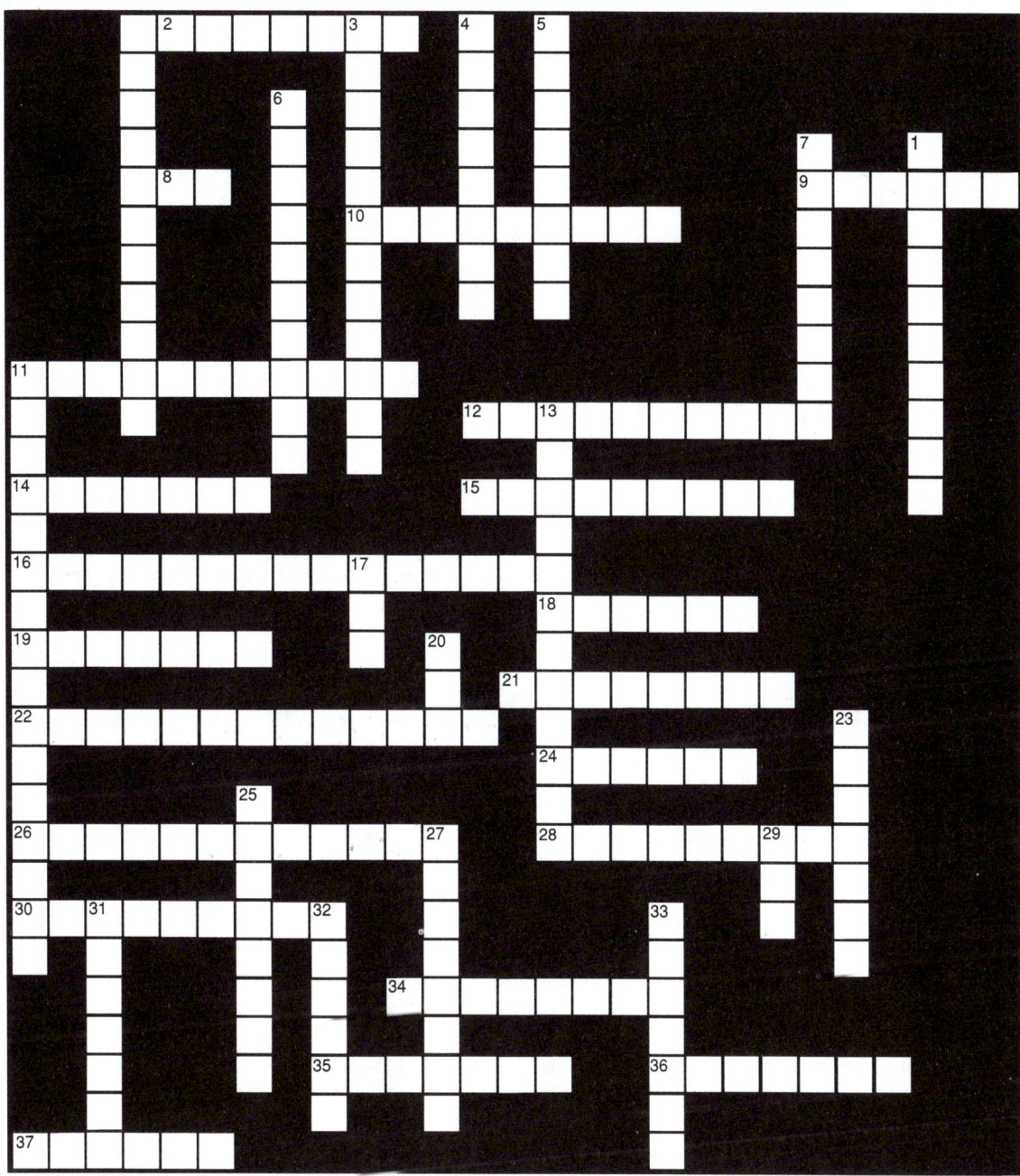

Across

2. A sudden, excruciating, or "thunderclap" _____ may indicate the presence of a subarachnoid hemorrhage.
8. The initials for a major warning sign of acute ischemic stroke. It looks like a stroke but resolves within 24 hours.
9. The Cincinnati Prehospital Stroke Scale identifies probable stroke victims based on evaluation of facial droop, arm drift, and _____.
10. What the "T" stands for in TIA.
11. A major category of stroke involves bleeding onto or into the brain.
12. Slurred speech.
14. A moving blood clot.
15. A main antihypertensive drug used in treating acute hypertensive emergencies in stroke patients. The pharmaceutical trade names for this drug are Normodyne and Trandate.

16. The arterial system that serves the posterior territory of the brain.
18. A term used to describe a deficit in coordination or trouble walking.
19. The pharmaceutical trade name for sodium nitroprusside.
21. This drug should be administered to all unconscious patients presenting with a history of malnourishment or alcoholism.
22. The subcategory of hemorrhagic stroke in which blood is found in the parenchyma of the brain.
24. Prophylactic use of this gas has not been shown to increase survival rates in stroke patients. Its use should be guided by measurement of blood saturation levels.
26. Any drug that breaks up a blood clot. One example is t-PA.
28. The first of the Hazinski's stroke chain steps. Early _____ of stroke is an educational problem for the public as well as health professionals. To identify. To recognize.
30. The term for a total blockage of a blood vessel by a thrombus or embolism. An _____ causes ischemia in the tissue distal to the blockage.
34. Double vision.
35. The term used when brain impairment leads to difficulty speaking or understanding speech.
36. Intravenous solutions containing _____ are contraindicated when initiating a lifeline unless low levels of this are documented.
37. A _____ onset of unconsciousness combined with focal neurologic deficits is a hallmark of stroke.

Down

1. The posterior-inferior portion of the brain that attaches to the brain stem and facilitates coordination.
2. If a stroke patient presents with _____, the clinician should search for causes other than intracerebral hemorrhage. Adults cannot lose enough blood in the cranial vault to cause this abnormality.
3. High blood pressure. Having to treat this abnormality aggressively to maintain normal limits is a contraindication to thrombolytic therapy.
4. The classification of solution normally started as a lifeline in strokes. The dissolved electrolytes are in the same proportion as is found normally in the bloodstream. This solution does not cause fluid shifts.
5. This type of headache mimics many of the signs and symptoms of subarachnoid hemorrhage. Sudden onset, intense pain, nausea, vomiting, and photophobia.
6. The _____ Hospital Stroke Scale. A large city in Ohio.
7. Shortage of oxygen at the tissue level. What occurs to distal brain or cardiac tissue when a blood clot totally occludes a vessel.
11. A short-term therapy to decrease ICP swiftly. Reducing the $PaCO_2$ to low levels by this method can result in cerebral ischemia.
13. The location of blood when it is on the surface of the brain, such as after an aneurysmal bleed
17. A 12-lead ECG is performed to rule out its presence. 5% of stroke victims have this occur concurrently. The initials of what happens when a coronary artery is occluded.
20. Initials for cerebrovascular accident
23. A _____ or sentinel bleed may herald a major rupture from an intracranial aneurysm.
25. A major sign of increased ICP. Patients exhibiting this phenomenon are in danger of losing airway control.
27. During the primary survey and again when contemplating pursuing the doll's eyes maneuver, the clinician should always exclude the possibility of trauma to the _____ spine.
29. Initials for intracranial pressure.
31. An anterior territory ischemic stroke involves the _____ artery.
32. Neck stiffness or _____ rigidity may indicate the presence of a subarachnoid hemorrhage.
33. The _____ Coma Scale is useful in documenting changes in levels of consciousness.

Comprehensive Posttest

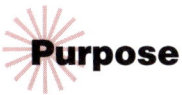
Purpose

The comprehensive posttest consists of 158 questions and answers. Two thirds of these questions are multiple choice questions, and the remaining one third are scenarios containing electrocardiograms (ECGs). There is only one correct answer for each question. Two answer sheets are provided so that you may take the test twice if you desire.

The comprehensive posttest is designed not only to provide practice but also to teach. Read each of the rationales in the answer section to learn why that response is correct. This approach will help you to understand, rather than just guess, the right answer. After you have completed the test, you can identify those areas in which you need more study and review.

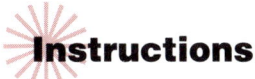
Instructions

Each question has only one correct answer. Should you need more information after reading the rationale, the appropriate pages in the *Advanced Life Support* textbook are provided at the end of each question.

Posttest Questions

Mark the correct answer.

1. Which of the following is *incorrect* for an oropharyngeal airway (OPA) (see ACLS text p. 2-2): _____

   _____ (a) It may cause gagging and vomiting in the semiconscious patient.
   _____ (b) It holds the tongue away from the rear of the oropharynx.
   _____ (c) It may be used in conjunction with an endotracheal tube.
   _____ (d) It removes the necessity for proper head–jaw positioning in the unconscious patient.

2. It is possible to have a pulse with ventricular fibrillation (see ACLS text p. 3-3). _____

   _____ (a) True
   _____ (b) False

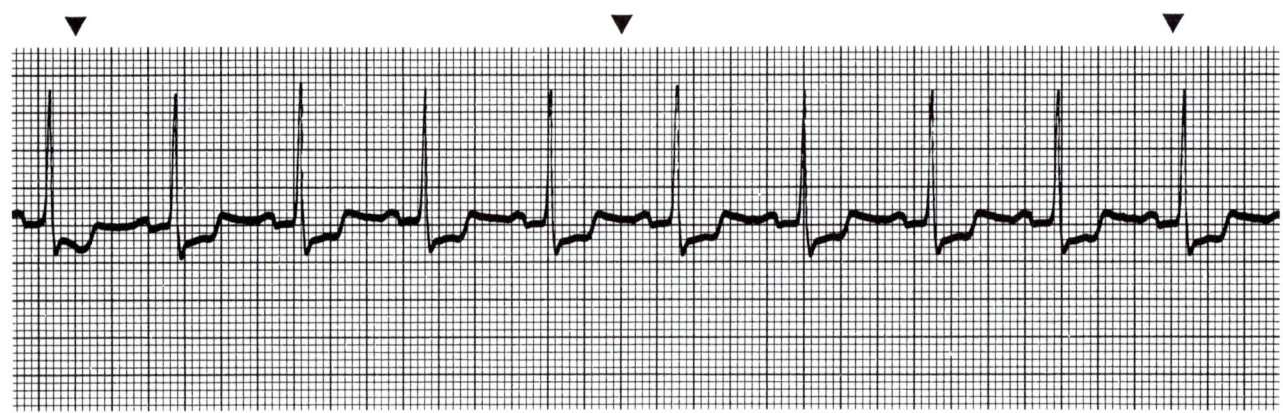

3. A 65-year-old woman arrives at the emergency department in full arrest. Her daughter relates that the patient has Alzheimer's disease and is taking oral verapamil. She notes that her mother's prescription was recently filled; however, the bottle found on the patient is now empty. The monitor reveals the above ECG. The patient is presently pulseless and apneic. Which protocol would you consider employing for this patient (see ACLS text pp. 1-21 to 1-23)? _____

4. The main difference between pseudo-electromechanical dissociation (EMD) and true EMD is the presence of an intermittently detectable carotid pulse throughout the code (see ACLS text p. 1-21). _____

   _____ (a) True
   _____ (b) False

5. Metabolic acidosis (see ACLS text pp. 7-14 to 7-16): (1) should be treated initially with sodium bicarbonate during a routine cardiac arrest; (2) occurs with increased anaerobic metabolism; (3) is a common occurrence in an aspirin overdose; (4) can be treated with sodium bicarbonate if the cause of the problem is tricyclic antidepressant (TCA) overdose. _____

   _____ (a) 1, 2, and 3
   _____ (b) 1, 3, and 4
   _____ (c) 2, 3, and 4
   _____ (d) 1, 2, and 4

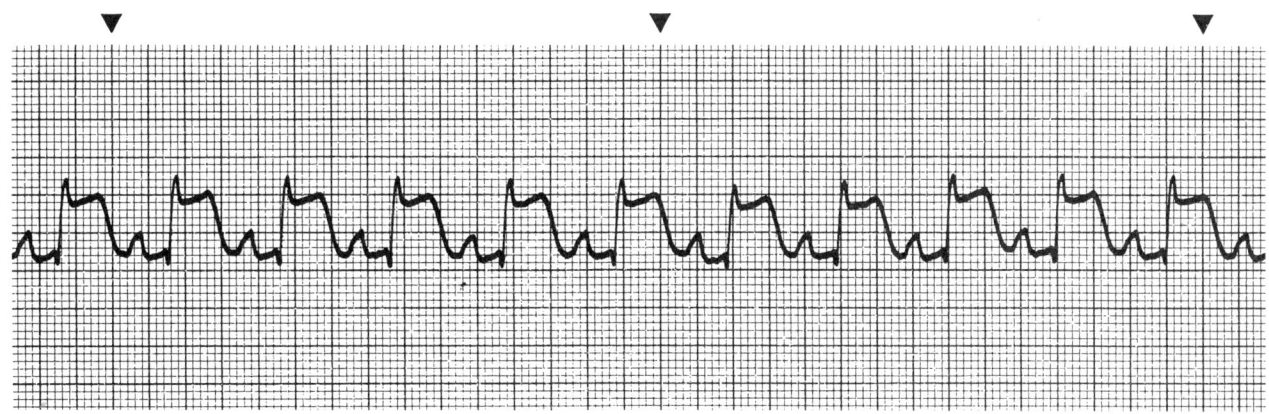

6. You arrive at the home of a 48-year-old man who is complaining of crushing chest pain. He describes the pain as radiating to the jaw and the left wrist. He has had many episodes of chest pain before, but they were always alleviated by resting and taking sublingual nitroglycerin. He is extremely apprehensive but relates a history of excessive smoking, poor exercise habits, and hypertension. His monitor reveals the above lead II ECG rhythm. Which protocol would you consider employing for this patient (see ACLS text pp. 9-3 to 9-5)? _____

7. Of the patients who die from an AMI, 50% will do so before they reach the hospital (see ACLS text p. 9-4).

    _____ True
    _____ False

8. In the bradycardia protocol, epinephrine is administered in which of the following manners (see ACLS text pp. 1-30 to 1-31 and 7-2 to 7-4): _____

    _____ (a) 1 mg in 250 mL of normal saline (NS) or D-5-W at 2 to 10 mcg/min.
    _____ (b) 1 mg of 1:1000 solution given by intravenous push slowly over 1 to 2 minutes.
    _____ (c) 1 mg of 1:10,000 solution given by intravenous push slowly over 2 to 4 minutes.
    _____ (d) 30 mg in 250 mL of NS or D-5-W at 2 to 20 mcg/kg/min.

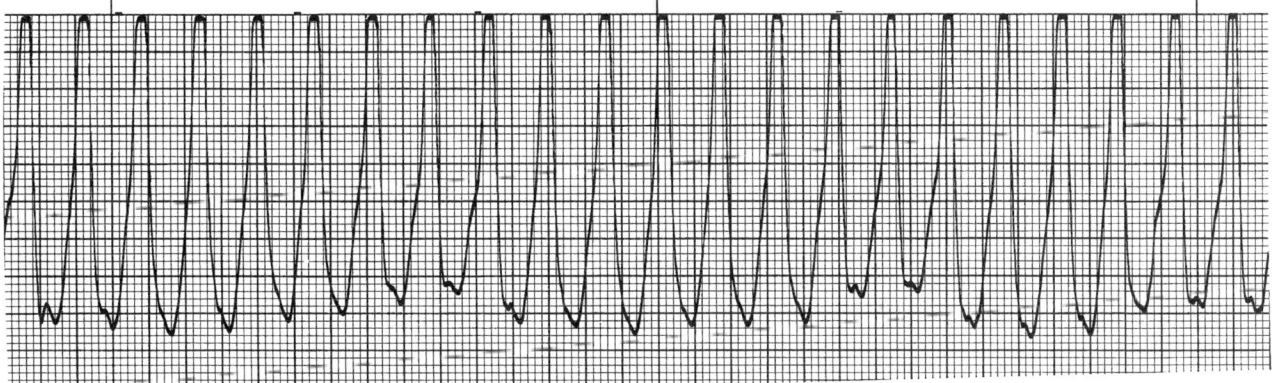

9. A 45-year-old woman was visiting her son on the medical floor of your hospital when she pulled the "help" cord. On arrival, a brief history and physical examination reveals that her heart started beating "all of a sudden." She denies both chest pain and difficulty breathing. Her rhythm appears in the above ECG. A 12-lead ECG was hastily ordered and an on-duty cardiologist verified it as ventricular. Her vital signs are as follows: pulse—250; respirations—22 (just apprehension, lung sounds are clear); and blood pressure (BP)—112/92. Which protocol would you consider employing for this patient (see ACLS text p. 1-39)? _____

10. You are treating a 34-year-old woman for stable supraventricular tachycardia (SVT) with 6 mg of adenosine. It has been 2 minutes since the initial dose, and she rolls her eyes up in their sockets and collapses to the gurney. Her pulse and cardiac rhythm have not changed from 190. Her blood pressure has dropped to 70/50, and she now responds only to painful stimuli. You should now consider (see ACLS text pp. 1-34 to 1-35): _____

  _____ (a) Lidocaine, 1.0 to 1.5 mg/kg
  _____ (b) Verapamil, 2.5 to 5.0 mg slowly given by intravenous push
  _____ (c) Synchronized cardioversion at 50 to 100 joules
  _____ (d) Precordial thump

11. Adenosine has no significant effect on ventricular rhythms (see ACLS text p. 7-13). _____

  _____ (a) True
  _____ (b) False

12. A 55-year-old man has been admitted for an acute myocardial infarction (MI) and is now experiencing the above rhythm. As you talk to him, he rolls his eyes back into their sockets and collapses to the gurney. He is now unconscious and diaphoretic. His vital signs are as follows: pulse—240; respirations—20 and shallow; and BP—80/60. Which protocol would you consider employing for this patient (see ACLS text pp. 1-35)? _____

13. A 48-year-old man is suddenly complaining of palpitations. The patient is alert and coherent and denies dyspnea or chest pain. The monitor rhythm appears to be ventricular tachycardia, and a 12-lead ECG confirms it. The patient's pulse is 140 and BP is 102/86. After placing the patient on oxygen, your next act would be to (see ACLS text pp. 1-33 and 1-39): _____

  _____ (a) Administer lidocaine, 1.0 to 1.5 mg/kg.
  _____ (b) Sedate and administer a synchronized cardioversion at 50 joules.
  _____ (c) Administer adenosine intravenously, 6 mg given rapidly.
  _____ (d) Administer procainamide, 20 to 30 mg/min.

14. The best airway for a deeply unconscious, acutely intoxicated patient is (see ACLS text p. 2-3): _____

  _____ (a) An oropharyngeal airway (OPA).
  _____ (b) A nasopharyngeal airway (NPA).
  _____ (c) A nasogastric tube
  _____ (d) An endotracheal tube

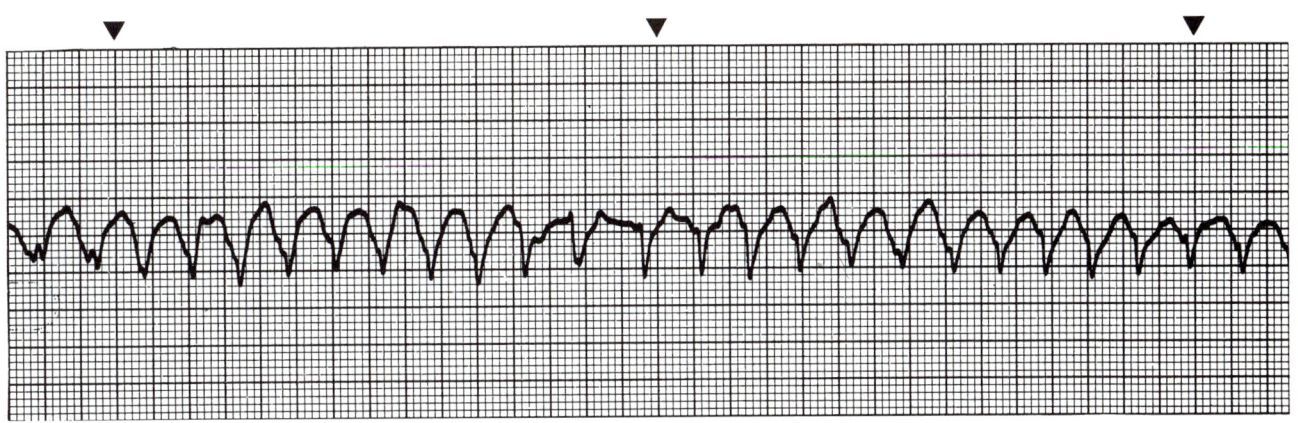

15. A 45-year-old man presents in the emergency room complaining of crushing chest pain radiating to the jaw and the left arm. As you are initiating treatment, his eyes roll up in their sockets, and he begins to seize. Seconds later, the seizure subsides, and the rhythm strip changes from a sinus tachycardia with an elevated ST segment to the above rhythm. The patient is found to be both pulseless and apneic. Which protocol would you consider employing for this patient (see ACLS text p. 1-38)? _____

16. Ventricular fibrillation (see ACLS text pp. 1-14 to 1-15 and 3-3): (1) can be mimicked by artifact on a monitor; (2) can occur with the presence of a peripheral pulse; (3) produces slight cardiac output; (4) should be treated with early defibrillation. _____

    _____ (a) 1 and 4
    _____ (b) 1, 3, and 4
    _____ (c) 1, 2, and 4
    _____ (d) All of the above

17. The key treatment strategy in the treatment of pulseless electrical activity (PEA) is (see ACLS text p. 1-23): _____

    _____ (a) finding an appropriate cause and treating it
    _____ (b) Performing cardiopulmonary resuscitation (CPR) until the PEA medications correct the neurotransmitter problem
    _____ (c) Putting the heart into asystole with epinephrine so that it can be defibrillated into a viable rhythm
    _____ (d) Allowing the PEA protocol sufficient time to correct the myoneural damage that has resulted in the pulseless condition

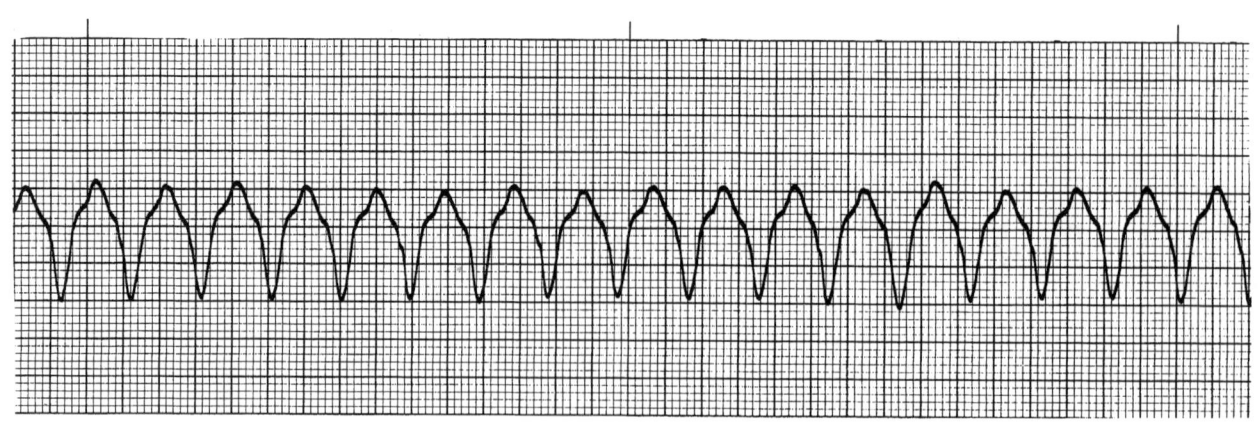

18. A 36-year-old man was admitted for hepatic surgery. Suddenly, his heart began to pound in his chest. He denies chest pain, difficulty breathing, or an altered level of consciousness. Lead II is noted above, but the 12-lead machine is broken. The patient's vital signs are are follows: pulse—200, respirations—18, and BP—132/88. Which protocol would you consider employing for this patient (see ACLS text pp. 1-36 to 1-38)? _____

19. Defibrillating a *true* asystolic heart can precipitate a massive _____ discharge, making the heart even more refractory to other therapy (see ACLS text p. 1-23).

    _____ (a) Adrenergic
    _____ (b) Parasympathetic
    _____ (c) Vasophrenic
    _____ (d) Nicorenergic

20. As long as a pulse oximeter documents that the patient's oxygen saturation is adequate, additional oxygen is not indicated when treating a suspected MI (see ACLS text p. 9-14).
    _____

    _____ (a) True
    _____ (b) False

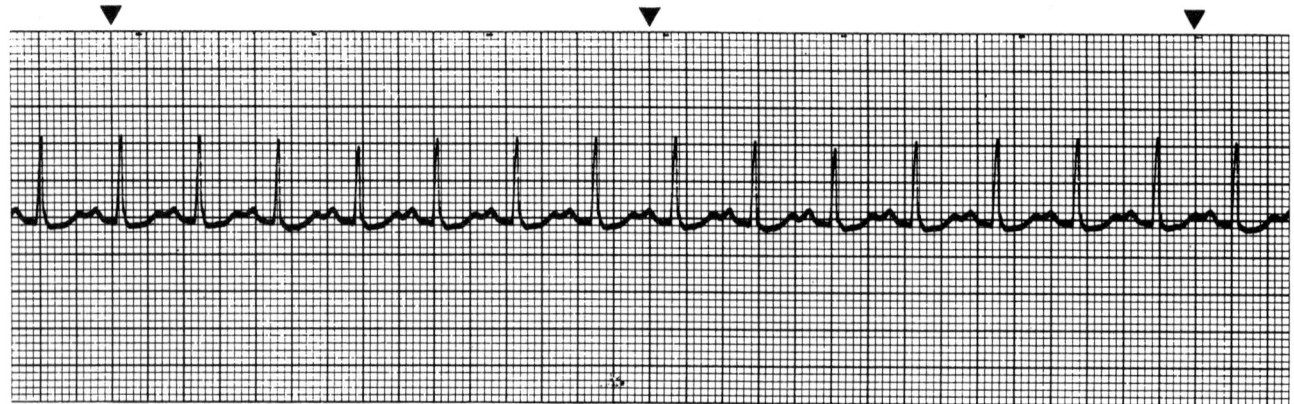

21. The paramedics have arrived at the home of a 70-year-old woman. She has been a heavy smoker for most of her life and has been on a ventilator in the past. When questioned, her husband states that she has had difficulty "getting her breath" for the past hour and that she quit breathing as the ambulance arrived. Her vital signs are pulse—140, respirations—0, and BP—100/80. What would you do (see ACLS text p. 1-11)? _____

22. Transcutaneous pacemakers (TCPs) are considered *bridge devices* to a more definitive transvenous pacemaker (see ACLS text p. 1-32). _____

_____ (a) True
_____ (b) False

23. A 43-year-old woman presents to you with a blood pressure of 70/50. She is diaphoretic, pale, and responds only to painful stimuli. Her ECG reveals a wide complex tachycardia at 200 beats/minute. Her husband relates a previous history of ventricular tachycardia. Your *initial* treatment after oxygen is started is (see ACLS text pp. 1-35 to 1-36): _____

    _____ (a) Verapamil, 5 mg given intravenously slowly
    _____ (b) Lidocaine, 1.0 to 1.5 mg/kg
    _____ (c) Adenosine, 6 mg given intravenously rapidly
    _____ (d) Synchronized cardioversion at 50 to 100 joules

24. The patient is rubbing his chest with his fist and is complaining of "crushing" substernal chest pain radiating down the left arm and the jaw. He is both cool and diaphoretic. His vital signs are: pulse—240, respirations—16 (clear bilaterally), and BP—110/90. The monitor shows the above rhythm. Which protocol would you consider employing for this patient (see ACLS text p. 1-35)? _____

25. All of the following are common side effects of adenosine *except* (see ACLS text pp. 7-13): _____

    _____ (a) Premature ventricular contractions (PVCs)
    _____ (b) Chest pain
    _____ (c) A short period of asystole
    _____ (d) Facial flushing

26. A 55-year-old man is brought in with a history of fainting spells in the past hour. He admits to epigastric distress just before this episode. As you examine him, you find his pulse irregular at 90 to 95. The ECG shows multifocal PVCs with runs of documented ventricular tachycardia. Your *initial* intervention is (see ACLS text pp. 7-7 to 7-8): _____

    _____ (a) Propranolol, 1.0 mg given by intravenous bolus
    _____ (b) Atropine, 0.5 mg given by intravenous bolus and repeated as needed
    _____ (c) Lidocaine, 1.0 to 1.5 mg/kg
    _____ (d) Infusion of lidocaine, 1 g in 250 mL D-5-W

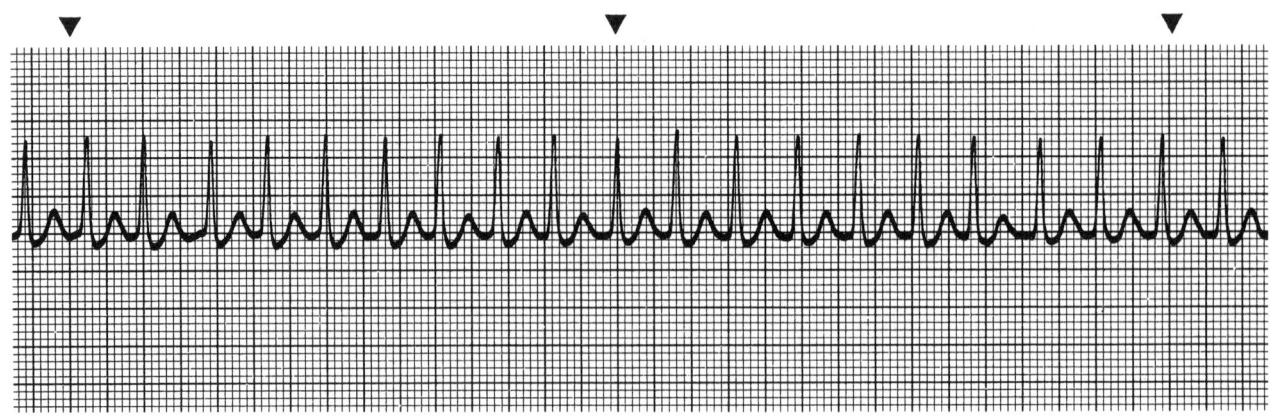

27. A paramedic unit responds to the home of a 43-year-old woman. She does not appear to be in any acute distress; however, she states that she has had a rapid heart rate for the past hour and is becoming apprehensive. She denies chest pain or breathing difficulty. Her rhythm is noted above, and her vital signs are as follows: pulse—210, respirations—16, and BP—130/94. Which protocol would you consider employing for this patient (see ACLS text pp. 1-36 to 1-38)? _____

28. Bag-valve-mask (BVM) devices (see ACLS text pp. 2-8 to 2-9): (1) should be used only by trained clinicians (2) can deliver close to 100% oxygen if the reservoir is used with 4 L/min of oxygen; (3) are often difficult for one person to apply effectively; (4) usually provide more tidal volume than mouth-to-mask resuscitation when applied effectively. _____

    _____ (a) 1, 2, and 4
    _____ (b) 2, 3, and 4
    _____ (c) 1 and 3
    _____ (d) All of the above

29. The most common arrhythmia noted in the first 60 seconds of an arrest is (see ACLS text pp. 1-5 and 9-4): _____

    _____ (a) Sinus bradycardia with PVC couplets
    _____ (b) Complete heart block
    _____ (c) Ventricular fibrillation
    _____ (d) Ventricular standstill

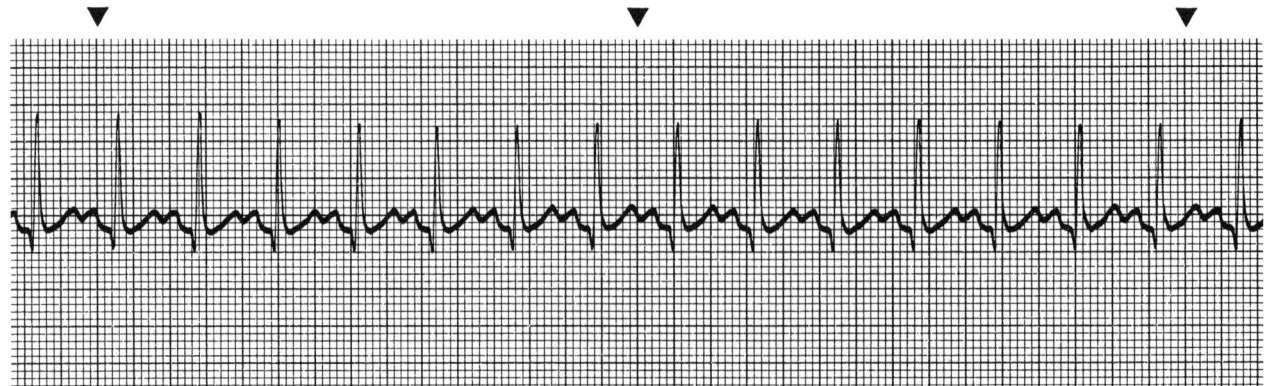

30. A 48-year-old woman presented in cardiac arrest. CPR was halted, and the above rhythm strip obtained. There was no palpable pulse or respirations; however, a Doppler gave you a systolic reading of 30. Which protocol would you consider employing for this patient (see ACLS text pp. 1-14 and 1-21 to 1-23)? _____

31. When treating PEA caused by pulmonary embolism, all of the following are signs, symptoms, or pertinent history *except* (see ACLS text p. 1-21): _____

    _____ (a) Hip fracture
    _____ (b) Oral contraceptives
    _____ (c) Renal failure
    _____ (d) Deep venous thrombosis

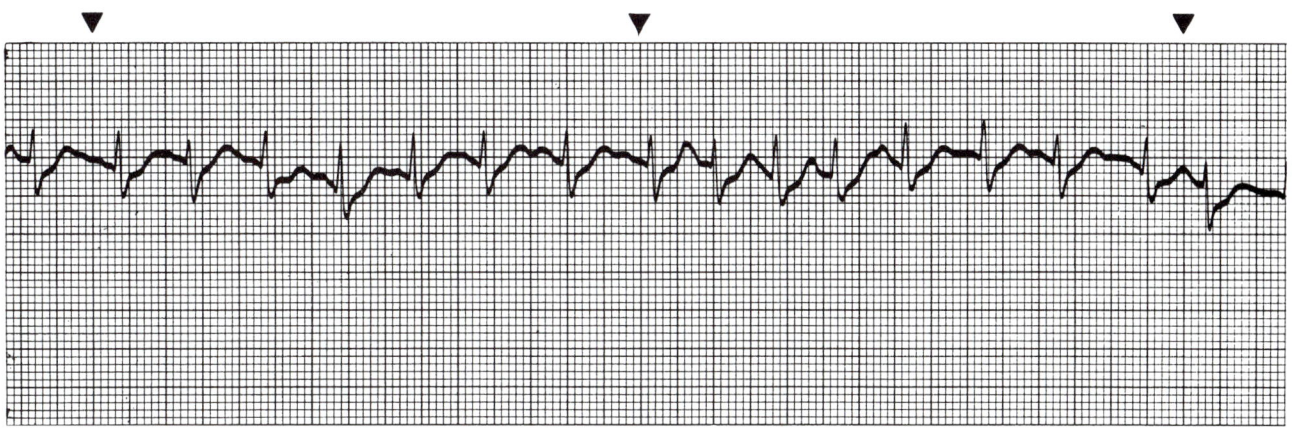

32. It is 4:00 AM and you are the sole person in the emergency room. You are evaluating a 44-year-old man who is responsive to verbal stimuli. He denies chest pain and difficulty breathing but is apprehensive about his fast, irregular heart rate. Lead II is noted above. His vital signs are as follows: pulse—150, respirations—22, BP—112/96. Which protocol would you consider employing for this patient (see ACLS text pp. 1-33 and 1-36)? _____

33. Epinephrine (see ACLS text pp. 7-2 to 7-4): (1) increases peripheral vascular resistance; (2) increases perfusion to the left ventricle; (3) increases automaticity; (4) increases myocardial contractility; (5) increases parasympathetic tone. _____

    _____ (a) 1, 2, 4, and 5
    _____ (b) 2, 3, 4, and 5
    _____ (c) 1, 2, 3, and 4
    _____ (d) All of the above

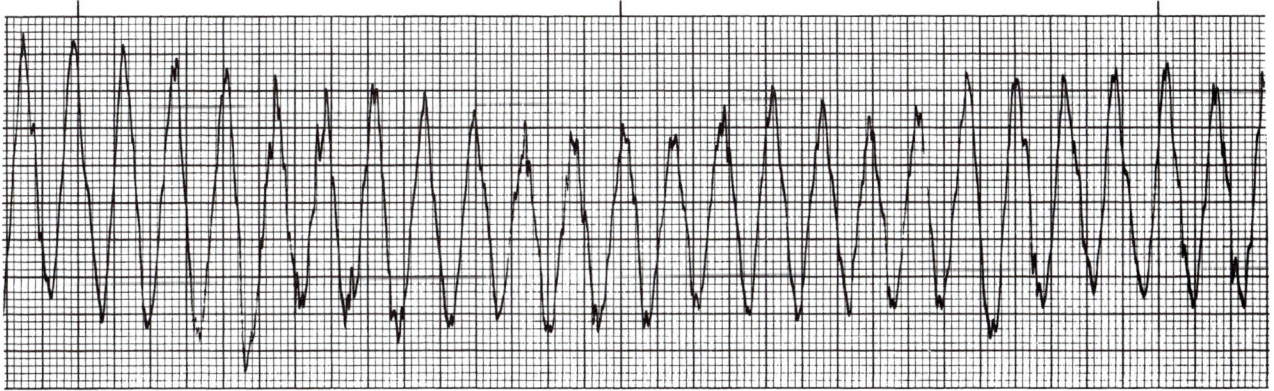

34. You encounter a 45-year-old man who was having pain in his lower lumbar region due to improper lifting. As you examine his spine, he sucks in his breath and states, "Whoa! My heart! It just started pounding rapidly." His rhythm appears above. A 12-lead ECG verifies that the rhythm is ventricular in nature. He denies both chest pain and difficulty breathing. His vital signs are as follows: pulse—180, respirations—20 (just apprehension, lung sounds are clear), and BP—106/90. Which protocol would you consider employing for this patient (see ACLS text p. 1-39)? _____

35. Which of the following selections is *inappropriate* for routine intravenous lifeline administration in suspected cardiac patients (see ACLS text pp. 1-10 to 1-11)? _____

   _____ (a) D-5-W
   _____ (b) NS (0.9%)
   _____ (c) Half NS (0.45%)
   _____ (d) None of the above

36. Although all may be employed separately or together, which of the following is the *definitive* therapy for a hemodynamically significant bradycardia of ventricular origin (see ACLS text p. 1-31)? _____

   _____ (a) Atropine given by intravenous push
   _____ (b) Transvenous pacemaker
   _____ (c) Dopamine drip
   _____ (d) Epinephrine drip

37. A 45-year-old man is brought by private car to the emergency room. His wife shouts for help as he is assisted to the nearest gurney. He is clutching his chest, obviously in great distress. As you hook up his electrodes to a bedside monitor, he passes out and becomes unresponsive, with no detectable pulse. The monitor reveals the above rhythm. What protocol would you consider employing (see ACLS text pp. 1-11 to 1-21)? _____

38. Although individual responses may vary, *in general*, at doses of more than 10 mcg/kg/min, treatment with dopamine may result in: (1) renal and mesenteric vasodilation; (2) increased inotropic activity; (3) respiratory depression; (4) renal arterial vasoconstriction (see ACLS text p. 8-3). _____

   _____ (a) 2 and 4
   _____ (b) 1
   _____ (c) 2, 3, and 4
   _____ (d) 1, 2, and 3

39. Stability versus instability of a tachycardia should be primarily based on a diagnosis of cardiac origin (supraventricular versus ventricular) (see ACLS text pp. 1-35 to 1-36): _____

   _____ (a) True
   _____ (b) False

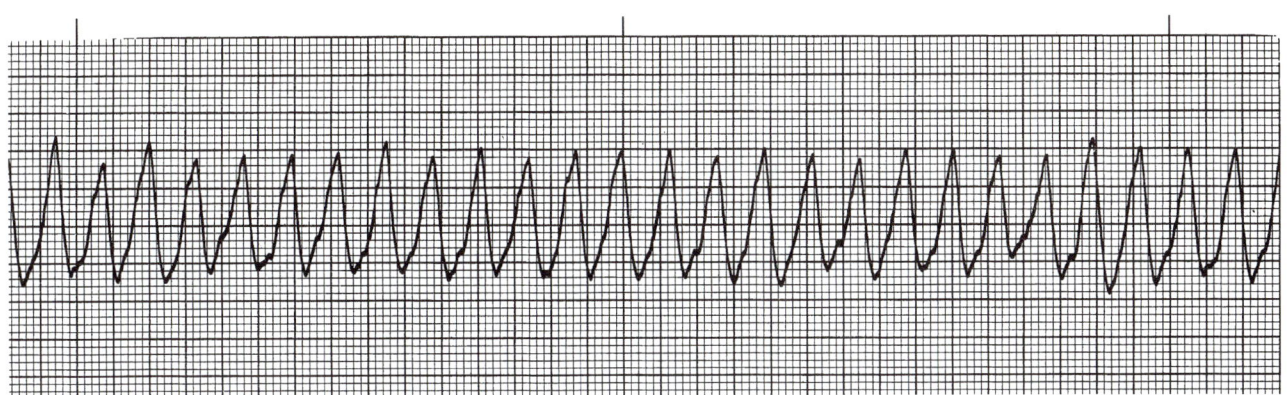

40. This is the rhythm of a 45-year-old man who presents to you with a spontaneous onset of tachycardia and concurrent crushing chest pain. He is alert and coherent with the following vital signs: pulse—260, BP—120/90, and respirations—14 and clear. He is both diaphoretic and pale. What protocol would you consider employing (see ACLS text p. 1-35)? _____

41. Lidocaine (see ACLS text pp. 7-6 to 7-8): (1) dosage in ventricular fibrillation should be 1.0 to 1.5 mg/kg; (2) rarely causes toxicity in doses under 5 mg/kg; (3) has no significant effect on contractility in therapeutic doses; (4) elevates fibrillation threshold of the ventricles. _____

    _____ (a) 1, 2, and 4
    _____ (b) 1, 3, and 4
    _____ (c) 2, 3, and 4
    _____ (d) All the above

42. During cardiac arrest, which of the following should be used on a patient with an endotracheal tube and BVM (see ACLS text pp. 2-8 to 2-9)? _____

    _____ (a) 12 L/min oxygen flow to the BVM
    _____ (b) BVM without supplementary oxygen
    _____ (c) 12 L/min oxygen flow to a BVM with a reservoir
    _____ (d) 6 L/min oxygen to BVM

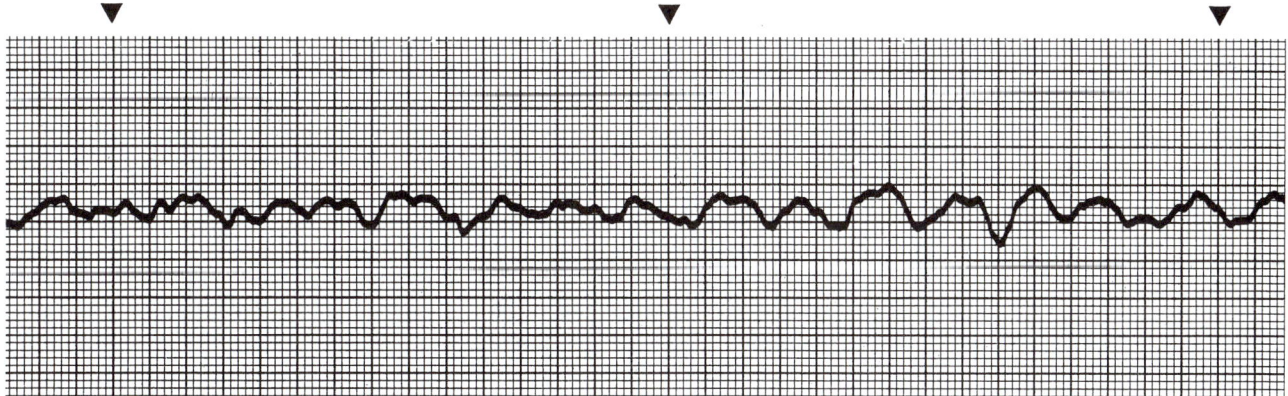

43. A 65-year-old woman was admitted to the critical care unit (CCU) to rule out an MI. She is on 60% oxygen. She is receiving NS intravenously and has received morphine for pain. She has a history of hypertension and is taking β-blockers. At your nursing station, her heart monitor alarm goes off and reveals the above strip. You find her both pulseless and apneic. What protocol would you consider employing (see ACLS text pp. 1-15 to 1-21)? _____

44. Which of the following is the *initial* treatment in a patient that had multifocal PVCs before progressing to ventricular fibrillation on your monitor-defibrillator screen? A quick assessment reveals that the patient is now pulseless and apneic (see ACLS text p. 4-1). _____
    _____ (a) CPR
    _____ (b) Immediate synchronized countershock at 200 joules
    _____ (c) Lidocaine, 1.0 to 1.5 mg/kg given by intravenous bolus
    _____ (d) Immediate defibrillation at 200 joules

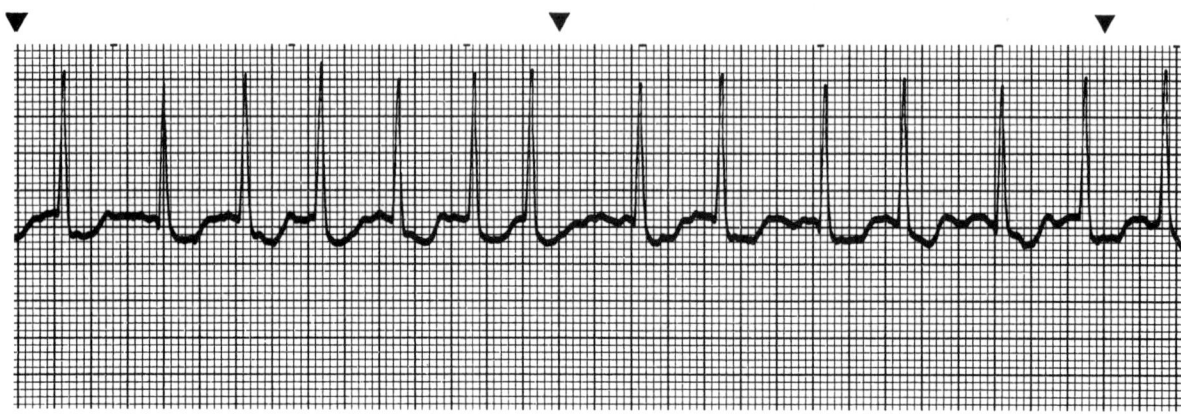

45. A 90-year-old man presents with a depressed level of consciousness secondary to the rhythm shown above. He has an irregular pulse of 130, BP is 80/40, and respirations are clear and 10. His skin is cool and clammy. Which protocol would you consider employing for this patient (see ACLS text pp. 1-35 to 1-36)? _____

46. PEA may be evidenced as all of the following rhythms *except* (see ACLS text p. 1-21): _____
    _____ (a) Bradyasystolic rhythm (a ventricular rate of 20 to 30 beats/minute)
    _____ (b) Ventricular tachycardia
    _____ (c) Idioventricular rhythm
    _____ (d) Sinus tachycardia

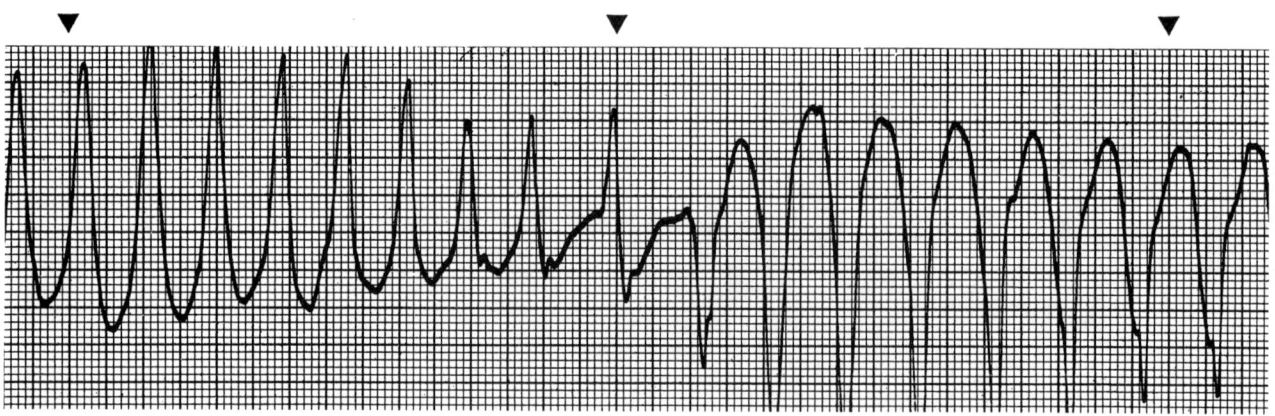

47. A 43-year-old man was placed in the intensive care unit after undergoing surgery on his left femoral artery. His heart monitor alarm goes off, and the above ECG is noted. The patient is conscious and alert with the following vital signs: pulse—160, respirations—18, and BP—132/88. He denies both chest pain and difficulty breathing. The 12-lead ECG technician is on break and a professional ECG analysis cannot be obtained, but you suspect torsades de pointes. What protocol would you consider employing (see ACLS text pp. 1-39 to 1-40)? _____

48. If you see asystole while monitoring the patient's rhythm through the "quick-look" paddles, it is acceptable to reverse your hand placement (i.e., sternum moves to apex and vice versa) to verify in a second lead (see ACLS text p. 1-23). _____

    _____ (a) True
    _____ (b) False

49. Procainamide should be avoided in which of the following situations (see ACLS text pp. 1-39 to 1-40)? _____

    _____ (a) Ventricular fibrillation refractory to normal therapy
    _____ (b) Lidocaine refractory ventricular tachycardia
    _____ (c) Torsades de pointes
    _____ (d) Wide complex tachycardias of uncertain type

50. A 70-year-old woman with a history of chronic obstructive pulmonary disease arrives in the emergency room. Her breathing is becoming progressively more labored. With great difficulty, she relates a four-pack-a-day smoking habit. As she tries to communicate further, she becomes unresponsive and ceases breathing. Her vital signs are as follows: pulse—130, respirations—0, and BP—98/70. What would you do (see ACLS text pp. 1-9 to 1-10)? _____

51. It is acceptable, and even encouraged, to administer atropine, start a TCP, and hang a dopamine drip simultaneously if the patient is beginning to decompensate quickly from a hemodynamically significant bradycardia (see ACLS text p. 1-30). _____

    _____ (a) True
    _____ (b) False

52. Endotracheal intubation: (1) should be performed before defibrillation in witnessed ventricular fibrillation; (2) reduces the risk of aspiration of gastric contents; (3) should not be attempted by inexperienced clinicians; (4) is always necessary for adequate lung ventilation (see ACLS text pp. 1-14 and 2-3). _____

    _____ (a) 2 and 3
    _____ (b) 2 and 4
    _____ (c) 3 and 4
    _____ (d) 1 and 3

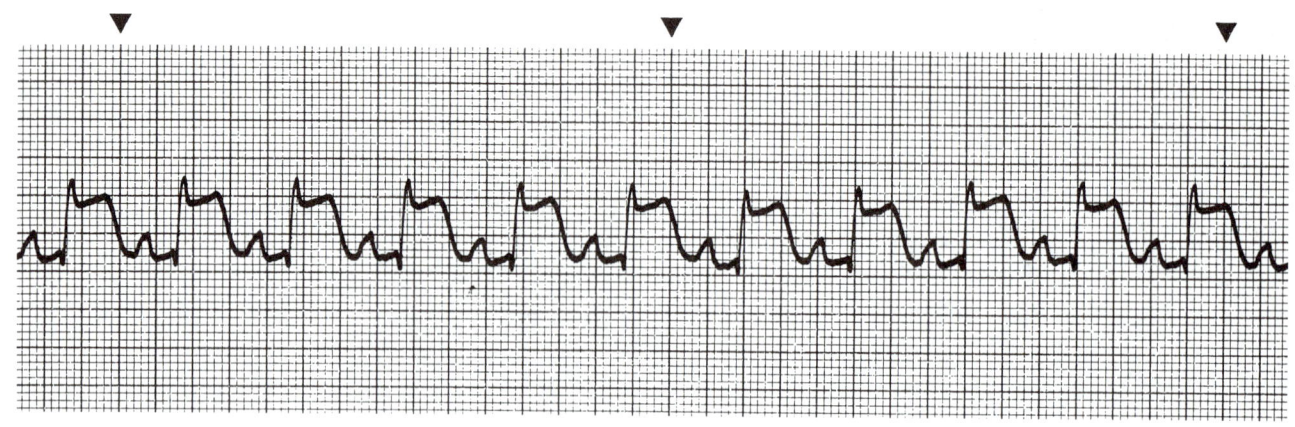

53. A 48-year-old male patient, complaining of epigastric distress with pain radiating to the jaw and the left arm, is brought to the emergency room by private car. When interviewed, he is pale and profusely diaphoretic. He is a nonsmoker and has hypertension controlled by β-blockers. He had an MI 2 years ago. Lead II reveals the above rhythm. What protocol would you consider employing (see ACLS text p. 9-5)? _____

54. A dopamine infusion of greater than 20 mcg/kg/min will likely result in (see ACLS text pp. 8-3): _____

    _____ (a) Mesenteric vasodilation
    _____ (b) Peripheral arterial vasoconstriction
    _____ (c) Renal arterial vasodilation
    _____ (d) Respiratory depression

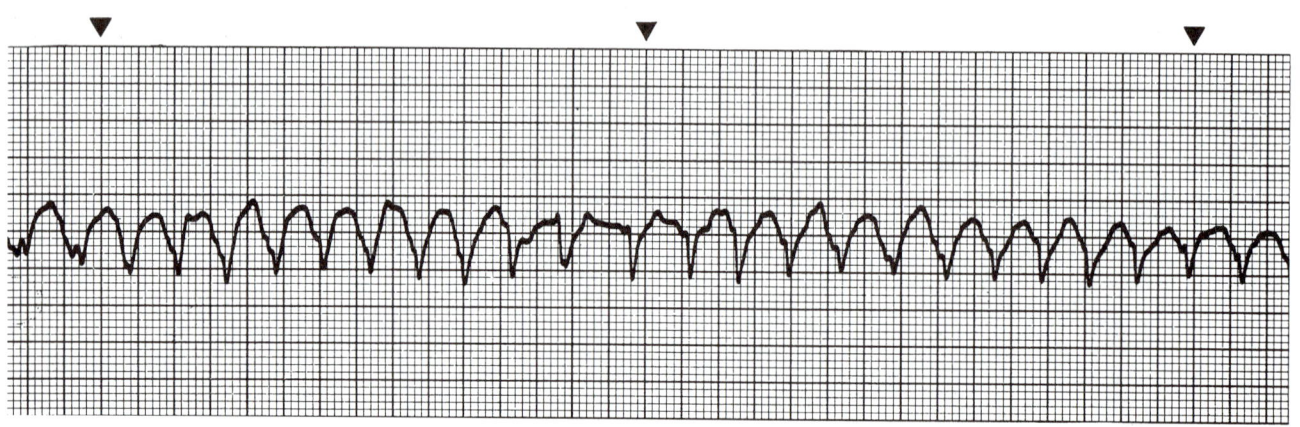

55. This is the rhythm of a 77-year-old woman who was admitted for a chronic kidney condition. As she relates it, "my heart started beating a mile-a-minute a few minutes ago." She is now experiencing difficulty breathing. Your thoracic examination reveals bilateral rales and rhonchi. Her vital signs are as follows: pulse—270, respirations—30 and labored, and BP—180/130. What protocol would you consider employing (see ACLS text p. 1-35)? _____

56. You are treating what appears to be a stable SVT with adenosine when the QRS complex suddenly becomes wide. Verapamil should be withheld and lidocaine employed (see ACLS text p. 1-38). _____

    _____ (a) True
    _____ (b) False

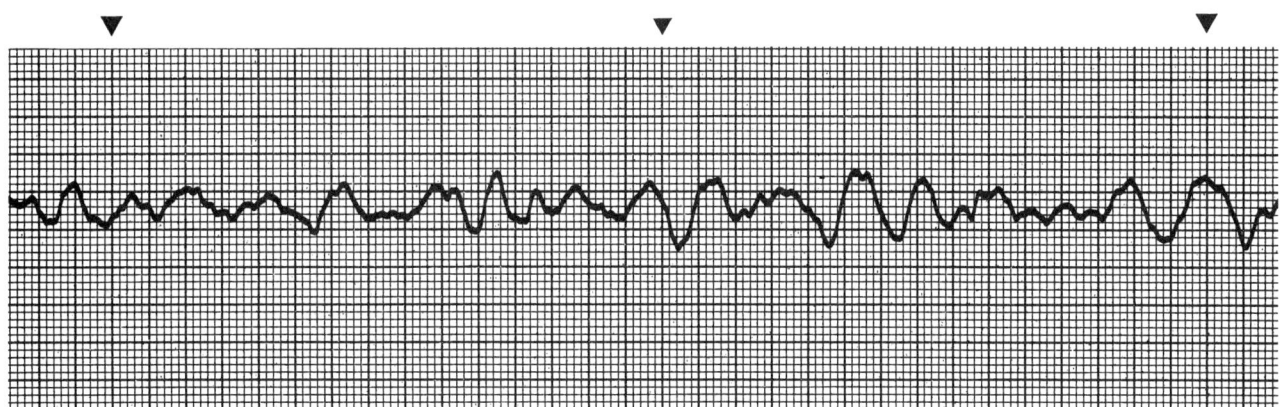

57. This is rhythm strip of a 55-year-old man who was found by his wife at home. She stated that she called 911 immediately and that the ambulance arrived within 5 minutes. Her son was performing adequate CPR in the interim. The paramedics call in and state that the patient is both pulseless and apneic and request instructions. What protocol would you consider employing (see ACLS text pp. 1-11 to 1-15)? _____

58. Regardless of how a lidocaine drip is mixed at your facility, the concentration (in mg/mL) commonly is (see ACLS text pp. 7-6 to 7-8): _____

    _____ (a) 1 mg/mL
    _____ (b) 2 mg/mL
    _____ (c) 3 mg/mL
    _____ (d) 4 mg/mL

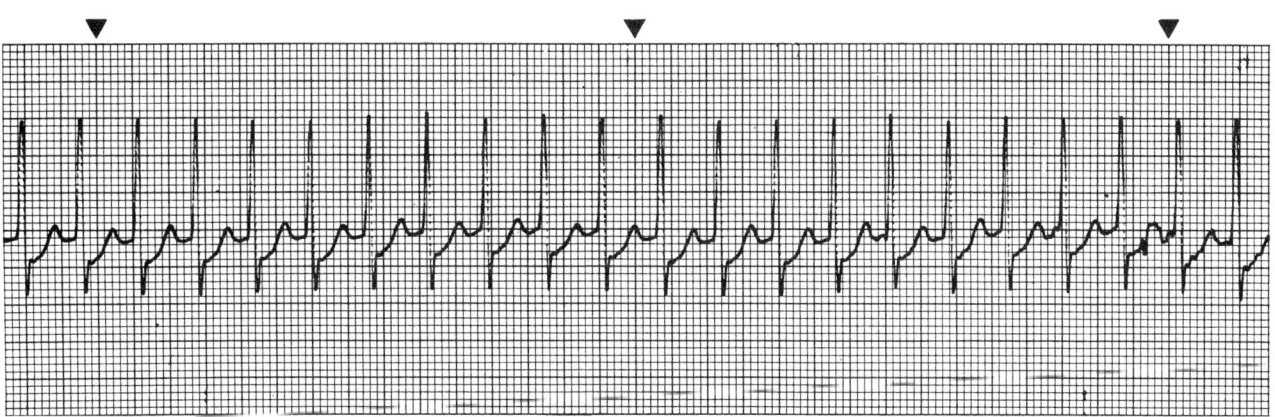

59. A 62-year-old man was in the intensive care unit with a diagnosis of pleurisy. He was resting quietly until he suddenly sat bolt upright and grabbed his chest and screamed with pain. When questioned, he gasped that his heart started palpitating and then crushing chest pain began. His rhythm is noted above. His vital signs are as follows: pulse—186, respirations—20, and BP—140/96. What protocol would you consider employing (see ACLS text p. 1-45)? _____

60. After endotracheal intubation, the clinician can hear lung sounds only on the right side but not on the left. The clinician should suspect (see ACLS text p. 2-6): _____

    _____ (a) Intubation of the esophagus
    _____ (b) Underinflation of the cuff
    _____ (c) Insertion of the tube into the right main-stem bronchus
    _____ (d) Laryngospasms caused by tube insertion

61. Transthoracic resistance to flow of defibrillating current (the impedance) may *increase* with which one of the following (see ACLS text p. 4-4)? _____
    _____ (a) Successive countershocks
    _____ (b) Lighter paddle pressure
    _____ (c) Increase in successively higher joule settings
    _____ (d) Lower body weight

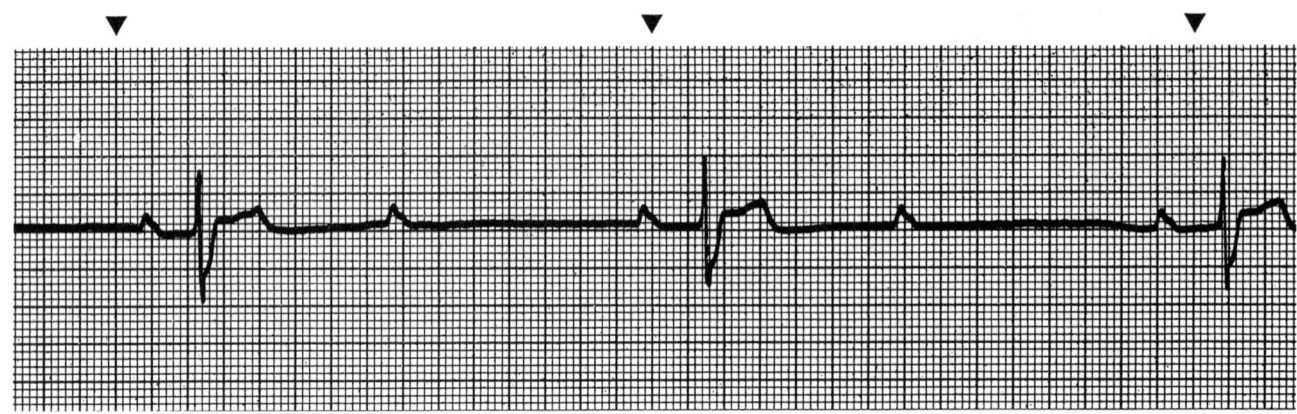

62. The aunt of a hospital in-patient is complaining of chest pain. She complains that she has had the pain for the last 2 hours but did not wish to mention it because her nephew was already in considerable pain. She is feeling faint with concurrent nausea, diaphoresis, and cool skin. Her vital signs are as follows: BP—80/60, respirations—12, and pulse—30. The monitor reveals the above rhythm. What protocol would you consider employing (see ACLS text p. 1-30)? _____

63. Sodium bicarbonate: (1) is used in the treatment of acute hyperkalemia; (2) is normally initiated within the first 5 minutes of an unwitnessed arrest; (3) should be administered as 1 mEq/kg bolus every 5 minutes if blood gas analysis and pH are unavailable; (4) neutralizes acidity generated in an aspirin overdose (see ACLS text pp. 7-14 to 7-16). _____
    _____ (a) 1, 2, and 3
    _____ (b) 2 and 4
    _____ (c) 1 and 4
    _____ (d) All of the above

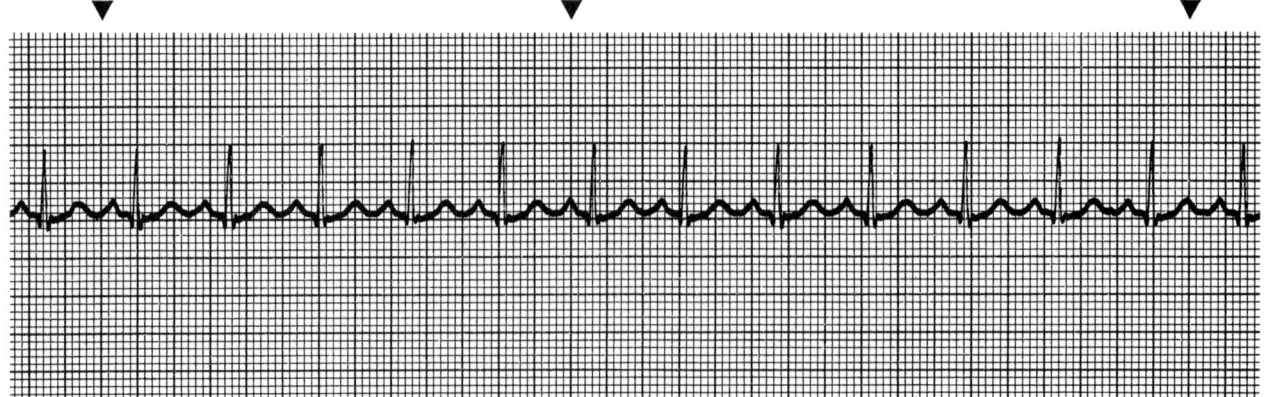

64. An 82-year-old man, admitted for urologic surgery the following day, is experiencing intense nausea and watery diarrhea, which he claims is from hospital food. However, he does not relate to you that he has had diarrhea and vomiting for the last 4 days and has not been able to keep anything down. He walks unsteadily to the commode and promptly vomits. He then feels an episode of diarrhea commencing, sits on the commode, and passes out. His vital signs are pulse—130, respirations—20, and BP—80/60. When a monitor is brought, the rhythm above is noted. Which protocol would you consider employing for this patient (see ACLS text p. 1-42)? _____

65. Atropine sulfate: (1) is of no value in treating ventricular tachycardia; (2) is always required if the heart rate is less than 60 beats/minute; (3) is usually given in 2-mg boluses up to a total of 0.04 mg/kg; (4) may be of value in the treatment of supraventricular bradycardias (see ACLS text pp. 7-4 to 7-6). _____

_____ (a) 1 and 4
_____ (b) 1 and 3
_____ (c) 2 and 3
_____ (d) 2 and 4

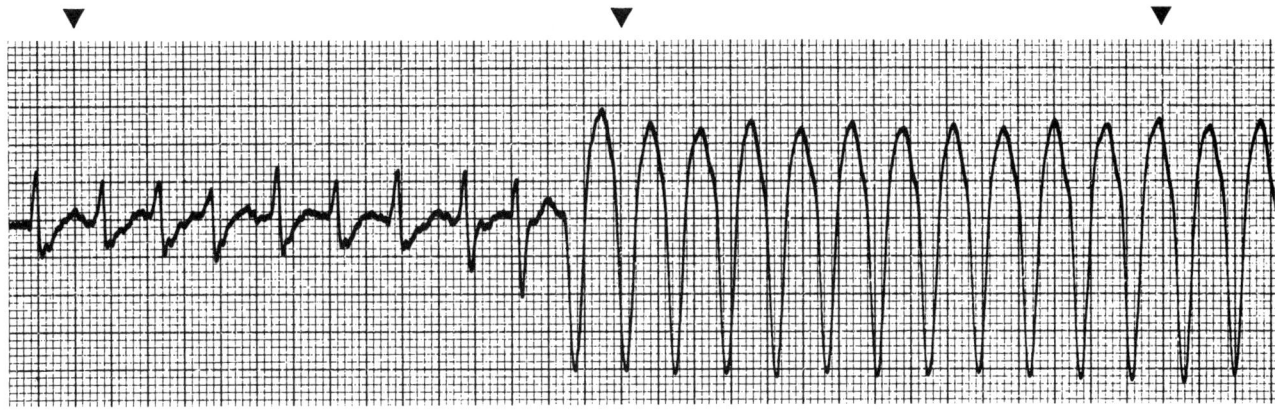

66. A patient was admitted to the CCU for a bout of uncontrolled atrial fibrillation. The admitting physician had just left the patient's bedside to sign the admitting orders at the nurse's station when he heard a loud clatter from the patient's room. On investigation, he finds his patient on the floor, pulseless and apneic. The bedside monitor recorded the above strip during the incident. What protocol would you consider employing (see ACLS text p. 1-38)? _____

67. When administered correctly, which of the following medications is either contraindicated or should be used with caution when treating suspected cardiac patients who exhibit hypotension: (1) morphine sulfate; (2) magnesium sulfate; (3) nitroglycerin; (4) β-blockers (see ACLS text pp. 9-12 to 9-16)? _____

_____ (a) 1, 3, and 4
_____ (b) 1 and 3
_____ (c) 2 and 3
_____ (d) All of the above

68. Regardless of which protocol in which it appears, atropine is given to rule out the possibility of vagal involvement (see ACLS text pp. 7-4 to 7-6). _____

_____ (a) True
_____ (b) False

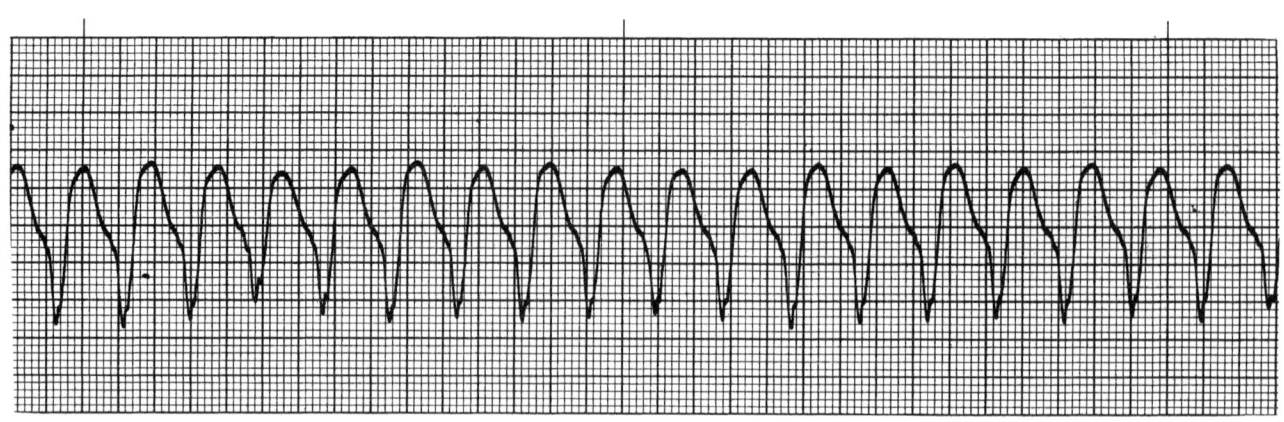

69. This is the rhythm of a 36-year-old man in mild respiratory distress. He denies chest pain, but his respiratory rate evidences apprehension. He states, "My heart is pounding in my chest!" He denies previous episodes or pertinent cardiac history. His vital signs are stable at the present moment, and his lung sounds are bilaterally clear. You order a 12-lead ECG but are unable to verify the origin of the rhythm. What protocol would you consider employing (see ACLS text p. 1-38)? _____

70. A 55-year-old man with SVT presents with a depressed level of consciousness. He is hypotensive with a pulse of 210 beats/minute. Can the patient be given adenosine while charging the paddles for a synchronized cardioversion (see ACLS text p. 1-35)? _____

    _____ (a) Yes
    _____ (b) No

71. When performing carotid massage, the most important thing to assess is (see ACLS text p. 1-37): _____

    _____ (a) The age of the patient
    _____ (b) A history of ischemic heart disease
    _____ (c) The presence of bruits
    _____ (d) A history of eye disease

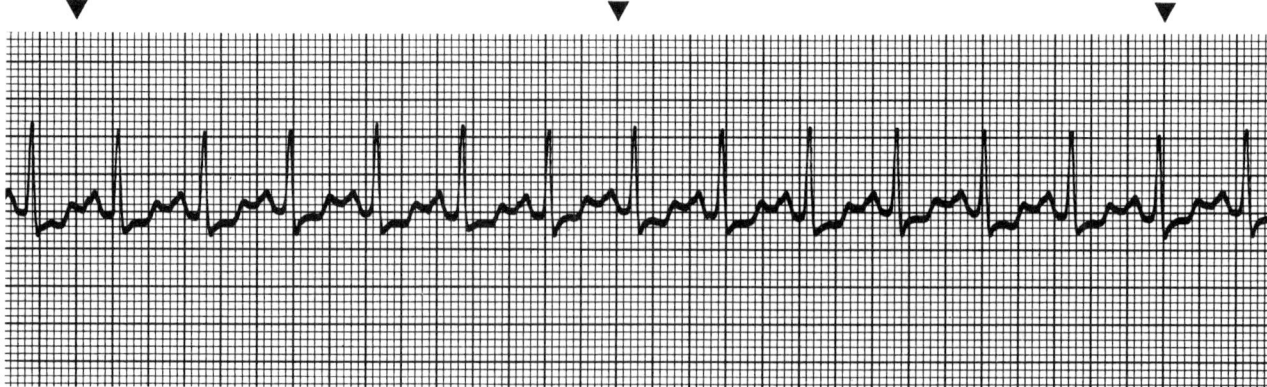

72. A 70-year-old woman has been admitted to the floor of your facility. She has been on a ventilator for chronic obstructive pulmonary disease on a semiregular basis. Her chart notes a long history of smoking, and the emergency staff note that her dyspnea began 2 hours ago. As you take your initial set of vital signs, she becomes both apneic and unresponsive: pulse—130, respirations—0, and BP—100/80. What would you do (see ACLS text pp. 1-9 to 1-11)?

    _____

73. The following are considered end points during the administration of procainamide: (1) the QRS interval widens by at least 75% of its pretreatment width; (2) hypotension develops; (3) a total of 1 g of the drug has been injected at a rate of 20 mg/min; (4) a total of 17 mg/kg of the drug is administered (see ACLS text pp. 7-8 to 7-10). _____

   _____ (a) 1 and 3
   _____ (b) 2 and 4
   _____ (c) 1 and 4
   _____ (d) 1, 2, and 3

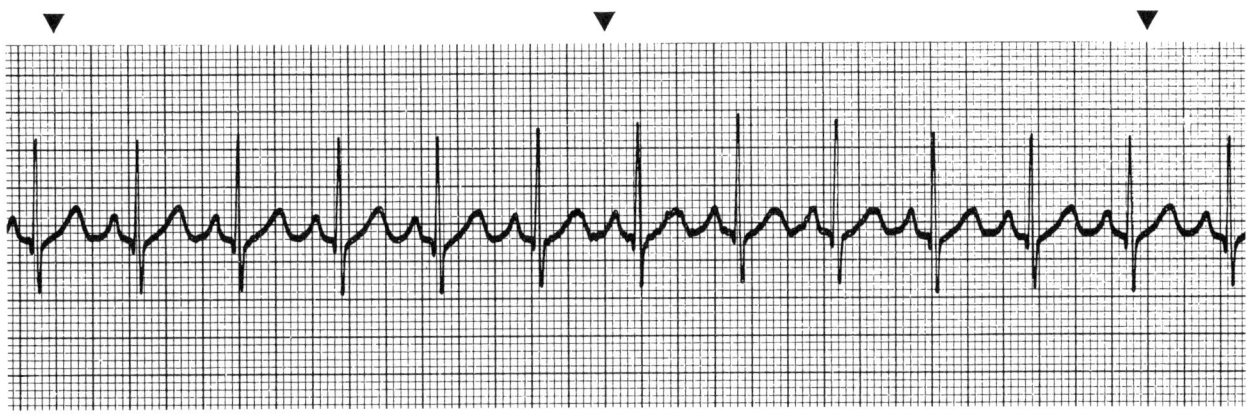

74. While making medication rounds, you enter the room of a 90-year-old man who was admitted for abdominal pain of unknown cause. You just answered his "buzzer" 5 minutes ago and he was alert, but now he responds only to verbal stimuli. Closer inspection discloses that his respirations are rapid and that he is both cool and diaphoretic. A quick set of vital signs reveal the following: pulse—120, respirations—26, and BP—80/50. The ECG appears above. Which protocol would you consider employing for this patient (see ACLS text p. 1-42)? _____

75. Both an OPA and NPA are contraindicated when a deviated septum is noted (see ACLS text pp. 2-2 to 2-3): _____

   _____ (a) True
   _____ (b) False

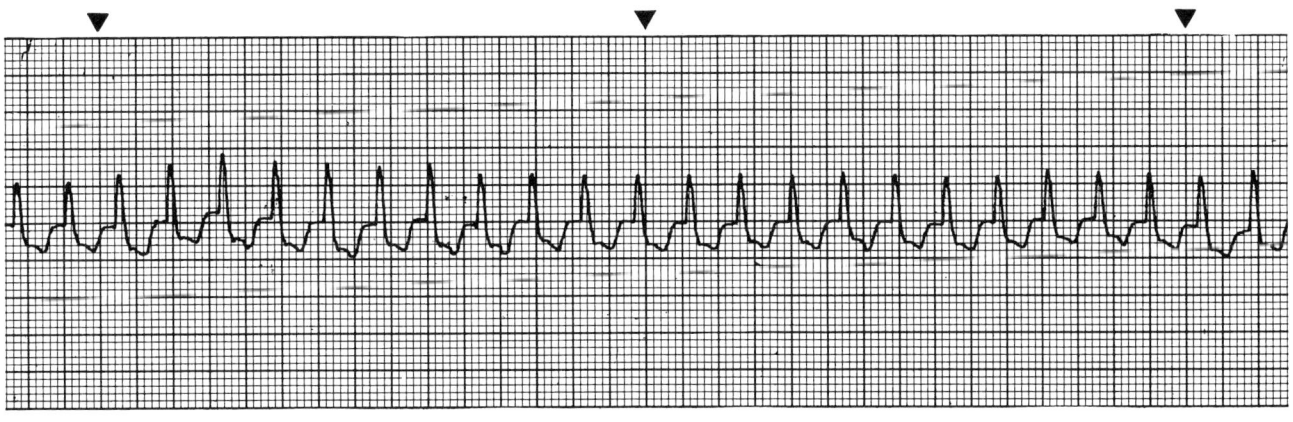

76. A 36-year-old man was admitted for gall bladder surgery. Suddenly, his heart began to pound in his chest. He denies chest pain, difficulty breathing, or an altered level of consciousness. His ECG is noted above. His vital signs are as follows: pulse—210, respirations—18, and BP—132/88. What protocol would you consider employing (see ACLS text pp. 1-36 to 1-38)?

   _____

77. In which of the following cases would endotracheal intubation be recommended: (1) a conscious patient with a suspected MI; (2) a patient unconscious from an aspirin overdose; (3) a normotensive patient with ventricular tachycardia; (4) a patient in cardiac arrest (see ACLS text pp. 2-3 to 2-6)? _____

    _____ (a) 2 and 3
    _____ (b) 1 and 4
    _____ (c) 2 and 4
    _____ (d) 3 and 4

78. An automated external defibrillator (AED) can *analyze* a cardiac rhythm while CPR is in progress (see ACLS text pp. 4-9 to 4-10). _____

    _____ (a) True
    _____ (b) False

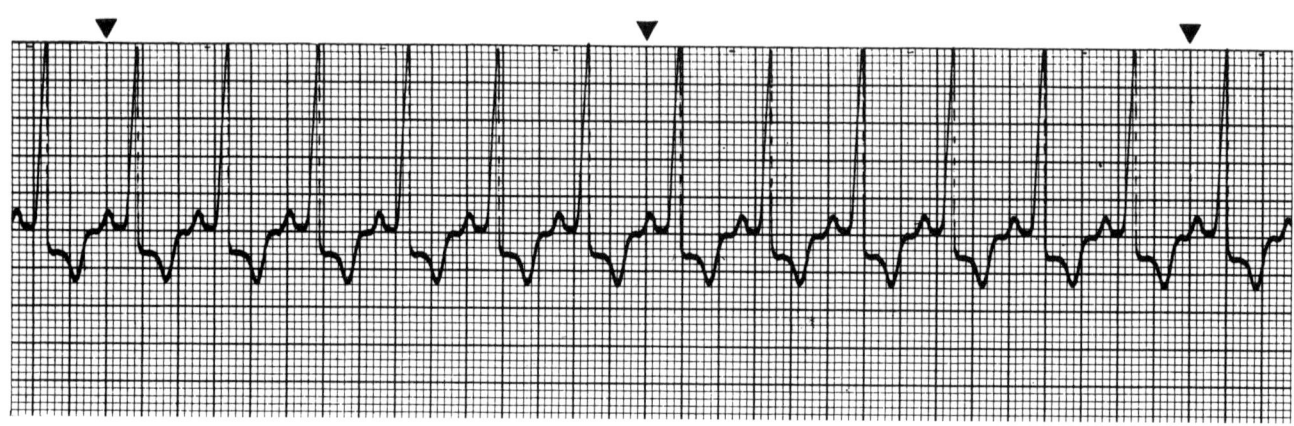

79. Paramedics respond to a home and arrive to find a 40-year-old man lying in a large pool of blood. There are no wounds, but they note congealed blood in the oropharynx. The patient's wife mentions that her husband is a long-term alcoholic. The patient is both pulseless and apneic. A "quick look" from the monitor reveals the above rhythm. What protocol would you consider employing (see ACLS text p. 1-23)? _____

80. In an adult, atropine, 0.5 to 1.0 mg given intravenously, may: (1) assist in accelerating sinus bradycardia; (2) decrease vagal tone; (3) be administered every 3 to 5 minutes to total of 0.04 mg/kg if required; (4) exacerbate, or may not have any effect on, a second-degree, type II or complete heart block (see ACLS text pp. 11-30 to 11-32). _____

    _____ (a) 1, 3, and 4
    _____ (b) 1 and 4
    _____ (c) 1, 2, and 3
    _____ (d) All the above

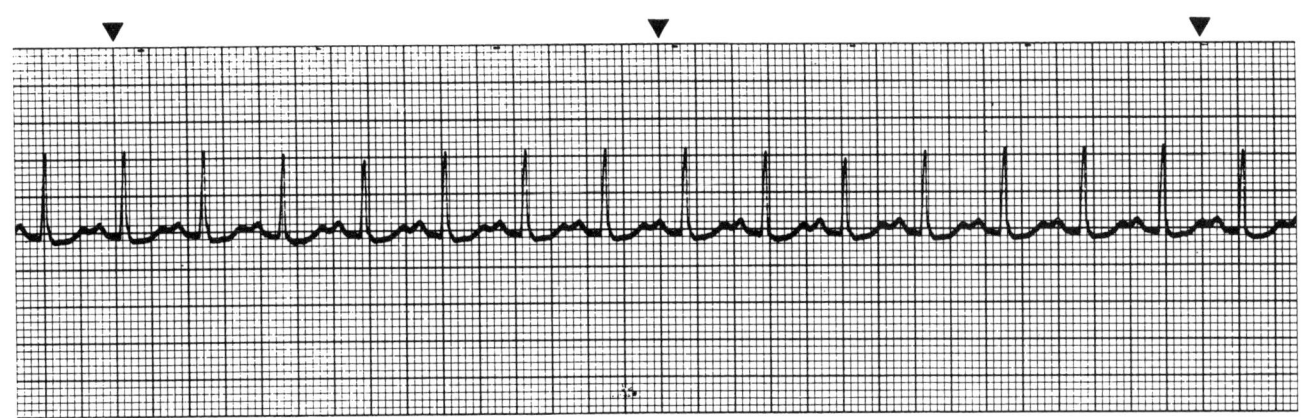

81. An unconscious 47-year-old man presents in the emergency room. His wife states that he had been hit with a baseball bat over his lower left rib margin yesterday. He did not seek medical care then, but 30 minutes ago he started to sweat and complain of intense abdominal pain. His vital signs are as follows: pulse—140, respirations—26, and BP—66/40. The patient's ECG appears above. Which protocol would you consider employing for this patient (see ACLS text p. 1-42)? _____

82. A TCP should always be initiated in rhythms presenting as asystole (see ACLS text p. 1-23). _____

    _____ (a) True
    _____ (b) False

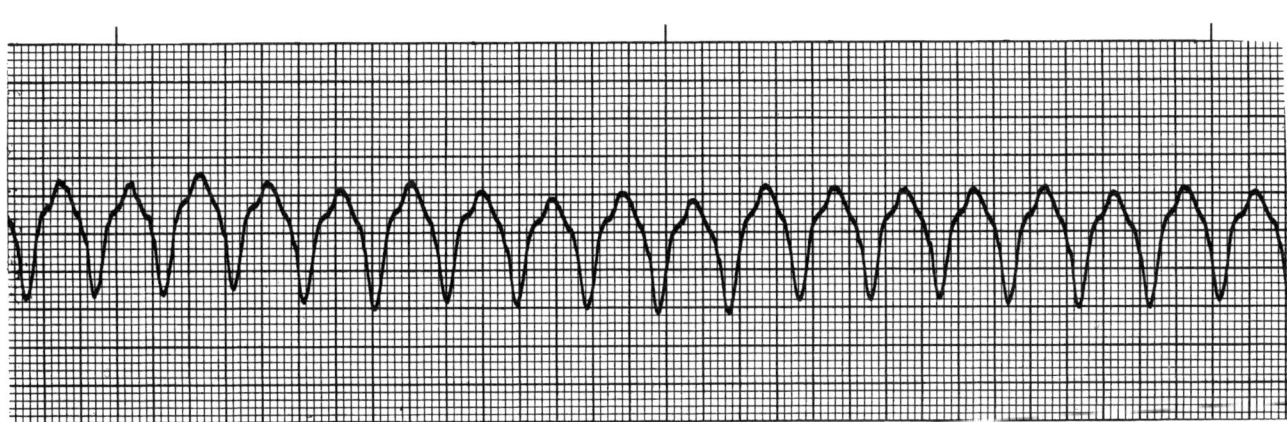

83. A 45-year-old man was being monitored in the CCU. His admitting diagnosis was a lateral MI. The monitor alarm went off, and you noticed the above rhythm on the monitor. The patient denies chest pain or pulmonary edema. A 12-lead ECG was performed and the rhythm verified as ventricular. His vital signs are as follows: pulse—150, respirations—22 (rate due to apprehension—lung sounds are clear), and BP—112/92. What protocol would you consider employing (see ACLS text p. 1-39)? _____

84. The most common cause of sudden death in men is (see ACLS text p. 17-1): _____

    _____ (a) Acute MI
    _____ (b) Coronary heart disease
    _____ (c) Foreign body airway obstruction
    _____ (d) Digitalis overdose

85. When dealing with a symptomatic bradycardia refractory to atropine, the definitive treatment modality would be an isoproterenol drip at 1 mg in 250 mL of D-5-W infused at 2 to 10 mcg/min (see ACLS text p. 1-30). _____

_____ (a) True
_____ (b) False

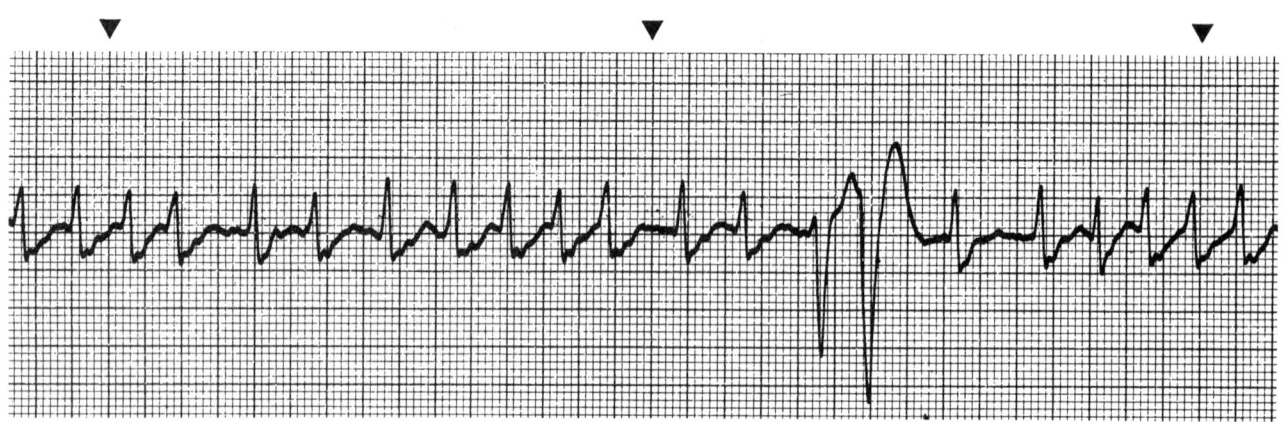

86. This is the rhythm of a 67-year-old woman who was brought into the emergency room by her husband. She has been taking digitalis for congestive heart failure (CHF) and atrial fibrillation. She is now cool and clammy and presenting with a depressed level of consciousness. Her vital signs are as follows: BP—80/60, pulse—180, and respirations—18. What protocol would you consider employing (see ACLS text p. 1-35)? _____

87. The difference between *emergent* and *elective* cardioversion is primarily *where* the procedure is accomplished (see ACLS text p. 1-35). _____

   _____ (a) True
   _____ (b) False

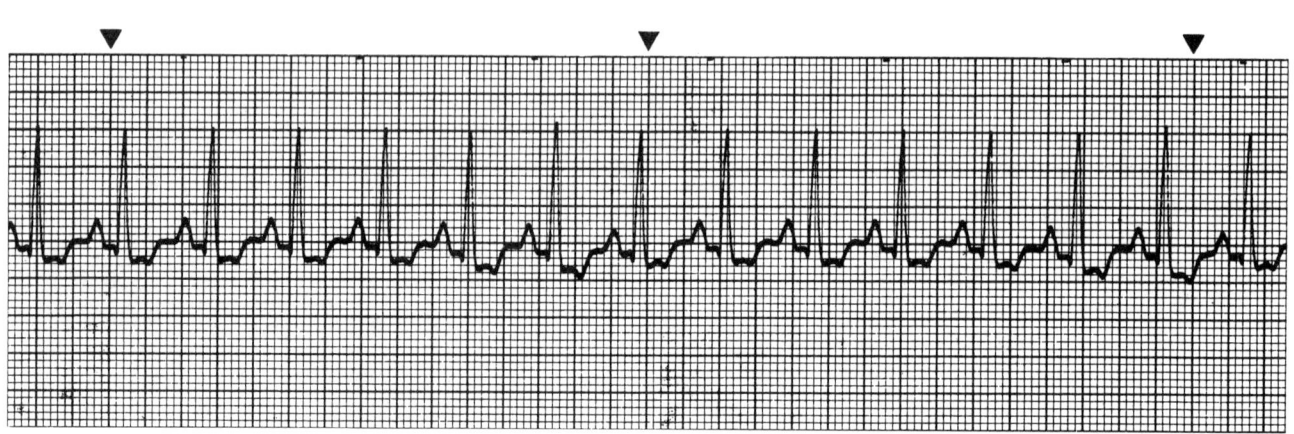

88. This is a rhythm of a 67-year-old woman complaining of difficulty breathing. Her tachycardic ECG is noted above. Her lungs reveal rales and rhonchi bilaterally. Her vital signs are as follows: pulse—130, respirations—36, BP—160/98. Which protocol would you consider employing for this patient (see ACLS text pp. 1-40 to 1-43)? _____

89. Calcium chloride is used as an antidote in all of the following *except* (see ACLS text pp. 7-16 to 7-17): _____

   _____ (a) Diltiazem overdose
   _____ (b) Adenosine overdose
   _____ (c) Verapamil overdose
   _____ (d) Hypocalcemia

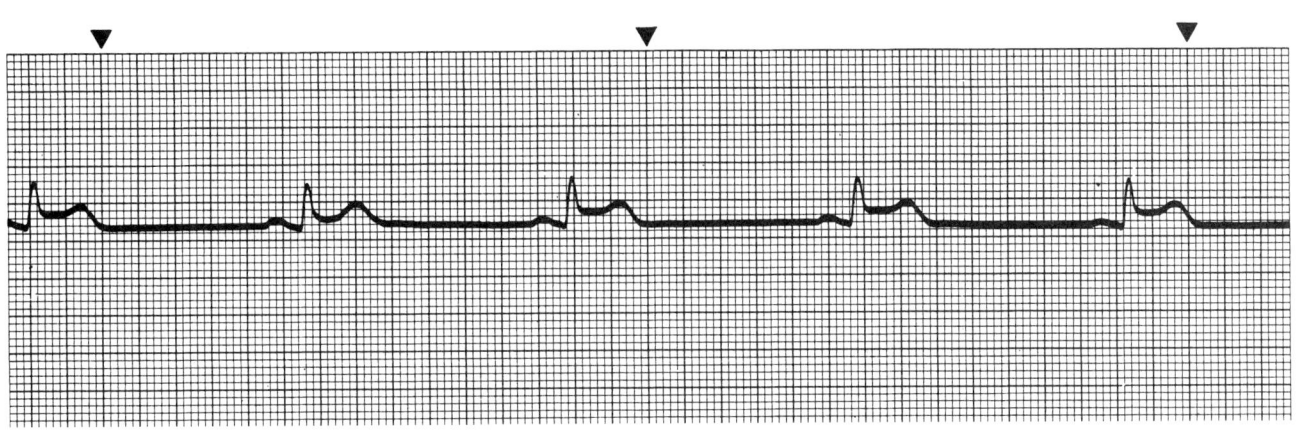

90. This is the rhythm of a 56-year-old woman who came into the emergency room complaining of "passing out" at home frequently over the last 2 days. She now presents to you with a depressed level of consciousness, cool extremities, and diaphoresis. Her vital signs are a palpated systolic BP of 60, pulse—45, and respirations—14. What protocol would you consider employing (see ACLS text pp. 1-30 to 1-31)? _____

91. The most common adverse reaction to bretylium when given for dysrhythmias other than ventricular fibrillation (see ACLS text pp. 7-10 to 7-11): _____

    _____ (a) Nausea and vomiting
    _____ (b) An initial bradycardic rate
    _____ (c) Postural hypotension
    _____ (d) Diuresis

92. Intubation should be performed during the secondary survey only (see ACLS text p. 1-9).
    _____
    _____ (a) True
    _____ (b) False

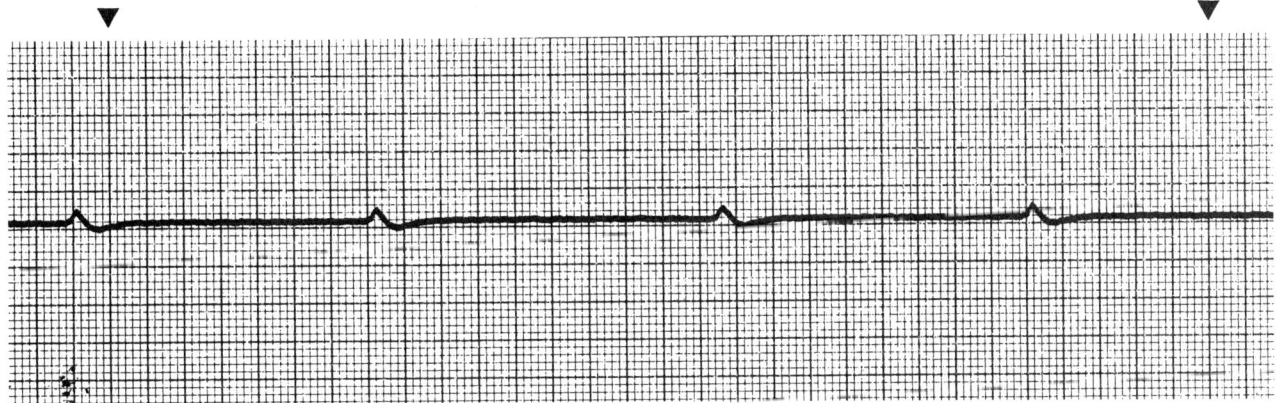

93. A 33-year-old woman was exhibiting narrow complex tachycardia at a rate of 190 beats/minute. She became uncomfortable after tolerating this rhythm for 1 hour. She was given intravenous NS and oxygen by nasal cannula. After checking for the presence of bruits, you begin carotid massage. After the second set, the patient collapses to the gurney unconscious. Her vital signs are absent, and the monitor reveals the above strip. What protocol would you consider employing (see ACLS text pp. 1-23 to 1-26)? _____

94. Infectious complications of intravenous cannulas can be minimized by (see ACLS text pp. 6-1 to 6-12): (1) careful aseptic technique during insertion; (2) systemic antibiotics in nearly all

patients; (3) removal of cannula after 3 days; (4) capping the stopcock when not in use (see ACLS text pp. 6-1 to 6-12). _____

_____ (a) 1, 2, and 3
_____ (b) 1, 3, and 4
_____ (c) 2, 3, and 4
_____ (d) All of the above

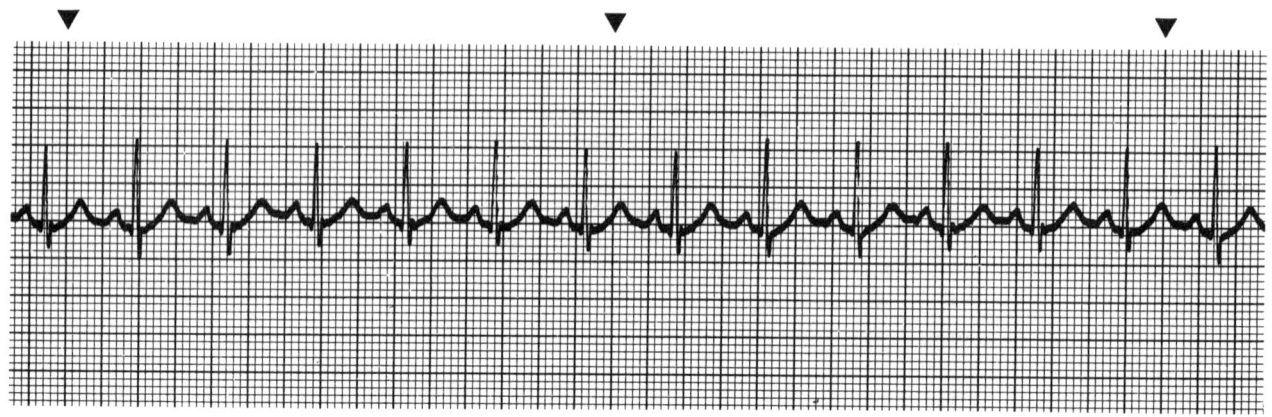

95. A 72-year-old man presents to the emergency room conscious and coherent but exhibiting acute pulmonary edema. His son states that he had a sudden onset of rapid, difficult breathing for the past hour. His vital signs are as follows: pulse—125, respirations—40, BP—140/100. Which protocol would you consider using (see ACLS text pp. 1-45 to 1-46)? _____

96. When performing the primary survey, the airway maneuver of choice in an emergency department is (see ACLS text p. 1-6): _____

_____ (a) Head-tilt, neck-lift
_____ (b) Head-tilt, chin-lift
_____ (c) Jaw thrust
_____ (d) Coma position (head in crook of arm)

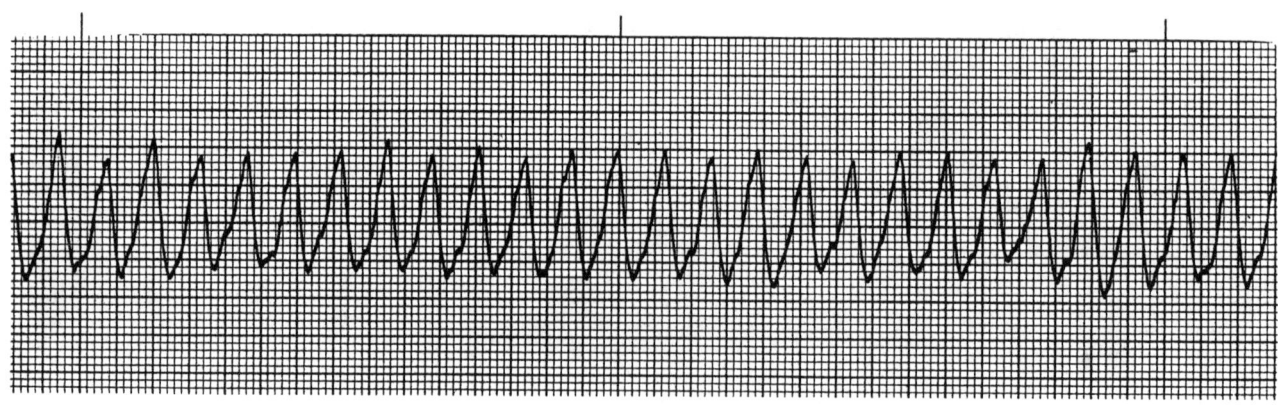

97. A 36-year-old woman is escorting her daughter through the emergency room to Labor and Delivery. As she walks past you, she confides that she has been experiencing an unusual bout of tachycardia for the last half hour. She is concerned that she is having a heart attack; however, she is not experiencing any chest pain or difficulty breathing and did not wish to alarm her pregnant daughter. You put her on a monitor, and the above rhythm is noted. Her vital signs are as follows: pulse—240, respirations—18, and BP—132/88. The 12-lead ECG is available, but no one qualified is nearby to read it. What protocol would you consider using (see ACLS text pp. 1-37 to 1-39)? _____

98. Assuming minimal charging time, how many shocks would you expect an AED-equipped rescuer to deliver to a patient within a 15-minute period of time (see ACLS text p. 1-13)? _____

   _____ (a) 3 to 9
   _____ (b) 10 to 22
   _____ (c) 22 to 45
   _____ (d) 45 or more

99. Cardiac tamponade (see ACLS text p. 1-21): (1) may profit initially from an increased preload; (2) results from excess fluid in the pericardium; (3) can be caused by intracardiac injection; (4) should be suspected if venous pressure is elevated and arterial pressure is low. _____

   _____ (a) 2 and 4
   _____ (b) 1, 3, and 4
   _____ (c) 1, 2, and 3
   _____ (d) All of the above

100. A 70-year-old woman has been removed from a ventilator. Her $Paco_2$ is now elevated, and her vital signs are deteriorating quickly. Her pulse is starting to drop into the bradycardic range noted on the above EC6. While you examine her, she ceases breathing. What would you do? _____

101. When gathering a history of an asystolic patient, which of the following histories would *not* point to hypothermia as the cause (see ACLS text pp. 11-1 to 11-4)? _____

   _____(a) History of exposure
   _____(b) History of alcoholism
   _____(c) History of diabetes
   _____(d) History of aspirin overdose

102. Large doses of morphine sulfate can result in transitional hypertension as well as respiratory depression (see ACLS text p. 7-16). _____

   _____(a) True
   _____(b) False

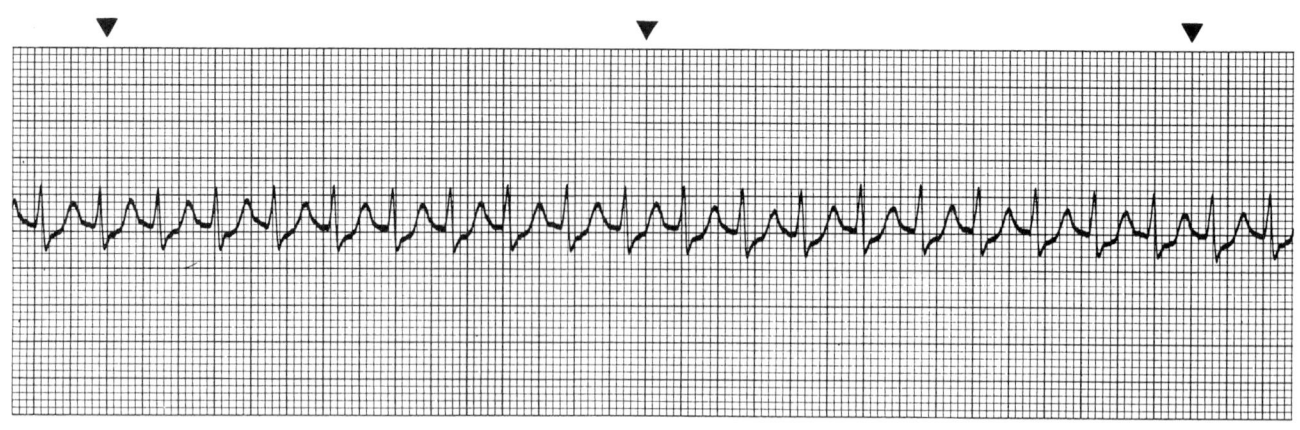

103. This is the rhythm of a 23-year-old woman who presents to you alert and coherent, complaining of a "sudden onset of rapid heart rate." The patient's vital signs appear stable, and she denies chest pain and difficulty breathing. She tolerated this rhythm for 2 hours before seeking help. What protocol would you consider using (see ACLS text pp. 1-36 to 1-38)? _____

104. After oxygenating the patient, which of the following is the *first* treatment for a hemodynamically significant bradycardia (see ACLS text p. 1-30)? _____

    _____ (a) Epinephrine
    _____ (b) Dopamine
    _____ (c) Atropine
    _____ (d) Isoproterenol (Isuprel)

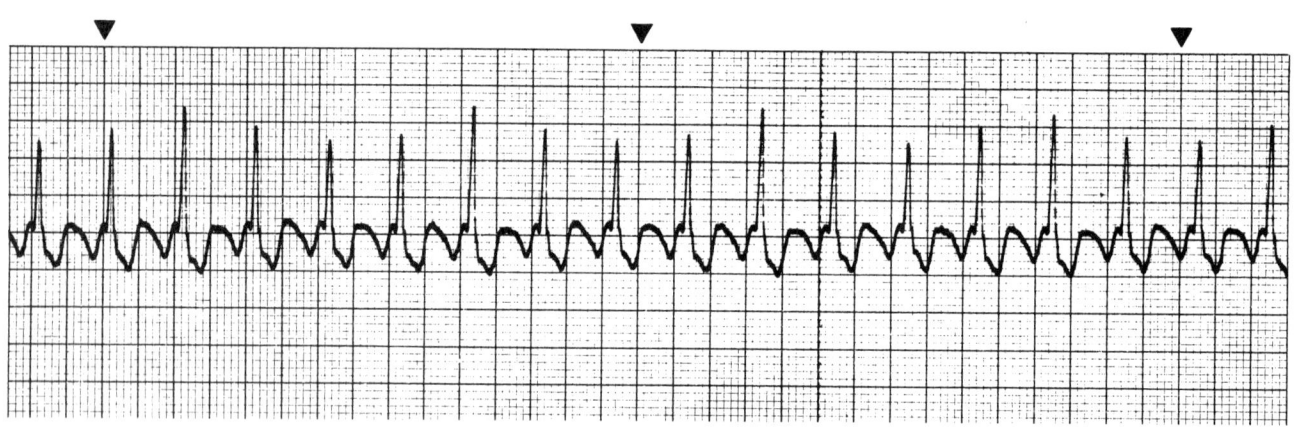

105. A 55-year-old man was admitted to the CCU for a suspected MI. Although apprehensive, he appeared to be tolerating the above rapid rhythm. After 1 hour, however, he became unconscious. His vital signs are as follows: pulse—150, respirations—12, and BP—70/60. Which protocol would you consider employing for this patient (see ACLS text p. 1-36)? _____

106. If the monitor-defibrillator has difficulty synchronizing on an R wave in an *unstable* polymorphic ventricular tachycardia (irregular morphology and rate), it is perfectly acceptable to turn off the synchronizer and defibrillate (see ACLS text p. 1-39). _____

    _____ (a) True
    _____ (b) False

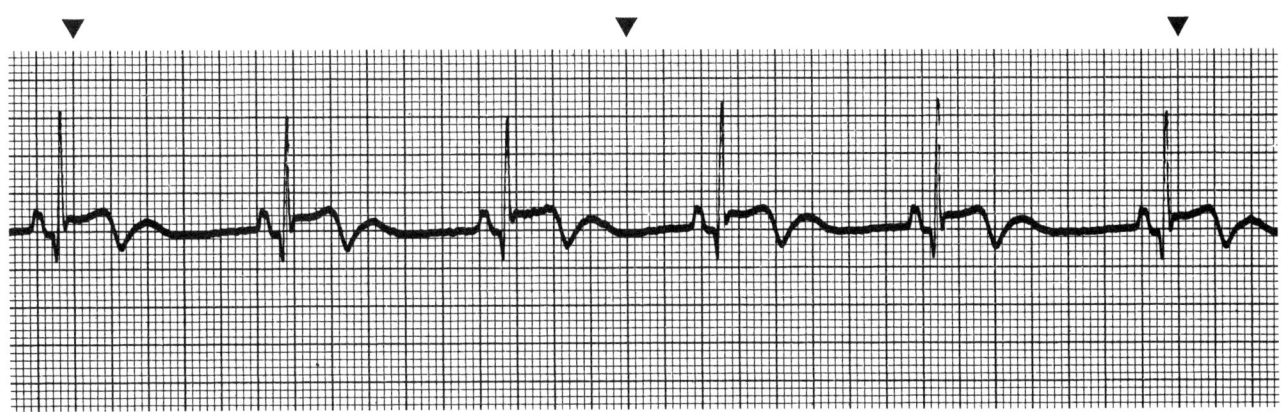

107. A 45-year-old man was admitted for chest pain. During your medication rounds to his CCU room, you note that the patient is both pulseless and apneic. When the monitor arrives, it reveals the above rhythm. What protocol would you consider using (see ACLS text pp. 1-21 to 1-23)? _____

108. All QRS complexes that are wide and rapid can be assumed to represent ventricular tachycardia (see ACLS text p. 1-38). _____

   _____ (a) True
   _____ (b) False

109. An adult victim who needs continued CPR has had an endotracheal tube inserted. In conjunction with the endotracheal tube, it is acceptable to use: (1) a manually triggered, time-cycled ventilation device (a demand valve); (2) a pressure-cycled automatic resuscitator (Bird or Bennett); (3) a BVM; (4) an OPA (see ACLS text pp. 1-9 to 1-10). _____

   _____ (a) 1, 2, and 3
   _____ (b) 2, 3, and 4
   _____ (c) 1, 3, and 4
   _____ (d) 1, 2, and 4

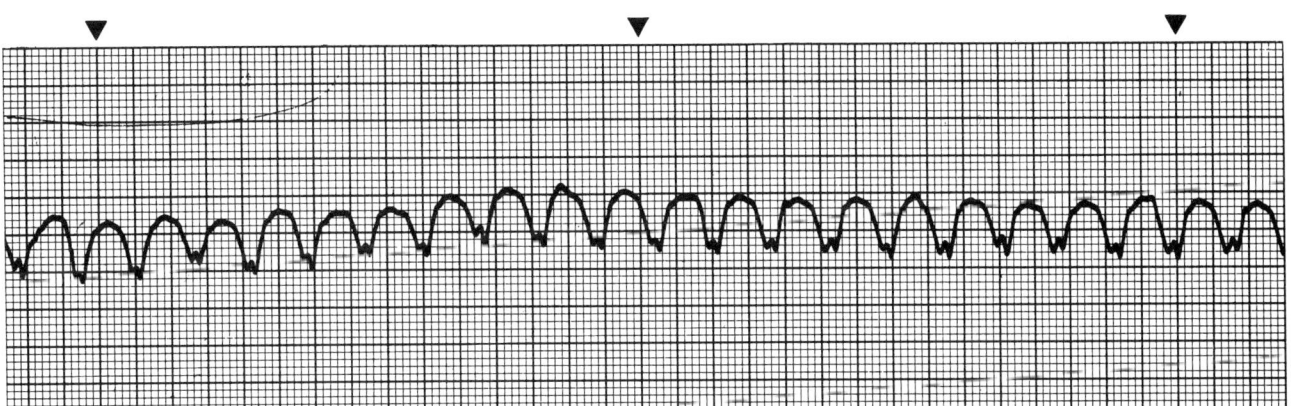

110. A 45-year-old man was lying on the gurney in the emergency room. His chief complaint was left lower quadrant abdominal pain. As you are taking a history and performing a physical examination, he grasps your arm and states that his heart just started palpitating. He denies chest pain and difficulty breathing. His rhythm appears above. A 12-lead ECG verifies it as a ventricular rhythm. His vital signs are as follows: pulse—180, respirations—22 (just apprehension—lung sounds are clear), and BP—102/90. What protocol would you consider using (see ACLS text p. 1-39)? _____

111. The basic difference between the primary and secondary surveys is that the rescuer's responsibilities during the secondary survey are targeted at mainly reverifying the primary survey (see ACLS text pp. 1-4 to 1-11). _____
   _____(a) True
   _____(b) False

112. The primary reason that defibrillation must be employed within 10 minutes after onset of ventricular fibrillation is (see ACLS text pp. 1-15): _____
   _____(a) Past that time limit, hypoxia has resulted in a nonneutralizable systemic acidosis.
   _____(b) Excessive fibrillation causes cardiac muscle to burn up the finite supply of neurotransmitters.
   _____(c) Fibrillation consumes high-energy phosphates (adenosine triphosphate [ATP]) more rapidly than other cardiac rhythms.
   _____(d) After 10 minutes, the transthoracic resistance becomes too much to overcome with 360 joules.

113. This is the rhythm of a 22-year-old man who was involved in a gang fight. He was struck with a baseball bat on the left lower rib margin. He did not seek medical aid for 2 days, but when his condition worsened, he called 911. He now presents to you with a BP of 70/40, pulse of 130, diaphoresis, and cool extremities. His respiratory rate is 26, and his monitor reveals the above rhythm. What protocol would you consider using (see ACLS text p. 1-42)? _____

114. Whenever trauma has been noted as a cause of a life-threatening emergency, the practitioner should look specifically for the presence of (see ACLS text p. 1-21): (1) tension pneumothorax; (2) hypocalcemia; (3) cardiac tamponade; (4) pulmonary edema. _____
   _____(a) 1 and 2
   _____(b) 2 and 4
   _____(c) 3 and 4
   _____(d) 1 and 3

115. The term *door-to-drug interval* implies (see ACLS text p. 9-18): _____
   _____(a) The interval necessary for a drug dealer to remove narcotics from the emergency room and sprint for the door
   _____(b) The time interval for a cardiac patient to receive narcotics when brought into the emergency room
   _____(c) The amount of drug necessary to alleviate pain before discharging a patient from the emergency room
   _____(d) The interval between when a patient comes into the emergency room and when he receives thrombolytic therapy

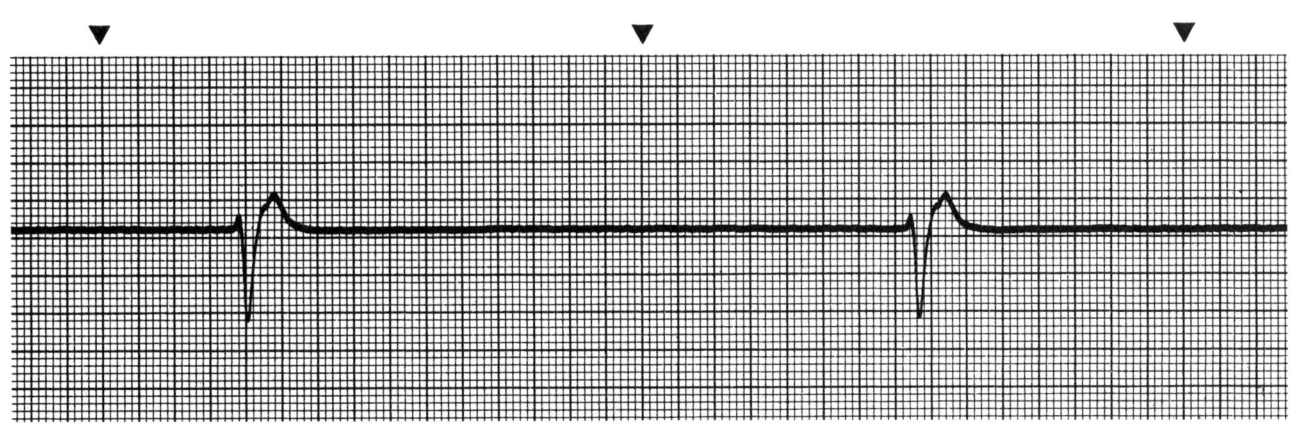

116. This is the rhythm of a 65-year-old man who was found in the intensive care unit in cardiac arrest. What protocol would you consider using (see ACLS text p. 1-23)? _____

117. A 45-year-old woman with a history of angina claims to have had severe chest pain for 45 minutes. She was initially alert but is now drowsy, cool, and diaphoretic. Her vital signs are as follows: pulse—45, BP—80/60, and respirations—12. Her ECG reveals a sinus bradycardia with occasional ventricular escape beats. The first drug to consider is (see ACLS text p. 1-30): _____

　　___(a) Lidocaine, 50 mg given by intravenous bolus
　　___(b) Isoproterenol, 1 to 2 mg in 500 mL of D-5-W; titrate to a pulse of 60 beats/minute
　　___(c) Epinephrine, 1.0 mg given intravenously slowly over 1 to 2 minutes
　　___(d) Atropine, 0.5 to 1.0 mg given intravenously

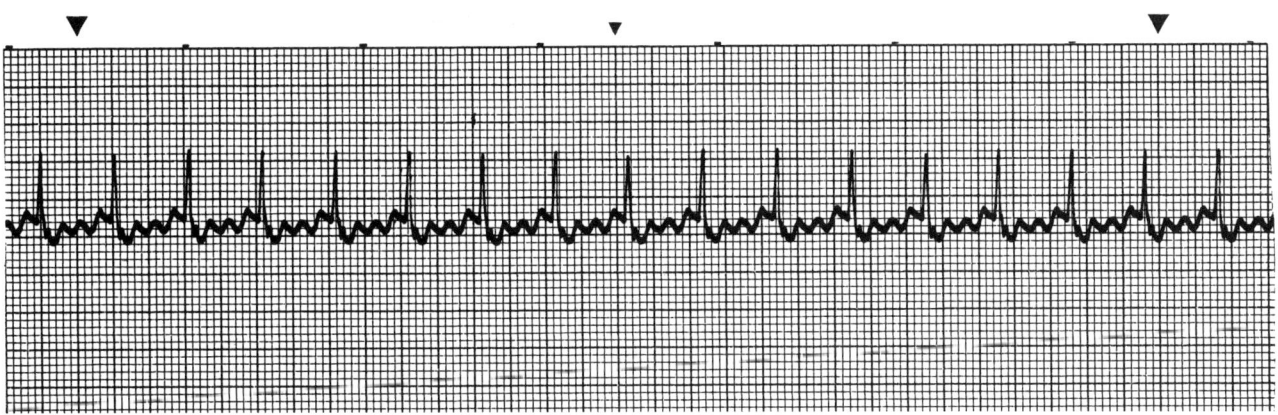

118. A 68-year-old man has been tolerating the above rhythm for 2 days and now presents to you in the hospital. He is alert and coherent but is becoming apprehensive that the tachycardia will never stop. His vital signs are as follows: pulse—145, respirations—20, and BP—180/98. Which protocol would you consider employing for this patient (see ACLS text p. 1-36)? _____

119. A monitor-defibrillator may fail to synchronize for all of the following reasons *except* (see ACLS text pp. 1-32 to 1-36 and 1-39 and 4-7): _____

　　___(a) Your machine may be switched over to the "only synchronize on the P wave" mode.
　　___(b) The rhythm may not have an obvious R wave.
　　___(c) The operator is not constantly holding down the firing buttons.
　　___(d) The ECG amplitude (size) is too small.

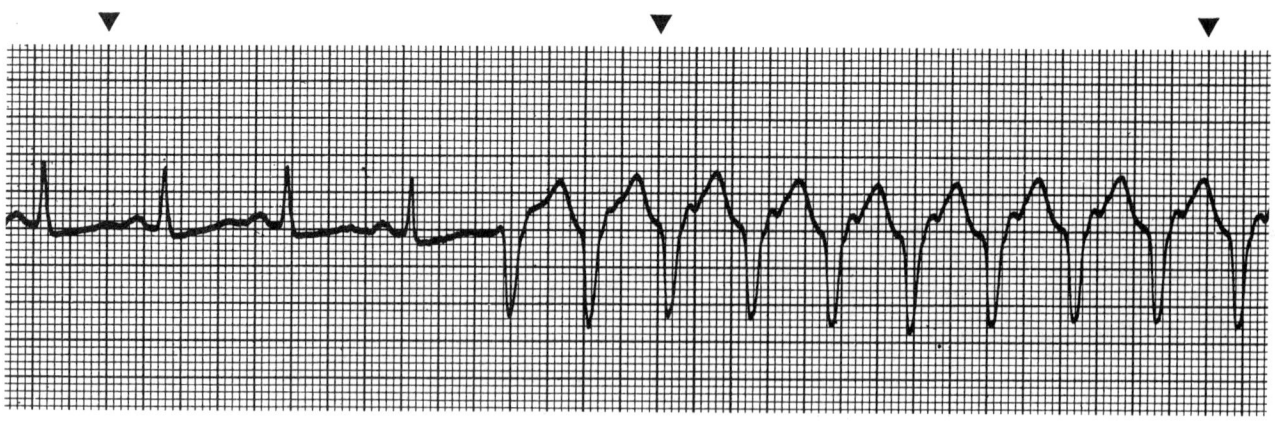

120. A paramedic unit responds to a doctor's clinic. The physician relates to you that while a 43-year-old woman was being hooked up to a one-lead ECG, she started complaining of a pounding in her chest. The rhythm is noted above. She is presently alert and coherent and denies any chest pain or pulmonary edema. There was not a 12-lead machine in the clinic. Her vital signs are as follows: pulse—150, respirations—24 (apprehension only), and BP—108/88. Which protocol would you select for this patient (see ACLS text p. 1-38)? _____

121. Adenosine: (1) has a 5- to 10-second half-life; (2) is an exogenous synthetic nucleoside that accelerates entry through the atrioventricular (AV) node; (3) is not effective in AV nodal *reentry* arrhythmias; (4) has chest pain as one of the more frequently observed side effects; (5) is the preferred treatment for narrow complex SVT (see ACLS text p. 7-13). _____

　_____(a) 1, 3, 4, and 5
　_____(b) 1 and 2
　_____(c) 1, 4, and 5
　_____(d) 2

122. All of the following are acceptable for endotracheal tube administration *except* (see ACLS text p. 1-10): _____

　_____(a) Lidocaine
　_____(b) Atropine
　_____(c) Sodium bicarbonate
　_____(d) Epinephrine

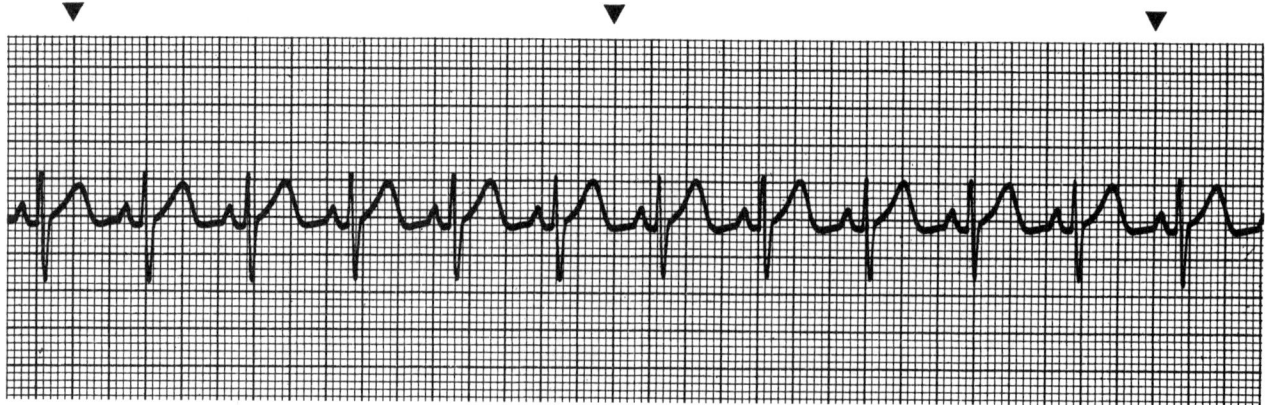

123. A 34-year-old woman is found at home both pulseless and apneic. On physical examination, you note needle marks on her abdomen. When ventilated, her exhalation smells fruity. Her skin is hot to the touch, and your search of the refrigerator reveals bottles of insulin. A "quick look" from the monitor reveals the above rhythm. What protocol would you consider using (see ACLS text pp. 1-21 to 1-23)? _____

124. During two-person CPR, it is necessary to stop compressions while ventilating an intubated patient (see ACLS text p. 2-3): _____

   _____(a) True
   _____(b) False

125. Research statistics note that AEDs deliver a shock when monitoring artifact in a statistically significant percentage of patients (see ACLS text pp. 4-8 to 4-9). _____

   _____(a) True
   _____(b) False

126. A 45-year-old husband of an in-patient has just been informed that his wife has been diagnosed with an inoperable brain tumor. At the nurse's desk, he grabs his chest and collapses to the floor unconscious. Your nearby monitor-defibrillator reveals the above rhythm. He is both pulseless and apneic. What protocol would you consider using (see ACLS text pp. 1-14 to 1-16)? _____

127. Intracardiac injection of epinephrine may cause various complications. Which of the following is not normally a complication (see ACLS text p. 14-4)? _____

   _____(a) Pneumothorax, simple or tension
   _____(b) Hyperpnea
   _____(c) Cardiac tamponade
   _____(d) Injection of epinephrine into the myocardial muscle

128. Clinical benefits, at any level, are noted if thrombolytics are administered within: (1) onset of symptoms to 90 minutes; (2) 90 minutes to 6 hours; (3) 6 hours to 24 hours; (4) 24 hours to 36 hours (see ACLS text p. 9-17). _____

   _____(a) 1 and 2
   _____(b) 1, 2, and 3
   _____(c) 1, 2, 3, and 4
   _____(d) None of the above selections

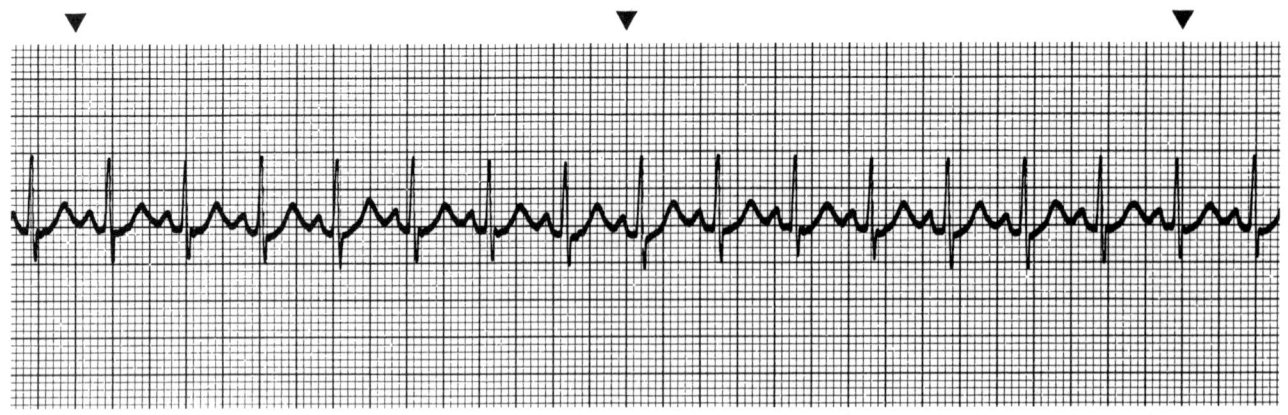

129. This is the rhythm of an 85-year-old man who has been bedridden for the past 2 weeks with a bad back. He is diaphoretic and experiencing acute breathing difficulty. When questioned, he barely responds and has a depressed level of consciousness, peripheral cyanosis, and pink frothy sputum bubbling from his mouth. His vital signs are as follows: pulse—150, respirations—24, and BP—130/100. His rhythm appears above. What protocol would you consider using (see ACLS text pp. 1-45 to 1-46)? _____

130. A mobile unit is bringing in a 46-year-old, 220-pound man. He has severe chest pain and a sinus bradycardia of 45 beats/minute, which responded to atropine initially. After 2.0 mg and 10 minutes later, the unit personnel reports a pulse of 40 and a blood pressure of 70/50. You would advise (see ACLS text pp. 1-30 to 1-31): (1) epinephrine drip, 2 to 10 mcg/min; (2) dopamine, 2 to 20 mcg/kg/min; (3) isoproterenol, 2 to 10 mcg/min; (4) additional atropine until a total dose of 4 mg is reached. _____

_____(a) 2
_____(b) 1
_____(c) 2, 3, and 4
_____(d) 2 and 4

131. When making a clinical judgment about a patient's stability, which of the following *usually* differentiates stable from unstable tachycardias most of the time: (1) level of consciousness; (2) pacemaker cell origin; (3) hypotensive vital signs; (4) other signs of cardiovascular compromise (e.g., chest pain, pulmonary edema) (see ACLS text pp. 1-35 to 1-37)? _____

_____(a) 1, 3, and 4
_____(b) 1, 2, and 3
_____(c) 3 and 4
_____(d) All of the above

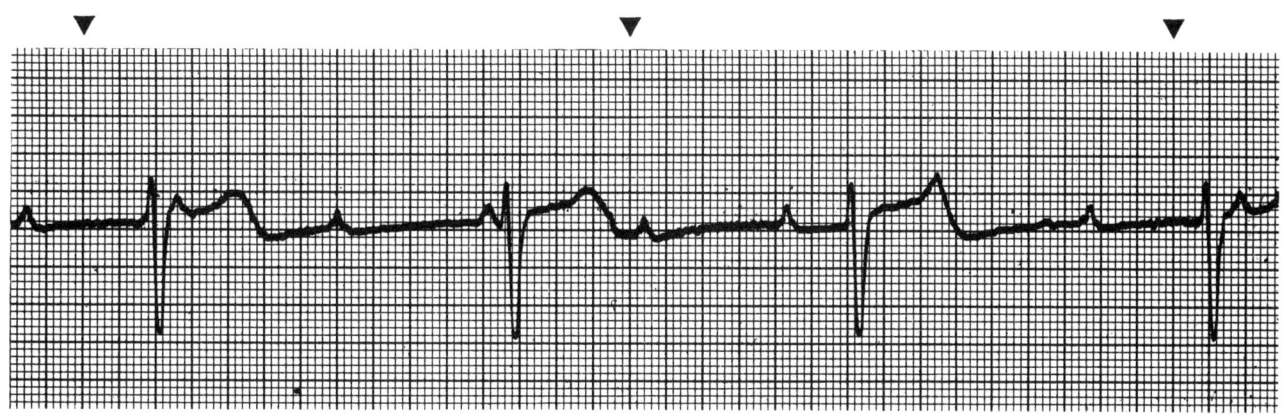

132. You are called to respond to a 66-year-old woman at a nursing home. On arrival, you note that she responds only to painful stimulation. She is both cool and clammy, and her skin is pale. Her vital signs are as follows: BP—76/60, respirations—10, pulse—38. Her monitor reveals the above. What protocol would you consider using (see ACLS text pp. 1-30 to 1-31)? _____

133. The purpose of the endotracheal tube stylet is to (see ACLS text p. 2-4): _____
    _____(a) Manipulate the vocal cords
    _____(b) Make the endotracheal tube firmer and conform more easily
    _____(c) Push the walls of the trachea apart
    _____(d) Secure the tube to the laryngoscope blade

134. Complications seen with the catheter-through-needle (Intracath) system include (see ACLS text pp. 6-2 to 6-3): (1) infection; (2) hematoma; (3) shearing off the catheter tip if the catheter is withdrawn back through the needle; (4) extravasation of the infused fluid. _____
    _____(a) 1, 2, and 4
    _____(b) 1 and 3
    _____(c) 2, 3, and 4
    _____(d) All of the above

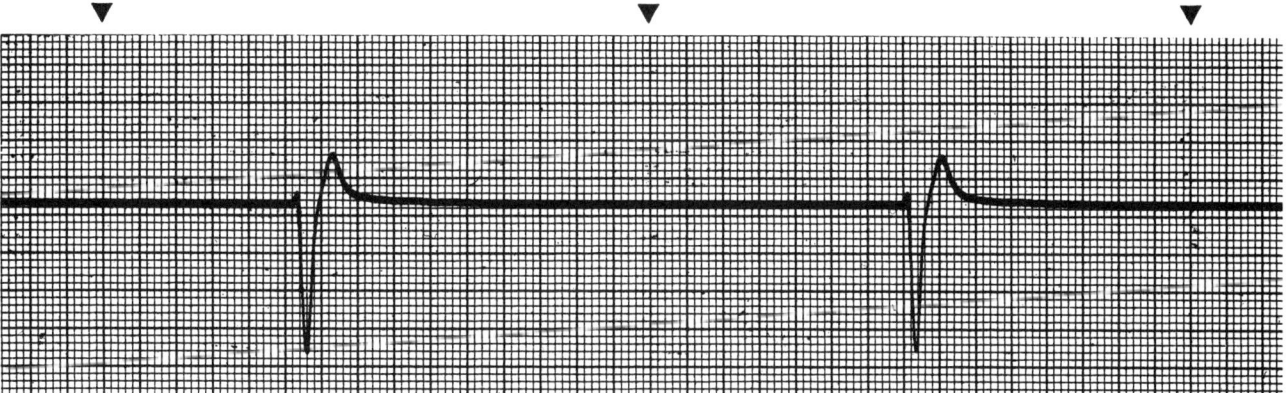

135. The emergency medical technicians have responded to an alleyway, where a 55-year-old man is lying on the street. Although it is not quite winter, the patient is unprotected from the chilly environment—his coat and shoes apparently stolen when he passed out. His skin is cold to the touch, and his respirations are 6 and shallow. When placed on the gurney, he immediately arrests. His monitor reveals the above rhythm. What protocol would you consider using (see ACLS text pp. 1-22, 1-24, and 11-2)? _____

136. Which of the dosing schemes of epinephrine are correct (see ACLS text p. 1-16)? _____
    _____ (a) Standard dosage of 2 mg given intravenously every 7 minutes
    _____ (b) Intermediate dosage of 1 mg—3 mg—7 mg given intravenously every 3 to 5 minutes
    _____ (c) Escalating dosage of 3 mg—7 mg—10 mg every 3 to 5 minutes
    _____ (d) High dosage of 0.1 mg/kg every 3 to 5 minutes.

137. In ventricular fibrillation, sodium bicarbonate may be administered before ventricular antiarrhythmics when the patient is suspected to be suffering from bicarbonate-responsive situations such as a TCA overdose or acute hyperkalemia (see ACLS text p. 7-15). _____
    _____ (a) True
    _____ (b) False

138. This is the rhythm of a 48-year-old man who presented to you with "heart palpitations." He is alert and coherent. His vital signs are BP—106/90, pulse—210, respirations—20 and clear. He denies chest pain and difficulty breathing but is extremely apprehensive. What protocol would you consider using (see ACLS text pp. 1-36 to 1-37)? _____

139. The maximal benefits of thrombolytics are obtainable if the time interval (infarct onset to thrombolytic administration) is kept to (see ACLS text pp. 9-9 to 9-12 and 9-17): _____
    _____ (a) Less than 90 minutes
    _____ (b) Within 6 hours
    _____ (c) Within 24 hours
    _____ (d) Within 36 hours

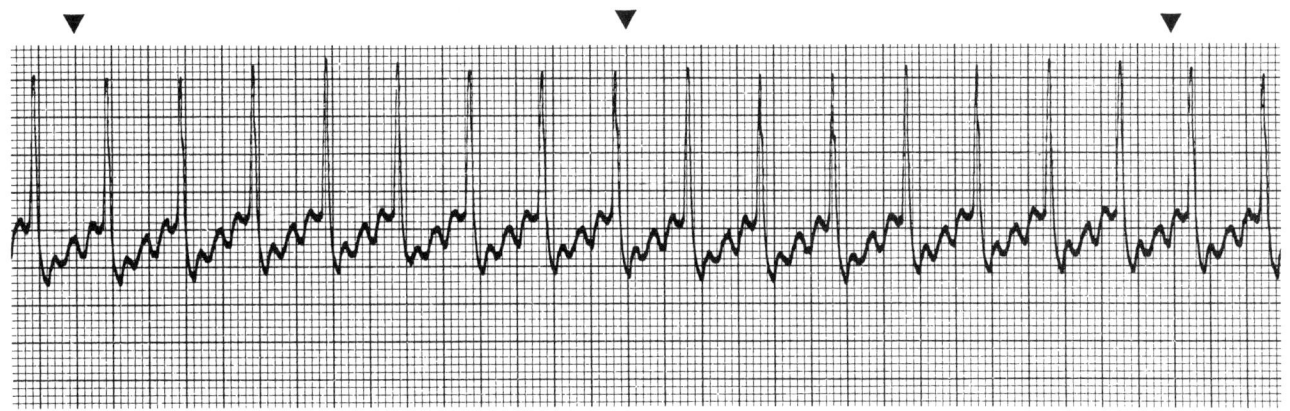

140. This is the rhythm of a 35-year-old woman who presents to you with a depressed level of consciousness only arousable with painful stimuli. Her husband relates that she has been been complaining about her rapid pulse all morning. Her vital signs are as follows: pulse—150, respirations—12, BP—78/60. What protocol would you consider employing (see ACLS text p. 1-36)? _____

141. At dosage ranges of 1 to 2 mcg/kg/min, dopamine can be expected to cause (see ACLS text p. 8-3): _____

    _____ (a) Mesenteric and renal vasodilation
    _____ (b) Increased inotropic and chronotropic activity
    _____ (c) Vasoconstriction
    _____ (d) Renal shutdown

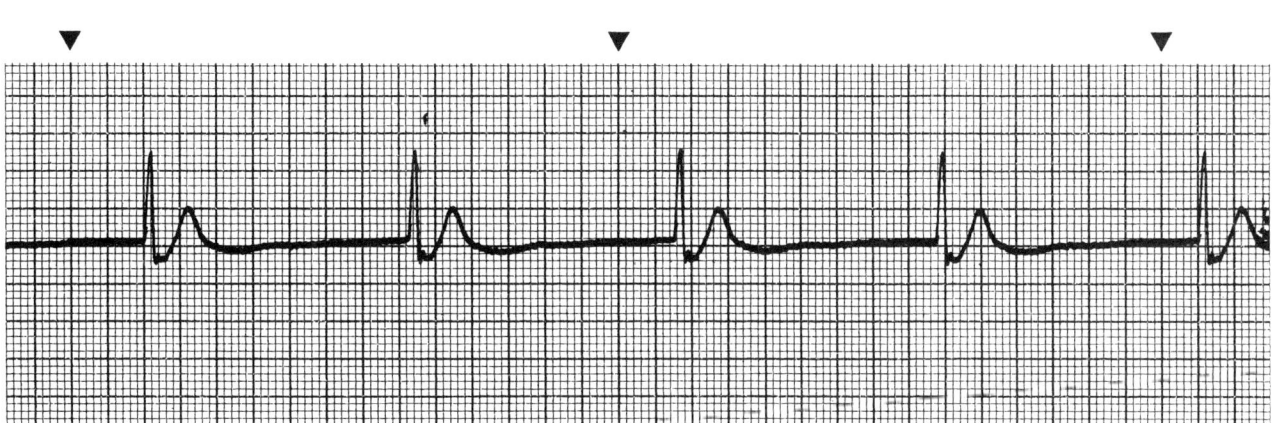

142. The paramedics respond to a request for help from a victim of gang violence. The 17-year-old boy has a single puncture wound just to the left of the sternum below the left nipple. Before your arrival, his girlfriend stated that he was having extreme difficulty breathing. She also was observant enough to tell you that the veins on his neck stuck out like tautly pulled cords. Currently, he is both pulseless and apneic. A "quick look" from the monitor reveals the above rhythm. What protocol would you consider using (see ACLS text pp. 1-21 to 1-23)? _____

143. The second dose of adenosine is (see ACLS text p. 7-13): _____

    _____ (a) 3 mg
    _____ (b) 4 mg
    _____ (c) 6 mg
    _____ (d) 12 mg

144. Using a standard adult oxygen face mask, it is possible to administer oxygen safely at 2 to 4 L/min (see ACLS text p. 2-7): _____

_____ (a) True
_____ (b) False

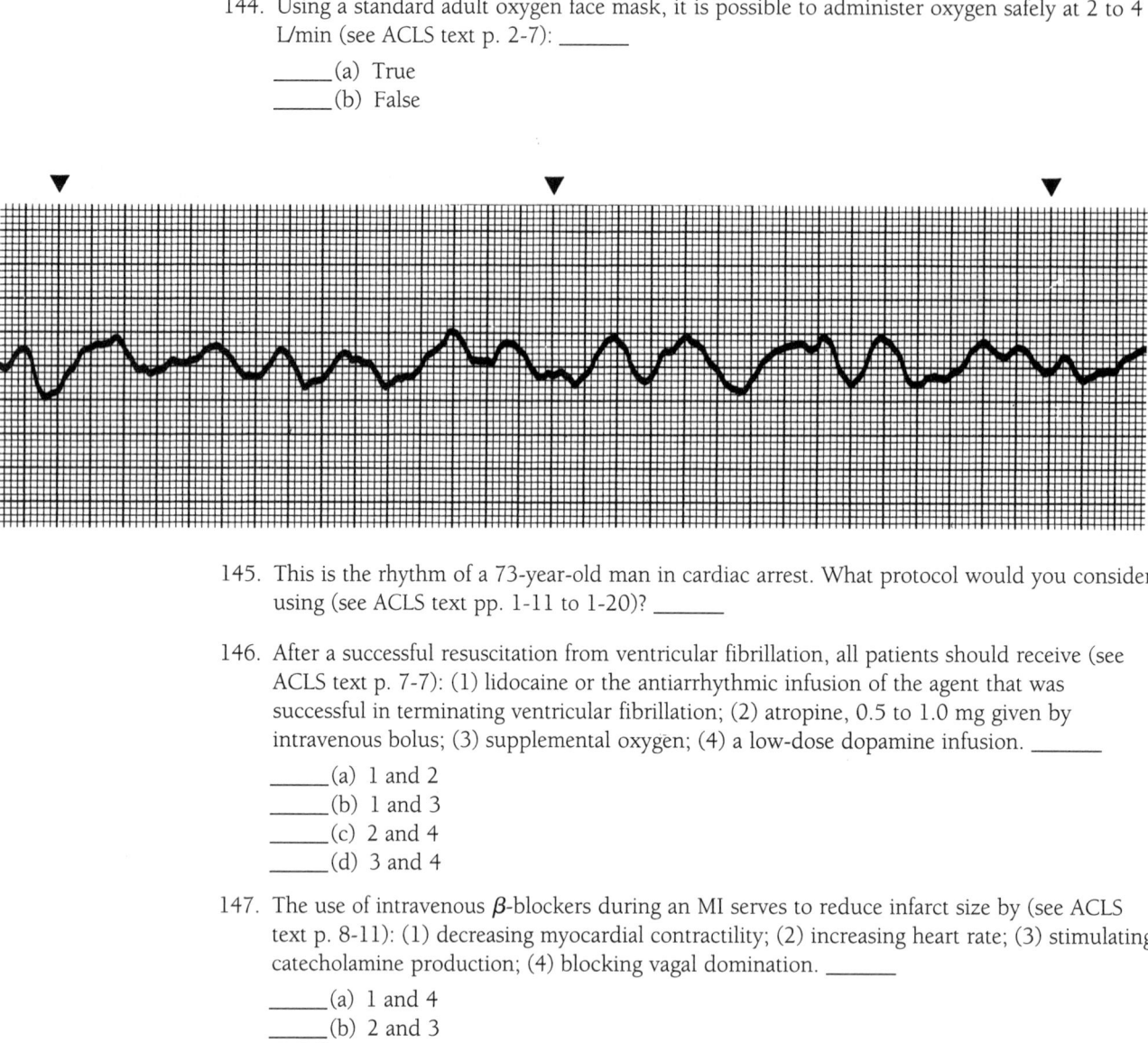

145. This is the rhythm of a 73-year-old man in cardiac arrest. What protocol would you consider using (see ACLS text pp. 1-11 to 1-20)? _____

146. After a successful resuscitation from ventricular fibrillation, all patients should receive (see ACLS text p. 7-7): (1) lidocaine or the antiarrhythmic infusion of the agent that was successful in terminating ventricular fibrillation; (2) atropine, 0.5 to 1.0 mg given by intravenous bolus; (3) supplemental oxygen; (4) a low-dose dopamine infusion. _____

_____ (a) 1 and 2
_____ (b) 1 and 3
_____ (c) 2 and 4
_____ (d) 3 and 4

147. The use of intravenous β-blockers during an MI serves to reduce infarct size by (see ACLS text p. 8-11): (1) decreasing myocardial contractility; (2) increasing heart rate; (3) stimulating catecholamine production; (4) blocking vagal domination. _____

_____ (a) 1 and 4
_____ (b) 2 and 3
_____ (c) 1 and 2
_____ (d) none of the above

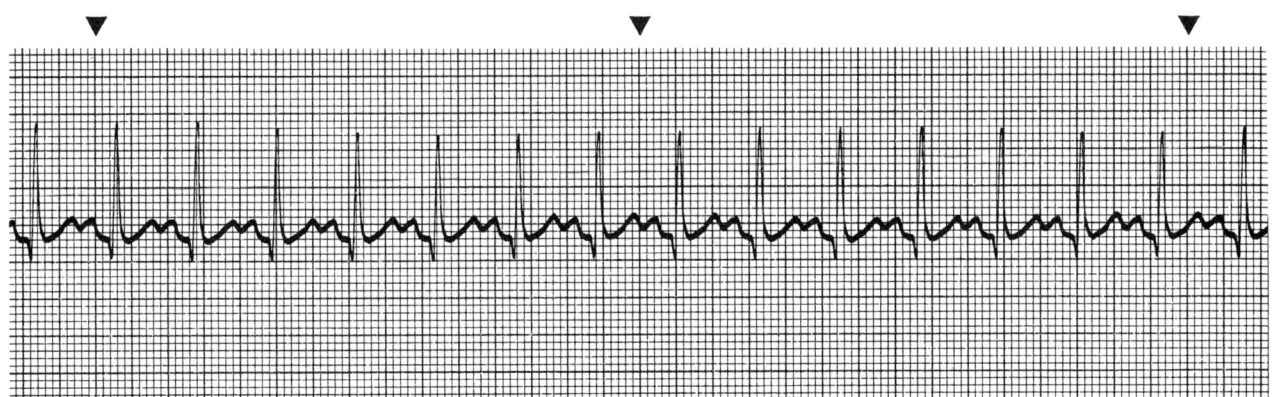

148. An 83-year-old patient is being observed for recurrent episodes of CHF. He received two doses of diuretics from the paramedics during transport and one dose in the emergency room before being admitted in the CCU. Although these doses were administered, they were not charted. During the first hour after admission, one more dose of a diuretic was administered before the arrival of the patient's physician. When the physician arrived, the patient became unconscious, pulseless, and apneic. The monitor revealed the above rhythm. What protocol would you consider using (see ACLS text pp. 1-21 to 1-23)? _____

149. Dopamine is an effective agent for the treatment of hypotension due to cardiogenic shock because it has α-adrenergic, β-adrenergic, and dopaminergic receptor stimulation (see ACLS text pp. 1-43 to 1-44). _____

    ____ (a) True
    ____ (b) False

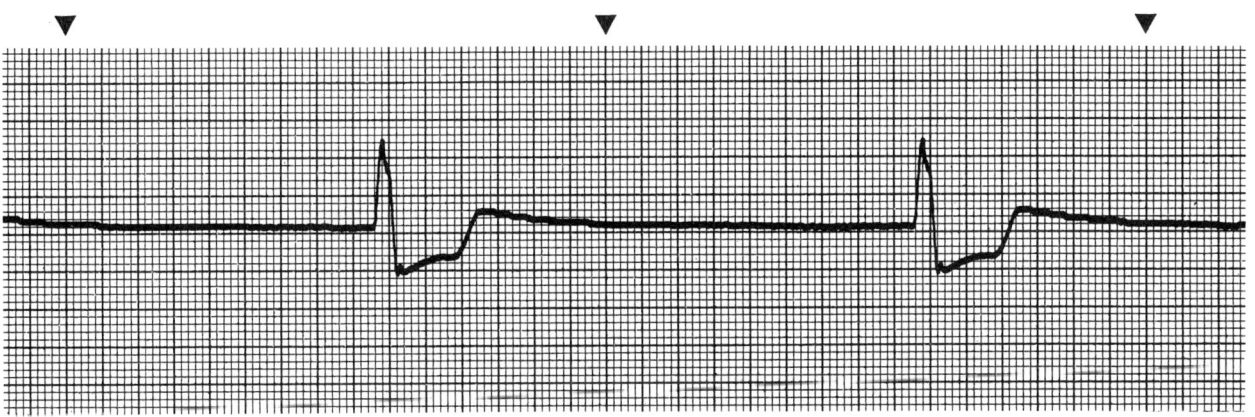

150. This is the rhythm of a 78-year-old woman who presented to you in cardiac arrest. What protocol would you consider using (see ACLS text p. 1-23)? _____

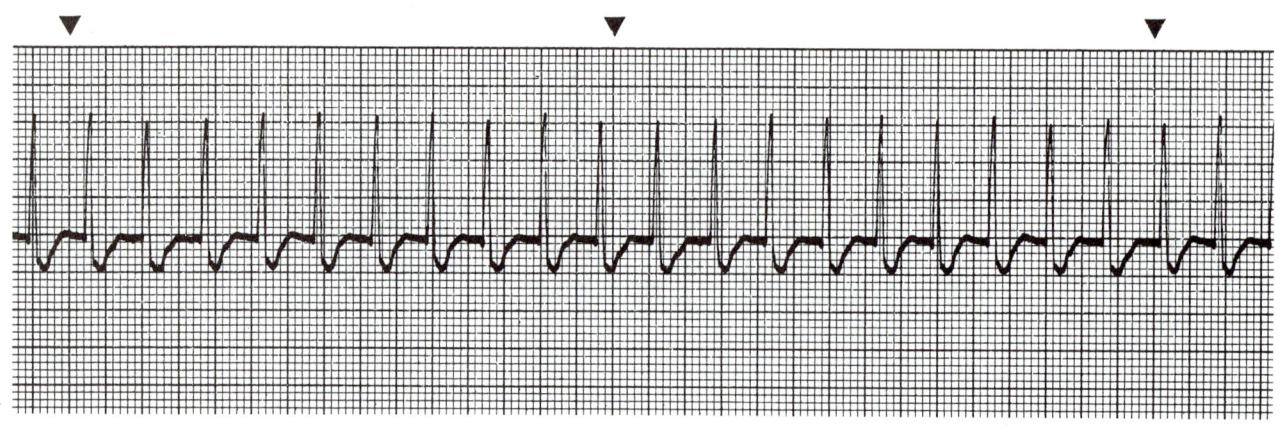

151. This the rhythm of a 48-year-old man who is experiencing an acute onset of rapid heart rate. He is experiencing acute dyspnea and is evidencing pulmonary edema. His vital signs are as follows: pulse—210, respirations—30, and BP—100/88. His rhythm appears above. What protocol would you consider using (see ACLS text pp. 1-34 to 1-35)? _____

152. In a routine cardiac arrest of a 170-pound adult, the initial dose of sodium bicarbonate would be about (see ACLS text pp. 7-14 to 7-15): _____

   _____(a) None
   _____(b) 50 mEq
   _____(c) 75 mEq
   _____(d) 100 mEq

153. Effects of intravenous nitroglycerin may be as powerful as thrombolytics in reducing infarct size and overall mortality rates in acute MI (see ACLS text p. 1-50). _____

   _____(a) True
   _____(b) False

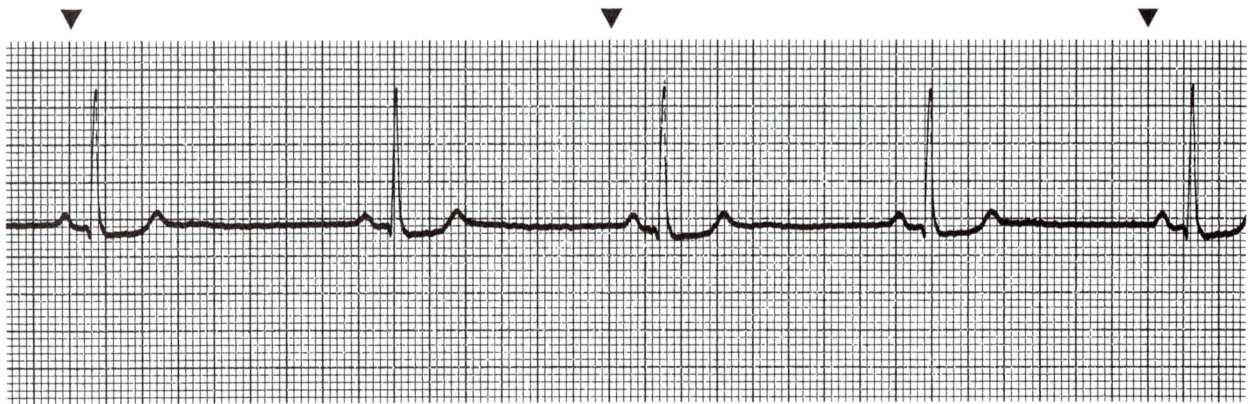

154. A 45-year-old man has been admitted to the CCU with a diagnosis of a lateral MI. He has an intravenous lifeline of NS and is receiving oxygen by nasal cannula. He has a depressed level of consciousness, a BP of 70/40, respirations of 12, and a pulse of 45. The monitor reveals the above rhythm. What protocol would you consider using (see ACLS text pp. 1-43 to 1-49)? _____

155. Magnesium sulfate should be withheld in ventricular fibrillation if a recent electrolyte panel documented a normal magnesium level (see ACLS text p. 1-20). _____

   _____(a) True
   _____(b) False

156. If, during your secondary assessment, you noted that the patient had a history of alcoholism, you might consider giving magnesium sulfate at what point in the ventricular fibrillation protocol (see ACLS text p. 7-14)? _____

_____ (a) After procainamide
_____ (b) After bretylium
_____ (c) After epinephrine
_____ (d) After lidocaine

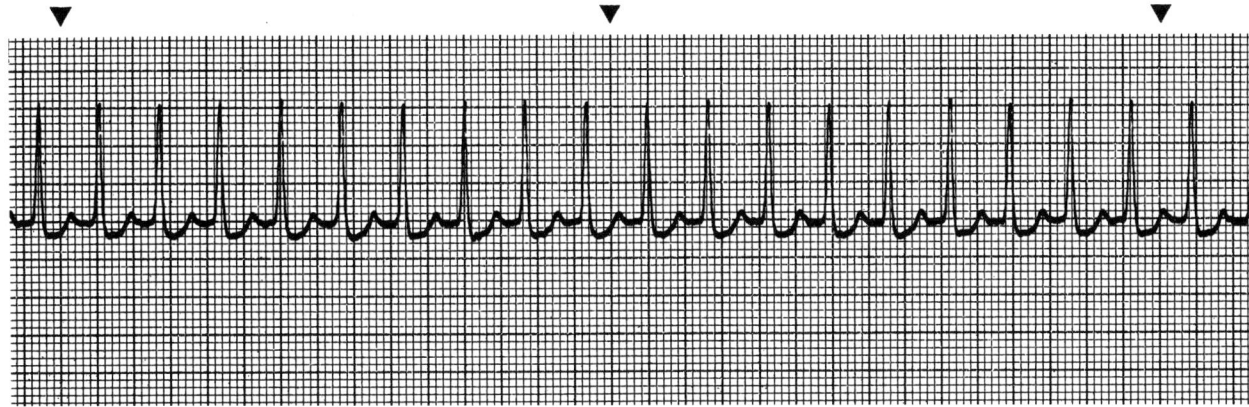

157. A 45-year-old man is visiting his wife after surgery. While he is talking to her, his heart starts to palpitate. He experiences crushing chest pain but not any other overt signs of cardiovascular compromise. The monitor shows the above rhythm. His vital signs are as follows: pulse—188, BP—130/90, and respirations—14. What protocol would you consider using (see ACLS text pp. 1-34 to 1-36)? _____

158. Intravenous nitroglycerin is contraindicated in unstable angina (see ACLS text pp. 8-9 to 8-11). _____

_____ (a) True
_____ (b) False

Unit Two
Learning Adjuncts

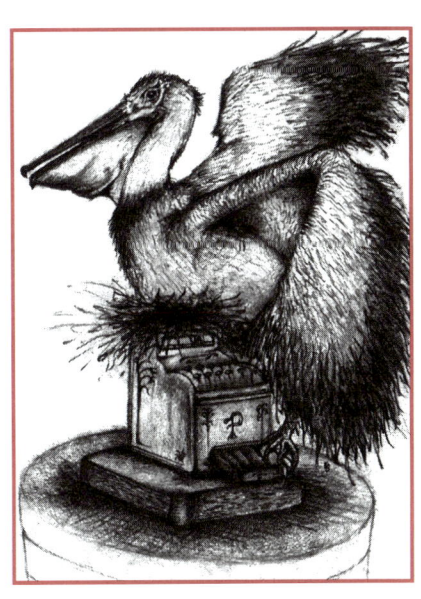

7 Megacode Survival Tips

Objectives

- Act as a team leader in cardiac arrest
- Be responsible for supervising and directing the team in a sequence that is most beneficial to the patient

During the mock code, the student is required to demonstrate proficiency in dysrhythmia recognition, defibrillator operation, and appropriate drug protocols, while at the same time supervising the team. Although the megacode may sound difficult, it is not hard if you are comfortable with the ACLS protocols.

The case study format, developed in conjunction with the 1992 revisions, is not nearly as difficult as in the past. The new standards mandate that each student be individually evaluated in all 10 case studies. Each case study highlights one, or a portion of one, of the ACLS algorithms. *Case studies 2 and 3 span initial and refractory ventricular fibrillation and together make up the megacode testing station*. For most ACLS courses, the ventricular fibrillation algorithm is *the main algorithm tested during the megacode*. In preparation, ask your course director if the megacode testing station is targeted *solely* on case studies 2 and 3 or if it includes algorithms from the other eight case studies.

During the megacode, the student's ability to treat the patient, as well as to monitor the team, is evaluated. The easiest way to approach the team leader role is to adhere to a plan. When initially confronting the patient, perform both a primary and a secondary survey. Reassess the patient any time the rhythm changes. By consistently checking and rechecking the airway, breathing, pulse, and blood pressure every time that the rhythm or situation changes, problems become immediately manageable.

Tips for Treating the Patient

One of the main objectives for the team leader during the megacode is to treat the patient. Although a variety of scenarios may occur, the team leader should adhere to a plan.

Regardless of how the patient presents, response to the patient is always the same. Begin with the primary survey and progress rapidly to the secondary survey.

Monitor the Patient's Consciousness

Begin by ascertaining the patient's level of consciousness. This shows cerebral perfusion patterns and ultimately indicates what treatment protocol, if any, is needed. Both wide complex tachycardia and supraventricular tachycardia (SVT) have stable and unstable protocols.

The protocols for a stable patient who is alert, coherent, and in no immediate danger encompass drug therapy. In an unstable tachycardic patient, the level of consciousness is hampered either by poor perfusion or by a deteriorating clinical status (e.g., chest pain, pulmonary edema). Intravenous therapy depends on adequate cerebral and vascular perfusion. Because unstable tachycardic patients have poor perfusion and commonly have an altered level of consciousness, electrical cardioversion is employed as the treatment protocol instead of intravenous therapy.

Monitor Airway and Ventilation

Consistently recheck the airway and verify ventilation throughout the code. Just giving instructions at the beginning and never monitoring later will not help a pneumothorax caused by cardiopulmonary resuscitation (CPR).

Monitor Pulse

IF THE PATIENT HAS NO PULSE, INITIATE CARDIOPULMONARY RESUSCITATION

If the patient has no pulse, the patient has either pulseless ventricular tachycardia, asystole, ventricular fibrillation, or pulseless electrical activity. Initiate CPR while ascertaining the length of time to obtain a monitor defibrillation.

IF THE PATIENT HAS A PULSE, CONSIDER PERFUSION

Avoid the assumption that because a patient has a pulse, perfusion is adequate. The American College of Surgeons ATLS Course notes some basic rules for perfusion. If the patient has a radial pulse, the systolic blood pressure is at least 80 mmHg. If the patient does not have a radial pulse but does have a brachial or femoral pulse, the systolic blood pressure is at least 70 mmHg. If the patient does not have a radial, brachial, or femoral pulse but does have a carotid pulse, the systolic blood pressure is at least 60 mmHg. Therefore, if the patient has a carotid pulse, systolic blood pressure is at least 60 mmHg.

Perfusion is not necessarily adequate when a patient has a carotid pulse. Although a thready pulse is obtained in the carotid artery, the patient may not be perfusing properly because of other predisposing factors. In addition, if the patient is normally hypertensive, a systolic blood pressure of 60 mmHg may not indicate adequate perfusion.

When there is a pulse, measure the blood pressure in the following manner. If the patient has a systolic blood pressure of 60 mmHg or more, CPR is probably not needed; the patient can tolerate that blood pressure for a limited time. If the patient has a systolic blood pressure of 40 mmHg less (probably obtainable only with Doppler), assume unacceptable perfusion and begin CPR. For systolic blood pressure readings between 40 and 60 mmHg, consider the age and clinical status of the patient. A young man may be able to tolerate this level of perfusion for a short time, whereas an elderly patient may have difficulty.

TREAT THE PATIENT, NOT THE MONITOR

If the patient's monitor shows a bradycardic pulse but the patient is not hypotensive, just monitor the patient. There is no need to treat the patient if there is adequate perfusion, regardless of the pulse rate.

If the patient's monitor shows wide complex tachycardia or SVT and the patient has a deteriorating clinical status, consider the unstable tachycardia protocols. If the patient has either of these rhythms but is alert and in no immediate clinical danger, employ the appropriate stable tachycardia treatment regimen.

Routinely, electrocardiogram (ECG) leads unsnap, causing the monitor to resemble ventricular fibrillation. If the patient has a pulse with ventricular fibrillation, assume that the leads are at fault.

TREAT HYPOTENSION WITH THE PULSE RATE AND THE ELECTROCARDIOGRAM

A systolic blood pressure of less than 90 mmHg, combined with an altered level of consciousness, defines a hypotensive patient. After checking for adequate ventilation and oxygenation, check whether the cardiac rhythm is too fast or too slow.

Slow Pulse Rate. Regardless of the QRS complex width, if the pulse rate is less than 60, consider hemodynamically significant bradycardia. Although a patient with an acute inferior or anterior myocardial infarction could present with bradycardia and would profit from a cautious fluid challenge, fluids are not a routine treatment. When the patient is hypotensive secondary to hypovolemia, the patient's pulse rate usually is tachycardic, not bradycardic. Only when approaching death does the patient become bradycardic. Giving a bradycardic patient large amounts of fluids to correct hypotension might cause pulmonary edema and later result in heart failure. For a better treatise on this subject, see case study 7.

Rapid Pulse Rate. If the patient's pulse is rapid, determine the patient's stability. If the patient is stable, check the width of the QRS complex. If the QRS complex is narrow and the rate is greater than 170 beats/minute, consider SVT. If the QRS complex is wide, consider wide complex tachycardia of unknown origin. If the width and rate are both narrow and less than 170, consider a compensatory tachycardia, such as hypovolemia or congestive heart failure.

If the patient is unstable, consider immediate cardioversion. There is no need to check the QRS complex width because all widths are cardioverted when they become unstable.

Assuming the patient is hypotensive and the pulse rate is either above 100 beats/minute with a wide QRS complex or above 170 with a narrow QRS complex, consider the unstable tachycardia protocol (see case study 8).

Two exceptions to the previous statement are atrial fibrillation and atrial flutter. Both of these dysrhythmias need to be treated with the stable or unstable tachycardia protocols (depending on their presenting symptoms) because the heart rates that cause significant cardiovascular compromise may not approach 160 to 170 in these cases. The clinician needs to recognize these two rhythms and not group them with most narrow QRS complex tachycardias. All hypotensive tachycardias with wide QRS rhythms are treated as wide complex tachycardias and subsequently cardioverted. With the exception of atrial fibrillation and atrial flutter, however, a narrow QRS complex with a rate above 170 is most likely *not* a compensatory tachycardia but an irritable atrial pacemaker cell. Treatment consists of immediate cardioversion.

With the exception of atrial fibrillation or atrial flutter, which have narrow QRS complexes and can have rates less than 170, if the rate is either above 60 but less than 100 with a wide QRS complex, or above 60 beats/minute but less than 170 with a narrow QRS complex, it could be a compensatory mechanism for hypovolemia; therefore, consider an immediate fluid challenge of 500 mL of normal saline. If the patient responds positively to the fluid challenge, continue fluids. The operative term here is *consider*. Depending on the patient's history and your physical examination, fluids may be inappropriate (e.g., congestive heart failure, kidney failure). The clinician, however, *must consider* a fluid challenge before considering other options.

If the pulse is in excess of 60 and you have considered fluids, or your challenge was unsuccessful, consider vasopressors. At this time, after considering both a rate and fluid problem, the most likely cause is a pump problem. Because the patient did not respond to the fluid challenge, hypovolemia can be ruled out. The appropriate drug to administer for a pump problem varies according to the patient's vital signs. If the patient's systolic blood pressure is less than 70 mmHg, consider using either norepinephrine or dopamine. Some clinicians prefer to start with norepinephrine until the blood pressure is raised above 70 mmHg, and then switch to dopamine. Other clinicians, however, initially employ dopamine, regardless of the blood pressure. A common dopamine dosage regimen can be found in the flash cards in the appendices. Titrate the drops per minute until the patient's systolic blood pressure reaches 90 mmHg. Consider starting at 2 to 5 mcg/kg/min and increase the dose over a period of 5 minutes to 8 to 12 mcg/kg/min.

Monitor Cardiopulmonary Resuscitation

Each time the rhythm changes, monitor breathing for equal, bilateral breath sounds. After continuing CPR and checking for breath sounds, monitor CPR. In the past, clinicians checked for the presence of a pulse during CPR to determine if basic life support was effective. Recent research (see ACLS text pg. 12-5), however, questions this axiom. Although the presence of a pulse during CPR does indicate some amount of forward blood flow, it does not give the clinician any information about aortic diastolic or myocardial perfusion pressures. When scrutinizing the effectiveness of the femoral pulse during CPR, note that because the inferior vena cava has no valves, retrograde venous blood flow may mistakenly be taken as a femoral pulse.

Capnometry, the measurement of the amount of CO_2 leaving the lungs, is an alternative method that shows some promise as an effective way to monitor CPR. Because there are no effective criteria for assessing the adequacy of CPR, the American Heart Association advocates the use of Doppler ultrasound, arterial line measurements, or capnometry, rather than relying solely on a pulse to determine the adequacy of CPR.

Monitor Medications

On arrival, an intravenous line should be inserted using normal saline or lactated Ringer's solution for the rapid administration of drugs. If an intravenous line is unavailable, consider endotracheal (ET) tube administration. If an intravenous line is delayed or no longer patent, certain drugs may be administered down endotracheally. A helpful mnemonic for remembering these drugs is NAEL: *n*aloxone, *a*tropine, *e*pinephrine, *l*idocaine. These drugs can be administered through a feeding tube or needle-through-catheter projecting past the end of the ET tube for adults. The dosages are 2 to $2\frac{1}{2}$ times the standard intravenous dosage. It is necessary to use a more concentrated solution of epinephrine (1:1000) diluted in 10 mL of normal saline or distilled water.

In resuscitating infants and children, the dosage of epinephrine should be *10 times* the intravenous or intraosseous dosage. Dilution of the drug with 1 to 2 mL of normal saline or with half normal saline may aid ET tube delivery in children.

Monitor Blood Gases

Ventilatory insufficiency may be a problem introduced during an emergency. To monitor ventilation, review blood gases. When you examine the blood gas results, look at the PaO_2; if it is less than 80 mmHg, the patient may require oxygen, although serious signs of poor oxygenation show up as the PaO_2 drops below 60 mmHg. The ET tube may have migrated into the right main-stem bronchus. Listen for breath sounds; if they are unequal, retract the tube and recheck. If the PaO_2 remains uncorrected, search for alternative causes of hypoxia, such as trauma, by performing a quick thorax assessment.

Scrutinize the $PaCO_2$; if it is greater than 45 or less than 35 mmHg, consider ventilation problems. A normal $PaCO_2$ is 35 to 45 mmHg. If the $PaCO_2$ is less than 35 mmHg, the patient is blowing off carbon dioxide by hyperventilating. If the $PaCO_2$ is above 45 mmHg, the patient is retaining carbon dioxide by hypoventilating. Regardless of the specific blood gas values, you should note that the patient is not ventilating appropriately and suggest appropriate treatment.

In cardiac arrest, patients should be hyperventilated. Hyperventilation creates a respiratory alkalosis to combat the acidosis as a consequence of PaO_2 retention in an arrest. Look at the pH. If the pH is less than 7.35, continue hyperventilating to correct the acidosis. If the patient's pH is neutral (7.35 to 7.45), decrease the ventilatory pattern to one ventilation for every five compressions. Make certain that the PaO_2 is still above 80 mmHg because oxygenation and ventilation are separate values.

In summary, check the PaO_2 first. If the PaO_2 is less than 60 mmHg, there may be a problem with the patient's oxygenation; immediately scrutinize the airway. The most likely cause is migration of the ET tube into the right main-stem bronchus. The ventilation team member's inefficiency using the bag-valve-mask (BVM) device, however, may result in poor blood gas values (e.g., the mask on the BVM device may be placed on backward, resulting in poor seal). Monitor the ventilation team member and correct anything that appears amiss. Continuously observe the airway.

Tips for Monitoring the Team

During the megacode evaluation station, the student is required to assume the role of the team leader and to monitor the team during a cardiac arrest. The ACLS team is composed of five members: the team leader, a CPR rescuer, a respiratory professional, a defibrillator expert, and an intravenous line expert. Although each team member is responsible for a different aspect of the patient's treatment, they all rely on the team leader for instructions and guidance.

Cardiopulmonary Resuscitation Team Member

The CPR team member knows how to perform CPR properly; however, it is impossible to tell if the patient has a pulse while CPR is being performed. When checking the patient for a pulse, the assessment focuses on the presence or absence of a perfusing pulse, rather than on the presence or absence of a pulse. A palpable carotid pulse does not necessarily indicate that the heart is generating a sufficient cardiac output to perfuse the patient adequately. A systolic blood pressure of 60 mmHg may be sufficient to perfuse a 20-year-old but would fail to perfuse a normally hypertensive 70-year-old adequately. After each treatment, a pulse check should be performed to evaluate the patient's status. With every glance at the monitor, the team leader should say, "Stop CPR, pulse check please." If the patient does not have a pulse, the team leader should say, "Continue CPR."

If the patient regains a pulse after not having one, something has changed, and a quick primary survey (ABCD) should be performed. If the patient has a pulse as checked before, perform an abbreviated secondary survey to ascertain what has changed. Many professionals make the error of relying solely on the monitor display, without rechecking the patient.

Respiratory Team Member

The respiratory team member focuses on airway maintenance and is knowledgeable in airway equipment. This member of the team possesses the ability to operate a BVM and intubate if requested. The team leader is responsible for monitoring the respiratory team member. A request for the patient to be ventilated is not adequate directions for respiration. The team leader should request that the patient be ventilated with 100% oxygen, auscultated bilaterally, and intubated when appropriate. The team leader should continue to monitor the respiratory member every 5 minutes. During the advanced airway section of the secondary survey, the team leader should instruct the respiratory team member to place an oropharyngeal airway (if not already accomplished), employ a BVM at 100% oxygen, hyperventilate for about 3 minutes, and intubate when ready. This brief statement results in an airway being placed; hyperventilation with 100% oxygen; preoxygenation for at least 3 minutes; and preinstruction to intubate when ready.

Always check to make sure that these instructions were followed correctly. The respiratory team member may not have made an adequate seal with the BVM face mask, thus resulting in inadequate ventilation. The team leader is ultimately responsible for all of the treatment performed on the patient and should instruct the respiratory team member to monitor the airway carefully and frequently.

The team leader should stop intubation if the respiratory team member takes longer than 30 seconds to intubate (measured from breath to breath), uses the patient's teeth as a fulcrum, or introduces the ET tube into the right main-stem bronchus.

The respiratory team member must secure the tube and perform asynchronous ventilation (ventilate 12 to 15 times per minute, disregarding the timing of the compressor) with the person performing CPR. If the patient fails to respond to this therapy, the team leader should remind the respiratory team member to recheck for bilateral breath sounds. Monitoring the respiratory team member is essential because hypoxia is common in these situations.

Defibrillator Team Member

The defibrillator team member notes which lead the machine is using. After locating both the power and the lead switch, the latter can be turned to P to select the paddles or leads I, II, or III. This selection allows the paddles to be employed as electrodes, permitting an initial quick look at the patient's cardiac rhythm without placing gel electrodes on the patient's chest. If the paddles lose contact with the chest, the monitor will display artifact. Even though the patient may have a pulse, the artifact may be misinterpreted as ventricular fibrillation and lead to unnecessary defibrillation of the patient.

After telling the defibrillator team member to place the leads on the patient, the team leader asks for a lead II selection. Again, the most common problem arises when the monitor indicates ventricular fibrillation, even though the patient has a strong pulse. This most often occurs because an electrode wire has fallen off. The team leader can avoid being fooled into shocking the patient for ventricular fibrillation by carefully checking the equipment.

The defibrillator can often be complex to operate. Practice removing the paddles from the machine, and learn the location and purpose of each switch. On a defibrillator with an attached monitor, the synchronizer switch is usually a button or switch labeled "synch" or "synchronizer." When this button is depressed, the machine searches the ECG rhythm for an R wave. On locating an R wave, the monitor flashes, beeps, or somehow signals that the R wave has been sensed. If the monitor does not flash or beep, it probably means that it is not sensing the R wave. No matter how much, how often, or how long you hold down the red buttons, it will not fire. It may be ventricular fibrillation, which does not have R waves, or the ECG size (amplitude) switch on the machine is set too low and therefore the defibrillator cannot sense the R wave.

When attempting to deliver a synchronized countershock and the machine does not fire, check to make sure that the patient's cardiac rhythm has not deteriorated. If ventricular fibrillation occurs, verify with a pulse check, turn off the synchronizer, and immediately defibrillate. However, if this is not the case, increase the ECG amplitude until the machine senses the R wave; if it still does not fire, and the patient is critical, turn off the synchronizer and defibrillate!

The procedure sequence for the team is clearly delineated in case studies 2 and 3. The defibrillator member, however, should verbalize that the defibrillation pads have been placed on the patient or that the paddles are being gelled before the first countershock is delivered. In addition, a pulse check should be requested from the person performing CPR, before the three shocks and immediately afterward. A pulse check should be performed immediately, however, if the ECG changes at any time.

After delivering the shock, the machine should be automatically recharged by a team member so that the next shock can be given immediately. Do not remove the paddles from the patient's chest after delivering the shock because it may be necessary to deliver more shocks, and repositioning the paddles results in time wasted. The team leader is ultimately responsible for what happens. If the defibrillator member does not perform the sequence correctly, the team leader should interrupt immediately!

Intravenous Line Team Member

The IV team member administers the medications to the patient, as instructed by the team leader. On arriving, the team leader should request that this team member start an IV using normal saline or lactated Ringer's solution. The team leader also should be informed after any drug has been administered and the line has been flushed.

After flushing the line with 20 to 30 mL, allow no more than 30 to 60 seconds for circulation. It is helpful in a cardiac arrest to raise the limb with the intravenous site, permitting gravity to enhance the drug's entrance into the cardiovascular system. If there is no assigned documentation member, assign the IV member to note what drugs are administered.

At a minimum, it is necessary for the team leader to know the actions, indications, and dosages of the following medications:

- Epinephrine
- Atropine
- Lidocaine
- Procainamide
- Bretylium
- Isoproterenol
- Dopamine
- Adenosine
- Verapamil
- Sodium bicarbonate
- Calcium chloride

Sodium bicarbonate should be administered only in cases of preexisting acidosis or of suspected bicarbonate deficits (e.g., aspirin overdoses, diabetic ketoacidosis, tricyclic antidepressant overdoses, and acute hyperkalemia).

Calcium chloride is recommended only in hyperkalemic patients, hypocalcemic situations, or as an antidote for calcium-channel blockers or magnesium overdoses.

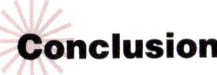
Conclusion

The team leader should approach any emergency as a chance to demonstrate his or her ability to treat the patient and guide the team. It is the team leader's responsibility to ensure that all of the members correctly follow the instructions. Did the respiratory team member intubate correctly and remember to auscultate afterward? Is the CPR team member initiating and stopping CPR when instructed? Did the defibrillator member clear the team in the proper manner? As the emergency progresses, remember to reassess the patient on a timely basis.

8 ACLS Drug Therapy

Adenosine

Actions	Indications	Dosage	Precautions
Depresses the atrioventricular (AV) node and, to a lesser extent, the sinoatrial nodes. Adenosine temporarily interrupts reentry mechanism tachycardias (supraventricular tachycardias)	• Paroxysmal supraventricular tachycardia (PSVT) refractory to vagal stimulation	PSVT and wide complex tachycardia of uncertain type:	The half-life is less than 5 to 10 seconds
		• **6 mg IV bolus (within 1 to 3 seconds)**	Common side effects:
	• Wide complex tachycardia of uncertain type when lidocaine has proved refractory	• Start IV line in the closest peripheral vein to the heart	• Facial flushing
Has a lesser or no significant effect on narrow complex tachycardias that do not employ a reentry mechanism (i.e., the rhythms that pass through the AV node: atrial fibrillation and atrial flutter)		• Chest pain
		• Period of asystole for 3 to 5 seconds
	• PSVT with accessory bypass tracts (Wolff-Parkinson-White syndrome)	• A separate syringe, filled with 20 mL of normal saline (NS) introduced in the same port, should be used to flush the drug immediately	All are usually transient.
		Greater than 90% success rate after 12 mg
		Consider increased doses if patient is currently taking theophylline or caffeine.
Will not harm, nor have any substantial effect in terminating, ventricular-origin rhythms	• May be helpful in elucidating the diagnosis of nonreentry tachycardias as a temporary block of the AV node	After 1 to 2 minutes, the drug may be repeated at 12 mg.	Dipyridamole (Persantine) is a platelet inhibitor blocking adenosine uptake.
		If still ineffective, an additional 12 mg may be introduced.	

225

Amrinone Lactate

Actions	Indications	Dosage	Precautions
A positive inotropic agent (increases cardiac function) distinctly different action from that of digitalis or catecholamines Reduces both preload and afterload through a potent vasodilatory effect on vascular smooth muscle Is *not* considered a β-adrenergic agonist.	Short-term management of congestive heart failure (CHF) that was not initially responsive to diuretics, digitalis, or vasodilators	**0.75 mg/kg (undiluted) slowly over 2 to 3 minutes followed immediately with IV infusion** Consider giving it over 10 to 15 minutes in patients predisposing to hypotension (e.g., those exhibiting marginal blood pressure or left ventricular dysfunction) IV infusion: • Drug comes in 20 mL ampules containing 5 mg/mL • Mix equal amounts of amrinone with NS (e.g., 60 mL [29 mL × 3 amps] of amrinone with 60 mL of NS. This will equal 2.5 mg/mL. Administer 2 to 5 mcg/kg/min titrated to effect (i.e., 10 to 15 mcg/kg/min).	The use of D-5-W is contraindicated. Furosemide precipiates in solutions with amrinone and is thus contraindicated. Constant monitoring of blood pressure and heart rate are required to optimize its use. Use of infusion pump is indicated. Contraindicated in severe aortic or pulmonic valvular disease in lieu of surgical intervention Patients receiving diuretics may have insufficient cardiac filling. Consider fluid therapy. Contraindicated in: • Thrombocytopenia • Allergy to sulfonamides May exacerbate ischemia, so use with caution in patients with ischemic heart disease Long half-life: 4 to 6 hours

Atropine

Actions	Indications	Dosage	Precautions
Parasympathetic nervous system (vagus nerve) blocking agent (i.e., vagolytic or parasympatholytic agent) If the vagus nerve was the predominating influence in the significant bradycardia, then introduction of atropine will cause an increase in sympathetic tone with resultant increase in heart rate and blood pressure. If atropine appears ineffective after the maximum dose is reached, vagal influence can be ruled out. Increases sinus node rate and improves AV conduction	Cardiac arrest: • Asystole • Pulseless electrical activity (PEA) Significant bradycardia: • Any form (but see precautions for second-degree, type II and third-degree blocks)	Asystole and PEA: • **1 mg every 3–5 minutes to a maximum dose of 0.04 mg/kg** Significant bradycardias: • **0.5 to 1.0 mg every 3–5 minutes to a maximum dose of 0.03–0.04 mg/kg** Endotracheal (ET) administration: • 1.0 to 2.0 mg diluted in enough NS for sterile water to make total of 10 cc.	Injection of subtherapeutic doses may cause reverse effects (bradycardia). Atropine will not work if the cause of the bradycardia did not involve increase in vagal tone. May precipitate acute tachydysrhythmias or ventricular fibrillation Watch for increasing oxygen demand as myocardial rate accelerates. Atropine may be ineffective or cause harm in certain infranodal blocks (second degree, type II and a new wide QRS complex with third-degree block) by paradoxically slowing the heart rate with resultant drop in blood pressure. However, because the above situation only occurs rarely, atropine should continue to be the first-choice pharmaceutical for significant bradycardia.

β-Blockers

Actions	Indications	Dosage	Precautions
Blockade of β-adrenergic receptors Competitive with adrenergic stimulants; level depends on level of stimulant Blocks catecholamines Causes decreases in: - Myocardial contractility (negative inotropic response) - Blood pressure - Heart rate (negative chronotropic response) - Myocardial oxygen consumption - Arrythmias Reduces creatine kinase–determined infarct size in patients with Q-wave MIs and can prevent reinfarction when given with thrombolytic agents	Appears to reduce the mortality in myocardial infarction (MI) by 25% when used in patients in whom no contraindications exist Indications: - Recurrent ventricular tachycardia (VT) or ventricular fibrillation (VF) - Refractory PSVT - Postinfarction	**Atenolol (Tenormin)** - 5 mg slow IV push over 5 minutes. If necessary, may repeat in 10 minutes **Esmolol (Brevibloc)** - A 250- to 500-mcg/kg loading dose administered over 1 minute. Comes prediluted in 100-mg vial - Follow with IV infusion at 25 to 50 mcg/kg/min administered over 4 minutes **Metoprolol (Lopressor)** - Slow IV push of 5 mg over 2 to 5 minutes. Continue at 5-minute intervals if necessary to total of 15 mg **Propranolol (Inderal)** - Total dose is 0.1 mg/kg. Administered slow IV push. The entire dose is divided into three equal doses and administered at 2- to 3-minute intervals. Common dosage is 1 to 3 mg by slow IV push over 2 to 5 minutes not to exceed 1 mg/minute.	All β-blockers should be avoided when treating patients with: - Bradycardia - Heart block - Hypotension - CHF - Lung disease with associated bronchospasm (e.g., asthma) Adverse effects may be precipitated with agents with similar actions: - Calcium channel blockers - Antihypertensive agents - Antiarrhythmic agents

Bretylium

Actions	Indications	Dosage	Precautions
Initially sympathomimetic activity (release of norepinephrine) causing: increase of heart rate and increase in blood pressure 20 to 30 minutes later, activity becomes largely sympatholytic (adrenergic blockade) causing: drop in heart rate, fall in blood pressure Elevates the VF threshold Suppresses ventricular ectopy refractory to lidocaine or procainamide	• VF or pulseless VT refractory to defibrillation and lidocaine • VT and wide complex tachycardia of uncertain type, both with pulses, refractory to both lidocaine and procainamide • Additionally, wide complex tachycardia of uncertain type was refractory to adenosine as well	VF or pulseless VT: • **5 mg/kg IV bolus followed by immediate defibrillation. If necessary, repeat drug every 5 to 30 minutes at 10 mg/kg to a maximum of 30–35 mg/kg** VT and wide complex tachycardia of uncertain type, both with pulses: • **5–10 mg/kg diluted in 50 mL of fluid and administered slowly over 8 to 10 minutes** IV infusion: • 1 g in 250 mL run at a rate of 2 mg/min after loading dose or after successful conversion with bretylium to a supraventricular rhythm	No contraindications in VF or pulseless VT In patients with pulses, postural hypotension is the most common side effect. The postural hypotension may be refractory to epinephrine. Nausea and vomiting are common if drug is administered too rapidly in conscious VT patients. Contraindicated in the presence of digitalis toxicity

Calcium Chloride

Actions	Indications	Dosage	Precautions
Positive inotropic agent	Considered a class II drug (probably helpful) in: • Hyperkalemia • Hypocalcemia • Overdose of calcium-channel blockers As a possible prelude to verapamil administration	Hyperkalemia and calcium channel overdose: • **8 to 16 mg/kg at a 10% solution. Repeat as necessary.** Prophylaxis of calcium channel blocker: • **2 to 4 mg/kg IV slowly** is usual dose. Dosage can be repeated at 10-minute intervals as needed.	Will precipitate if administered with sodium bicarbonate Caution should be exercised when administering with digitalis May result in bradycardia if given too rapidly IV

Digitalis

Actions	Indications	Dosage	Precautions
Naturally occurring plant. Names include: • Foxglove • Dead man's bells • Fairy's footprints Positive inotropic agent increasing cardiac output Negative chronotropic agent slowing conduction at AV node	• Hemodynamically significant rapid or uncontrolled atrial fibrillation and atrial flutter to slow ventricular response • Supraventricular tachycardia refractory to prior therapy • CHF	Loading dose is 10 to 15 mcg/kg Be aware that digitalis is rarely given as an emergency medication. The difference between toxic and therapeutic levels is very small.	Watch for the following adverse reactions: • Complete heart block • Hypotension • Bradycardia • Nausea and vomiting • Headache • Malaise • Drowsiness • Disorientation • Yellow or blurred vision • Diarrhea • Ventricular ectopy • Anorexia • Junctional rhythms Digitalis is contraindicated in patients with: • Hypokalemia • Hypercalcemia • Heart block • VT

Diltiazem

Actions	Indications	Dosage	Precautions
Slow channel calcium-channel blocker Slows AV nodal conduction time and prolongs AV nodal refractoriness, resulting in slowing of tachycardias involving the AV node (e.g., atrial fibrillation, atrial flutter, PSVT) Converts PSVT to sinus rhythm by interrupting the reentry circuit in AV nodal reentry tachycardias (e.g., Wolff-Parkinson-White syndrome) Decreases total peripheral resistance, resulting in decrease of systolic and diastolic blood pressures Controls rapid ventricular response in atrial fibrillation, atrial flutter, or PSVT Negative chronotropic agent with only mild negative inotropic effects	Controls atrial fibrillation and atrial flutter with a rapid or uncontrolled ventricular response Can control elevated ventricular rates associated with multifocal atrial tachycardia Can terminate and/or prevent PSVT	Initial dose of 0.25 mg/kg administered slowly IV over 2 minutes. A dose of 20 mg is acceptable for an average-sized patient. After waiting 15 minutes if response is still inadequate, a second dose of 0.35 mg/kg can be administered slowly IV over 2 minutes. A dose of 25 mg is considered acceptable IV infusion: • If initial loading dose is successful, administer a maintenance infusion at 5–15 mg/h. • Mix five vials (50 mg/vial) in 250 mL NS to achieve 0.83 mg/mL. 10 mg/h rate is 12 mL/h, and 15 mg/h is 18 mL/h.	Use may result in hypotension. Except in a functioning ventricular pacemaker, contraindicated in: • Sick sinus node syndrome • Second-degree block and third-degree block Should not be administered within a few hours of β-blockers Contraindicated in presence of Wolff-Parkinson-White syndrome Use with caution in patients exhibiting severe left ventricular dysfunction. Produces less myocardial depression than verapamil.

Dobutamine

Actions	Indications	Dosage	Precautions
Positive chronotropic agent using β-adrenergic receptor stimulation Increases: • Myocardial contractility balanced by increase in coronary blood flow at clinical doses • Stroke volume • Cardiac output • Renal perfusion due to increased cardiac output Mild increase in: • Heart rate • Hypertension • Arrhythmogenic effects • Vasodilative effects Does not increase epinephrine levels, as does dopamine	Indicated in: • Refractory CHF • Cardiogenic shock • Hypotension not related to hypovolemia	Infusion ranges: • Mix 500 to 1000 mg in 250 mL of NS. Dosage varies from 2.0 to as much as 40 mcg/kg/min in rare situations. Titrate to desired hemodynamic effect. Usual dosages ranges are 2.0–20 mcg/kg/min.	While titrating, endeavor to keep increase in heart rate to no more than 10%. Fluid deficits should be corrected before. May result in myocardial ischemia at high dosage ranges (>20 mg/kg/min) Less chronotropic effect than isoproterenol but still can cause tachycardias Do not mix with other chemicals, especially sodium bicarbonate. Taper off gradually, do not shut off. Use with caution in patients with coronary artery disease. Administer via infusion pump to ensure precise rates

Dopamine

Actions	Indications	Dosage	Precautions
Chemical precursor of epinephrine. It is dose dependent. See chart below. The colored boxes refer to what receptors are stimulated. On the *x* axis are the adrenergic receptors. The *y* axis contains the dosages.	• Hypotension secondary to significant bradycardia • Hypotension in the absence of hypovolemia • Cardiogenic shock • CHF (with other agents)	IV Infusion: • 400 mg (1 amp) in 250 mL = 1600 mcg/mL • Or a more concentrated dose, 800 mg (2 amps) in 250 mL = 3200 mcg/mL • Run the IV drip rate commensurate with the dosage that affects the receptors desired. Start at 1–5 mcg/kg/min and titrate to achieve a final range of 5–20 mcg/kg/min. • If dosage is increased beyond 20 mcg/kg/min to achieve desired effect, consider adding norepinephrine drip.	Contraindicated in: • Hypotension secondary to hypovolemia • Tachydysrhythmias • Pheochromocytoma Use cautiously in patients taking monoamine oxidase (MAO) inhibitors or diagnosed with pheochromocytoma. Do not shut off, taper gradually. Infuse through a central line or use a needle-through-catheter in a large peripheral vein to keep chances of extravasation low. If extravasation occurs, employ phentolamine (Regitine). Dose is 5–10 mg diluted in 10–15 mL of NS infiltrated into the area. If possible, use an infusion pump to deliver drug. Monitor patient for excessive vasoconstriction.

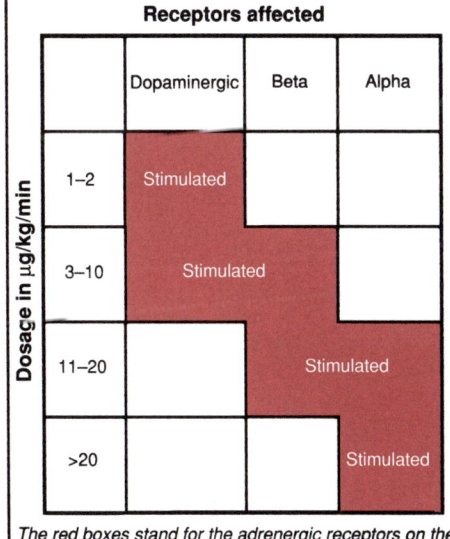

The red boxes stand for the adrenergic receptors on the x-axis that are stimulated at the dose on the y-axis

Epinephrine

Actions	Indications	Dosage	Precautions
An endogenous catecholamine that stimulates both β- and α-adrenergic receptors. Generally increases: • Systemic vascular resistance • Contractility • Automaticity • Arterial pressure • Heart rate • Myocardial oxygen demand • Cerebral blood flow • Myocardial blood flow During the bradycardia protocol, the β effects predominate, causing the heart to increase contractility and rate. However, during cardiac arrest, the α effects of vasoconstriction predominate. This vasoconstrictive effect increases the effectiveness of CPR by increasing perfusion to the cerebral arteries and the myocardium. No other agent produces greater cerebral blood flow.	IV push: • VF and pulseless VT • PEA • Asystole IV infusion: • Significant bradycardia • Cardiac arrest IV drip rather than constant bolus therapy every 3–5 minutes	Standard arrest dose: • **1 mg of 1:10,000 dilution IV push every 3–5 minutes** Megadose: *Intermediate* • 2–5 mg IV every 3–5 minutes Escalating • 1 mg—3 mg—5 mg every 3 minutes High • 0.01 mg/kg every 3–5 minutes Both the standard and the megadose regimens should be given routinely throughout the arrest sequence to keep up an acceptable therapeutic blood level. There is no maximum dose. IV infusion: *Bradycardia* • 1 mg in 250 mL titrated to pulse of 60 (2–10 mcg/min) Cardiac arrest • 30 mg in 250 mL initially run at 100 mL/h and titrate to hemodynamic end point ET administration: • 2–2.5 times the IV dosage of 1:1000 dilution. Add enough NS to make up the difference to 10 mL.	No specific contraindications in a cardiac arrest Megadose regimens of epinephrine are neither encouraged nor discouraged Cardiac arrest epinephrine drips should be administered through central lines to reduce chance of extravasation. Catecholamines such as epinephrine are inactivated when administered through the same line as alkaline solutions without flushing. If a VF has been defibrillated successfully and then rapidly deteriorates back into VF, consider withholding further doses of epinephrine because excessive amounts of epinephrine could be causing the problem. May induce ventricular ectopy in patients on digitalis

Furosemide

Actions	Indications	Dosage	Precautions
Potent diuretic Inhibits reabsorption in the loop of Henle and in the distal convoluted tubule Decreases preload by increasing venous capacitance	Indicated in: • CHF • Acute pulmonary edema • Cerebral edema	0.5–1.0 mg/kg slow IV push over 1 to 2 minutes. A usual adult dose is 40 mg. Initial dosage should be increased if the patient is currently taking furosemide.	Diuretics can cause: • Hypovolemia • Hypokalemia • Dehydration • Hypotension Cases of tinnitus have been reported when injecting too rapidly.

Isoproterenol

Actions	Indications	Dosage	Precautions
Pure β-adrenergic stimulator: • β$_1$-Adrenergic, positive chronotropic, and inotropic activity • β$_2$-Adrenergic, bronchodilation • Vasodilation Increases the myocardial oxygen consumption to the extent that any other dosage, other than low, is considered harmful (class III), causing myocardial ischemia	Significant bradycardia: • Only when atropine, dopamine, and epinephrine have proved refractory until a pacemaker is available In torsades des pointes: • Refractory to magnesium sulfate therapy, isoproterenol acts as a "chemical overdrive pacemaker" by increasing the ventricular rate faster than the torsades de pointes. After the pacemaker is captured, the rate is decreased.	Significant bradycardia: *IV infusion:* • 1 mg in 250 mL • 2–10 mcg/min titrating to achieving a pulse rate of 60 beats/min	Increases myocardial oxygen consumption and therefore increases myocardial ischemia Precipitates tachydysrhythmia and other dysrhythmias May precipitate hypokalemia Not indicated in cardiac arrest rhythms Use with caution when titrating to effect

Lidocaine

Actions	Indications	Dosage	Precautions

Elevates VF threshold
 	
Suppresses ventricular ectopic beats by depressing phase 4 of the action potential curve, thus shortening it
 	
Does not affect myocardial contractility in normal dosage ranges
	• VF
	• Pulseless VT
	• *Significant* premature ventricular ectopics in the acute cardiovascular compromise setting. This may include bursts or runs of VT. It does *not* include escape ventricular beats
	
	Routine prophylactic administration in acute MI is no longer recommended.
		VF or pulseless VT (any of following are acceptable):
		
		• **1.0–1.5 mg/kg repeated at 3- to 5-minute intervals to a maximum of 3 mg/kg**
		• **1.0–1.5 mg/kg repeated at 3- to 5-minute intervals at 0.5–0.75 mg/kg to a maximum of 3 mg/kg**
		• **Cardiac arrest patients may require only a single dose of 1.5 mg/kg**
		
		VT or wide complex tachycardia of uncertain type, both with pulses:
		
		• **1.0–1.5 mg/kg repeated every 5–10 minutes at half doses (0.5–0.75 mg/kg) to maximum of 3 mg/kg**
		
		IV maintenance infusion:
		
		• After loading dose in both stable situations or after return of pulse in cardiac arrest with supraventricular pacemaker
		• 1 g in 250 mL. Run at:
		  • 2 mg/min after 1 mg/kg conversion
		  • 3 mg/min after 2 mg/kg conversion
		  • 4 mg/min after 3 mg/kg conversion
		
		For non-cardiac arrest after stopping ectopics and starting maintenance drip:
		
		• Consider a second bolus of 0.5 mg/kg after 10 minutes to prevent therapeutic level decline
		
		ET administration:
		
		• 2 to 2.5 times the IV dose
			Contraindicated in ventricular escape rhythms
			
			If ventricular ectopic beats are part of a bradycardic rhythm, treat the rate *first*
			
			Signs of toxicity:
			
			• Hallucinations
			• Altered level of consciousness
			• Decreased hearing
			• Seizure disorders
			• Slurred speech
			• Paresthesia
			• Muscle twitching
			
			Lidocaine maintenance dosage should be limited to half the normal dose whenever the following is suspected or documented:
			
			• Decreased cardiac output
			• Decreased hepatic function
			• Patient age greater than 70 years

Magnesium Sulfate

Actions	Indications	Dosage	Precautions
Essential enzyme in sodium–potassium ATP pump Regulates calcium movement, thereby controlling cardiac contraction Hypomagnesemia is associated with high incidence of cardiac arrhythmias which include torsades de pointes Current literature is contradictory concerning the efficacy of using magnesium sulfate after an acute MI. However, the drug's introduction in a subset of acute MI patients who are not candidates for either thrombolytic therapy or PTCA (angioplasty) is encouraging.	Suspected or documented hypomagnesemia in: • VF or pulseless VT • Acute MI • Torsades de pointes	**VF or pulseless VT:** • 1 or 2 g (2–4 mL of a 50% solution) diluted in 10 mL of D-5-W administered by IV bolus **Torsades de pointes:** • 1 or 2 g (2–4 mL of a 50% solution) diluted in 10 mL D-5-W administered over 1–2 minutes • After initial infusion, follow with same amount spread out over 1 hour • Up to 5–10 g may be required to suppress torsades **Acute MI therapy:** • 0.5–1 g spread out over a 24-hour period after MI	*Hypo*magnesemia is associated with a high incidence of cardiac dysrhythmias Signs and symptoms of *hyper*magnesemia are: • Respiratory depression • Loss of deep tendon reflexes • Hypotension • Diarrhea

Morphine

Actions	Indications	Dosage	Precautions
Opiate-based analgesic or euphoric Decreases: • Preload • Afterload • Myocardial oxygen requirement Increases: • Venous capacitance • Pain threshold Pain causes an increased level of circulating catecholamines. The increased levels result in an increase in systemic vascular resistance, exacerbating myocardial ischemia. Morphine decreases anxiety and thus catecholamine release.	• Acute pulmonary edema • Ischemia chest pain	**Initial dose:** • 2–5 mg slow IV, titrated to patient's response. If pain is not curtailed, consider repeating same dosage every 5 minutes, titrating to either patient's pain level or desired hemodynamic response.	The definitive antidote of overdoses is naloxone (Narcan). Watch for signs of: • Respiratory depression • CNS depression • Hypotension • Nausea and vomiting Use with caution in volume-compromised patients.

Nitroglycerine

Actions	Indications	Dosage	Precautions
Smooth muscle relaxant. Has a vasodilatory effect on both peripheral arteries and veins Dilates coronary arteries The venous pooling decreases both preload and afterload, thereby decreasing myocardial oxygen requirement. Pulse rate may elevate when blood pressure decreases.	• Ischemic chest pain • Acute MI • Angina pectoris • Esophageal spasms • Cardiogenic pulmonary edema	Sublingual: • **0.3–0.4 mg.** May repeat at 5-minute intervals. Maximum of three total doses IV infusion: • **Mix 50 mg in 250 mL of NS.** Resulting concentration is 200 mcg/mL. Initial dosage should be 10–20 mcg/min delivered through an infusion pump. Initial titration should be in 5- to 10-mcg/min increments, with increases every 5–10 minutes until some response is noted. Be cautious if blood pressure is less than 100 mmHg. Endeavor to keep the mean arterial blood pressure above 80 mmHg. Once the desired hemodynamic response is noted, dose increase should be reduced and time intervals between doses lengthened.	*Hypotension* is the main precaution to guard against. • Monitor vital signs during and after administration • Decreasing mean arterial blood pressure can further exacerbate myocardial ischemia. • Consider fluid replacement therapy to correct hypotension. Other common side effects include: • Headache • Transient episodes of lightheadedness • Syncope • Tachycardic response to blood pressure decrease • Reperfusion dysrhythmias

Norepinephrine

Actions	Indications	Dosage	Precautions
An endogenous catecholamine that primarily stimulates α-adrenergic receptors; however, some β-adrenergic receptor stimulation is noted. Profoundly increases: - Systemic vascular resistance - Arterial pressure - Myocardial oxygen requirement *without* a compensatory increase in myocardial blood flow	- As a temporary measure in cardiogenic shock - Absense of peripheral vasoconstriction with hypotension	IV infusion: - One vial containing 4 mg added to 250 mL NS achieving a concentration of 16 mcg/mL. A central line would minimize chance of extravasation. - Infuse at a rate of 0.5–1.0 mcg/min to start, and titrate to the desired hemodynamic response. - To discontinue drug, taper slowly to avoid abrupt and severe hypotension.	Contraindicated in hypovolemia Use with caution in: - Hypertension - Arrhythmias If extravasation occurs, employ phentolamine (Regitine). Dose is 5–10 mg, diluted in 10–15 mL of NS infiltrated into the area. Temporary medication. It should not be considered long-term. Consider switching to dopamine when systolic blood pressure reaches 70 mmHg.

Oxygen

Actions	Indications	Dosage	Precautions
Increases oxygen tension, content, and hemoglobin saturation Hypoxia shifts the oxyhemoglobin curve to the left. Oxygen restores it, moving it back to the right. Poor oxygenation results in right-to-left shunting with resultant ventilation–perfusion mismatching.	Hypoxemia: - Chest pain due to myocardial ischemia - Any suspected hypoxemia - Cardiopulmonary arrest	By appropriate passive delivery device if patient is breathing spontaneously By positive pressure with 100% oxygen if patient is apneic or needs to be assisted	Caution in chronic obstructive pulmonary disease (COPD) However, *never* withhold oxygen if signs or symptoms of hypoxia are present. If COPD is causing cardiovascular decompensation, titrate oxygen flow upward cautiously. Be prepared to assist ventilations if necessary.

Procainamide

Actions	Indications	Dosage	Precautions
Elevates VF threshold Suppresses ventricular ectopics Prolongs refractory period and duration of action potential curve by suppressing phase 4. This reduces automaticity of pacemaker, slowing AV conduction.	Employed when lidocaine has proved refractory in: • VF or pulseless VT • VT • Wide complex tachycardia of uncertain type • *Significant* ventricular ectopic beats Adjunct drug: • Atrial fibrillation • Atrial flutter	**20 mg/min** until any of the following occurs: • Dysrhythmia is suppressed • A total of 17 mg/kg is administered • The QRS complex increases by more than 50% of pretreatment width **Higher infusion rates of 30 mg/min may be administered in time-critical situations** IV infusion: • 1 g in 250 mL and run at 1–4 mg/min	Limit maintenance infusion in liver impairment (CHF, elderly [>70 years], cirrhosis, and hepatitis and renal dysfunction) Administering too rapidly may result in hypotension. Use cautiously in acute MI. Refrain from using drug in torsades de pointes or any rhythm suffering from prolonged Q-T intervals Constantly observe for hypotension and widening QRS intervals Consider only after lidocaine and bretylium have proved refractory in the VF and pulseless VT protocol because its administration time is extremely lengthy.

Sodium Bicarbonate

Actions	Indications	Dosage	Precautions
Shifts oxyhemoglobin dissociation curve to left, decreasing oxygen's ability to leave hemoglobin for the tissues If not hyperventilated off during a cardiac arrest, carbon dioxide is retained, which can diffuse across cell membranes, resulting in intracellular acidosis. Restores buffering capacity of body and corrects bicarbonate-responsive problems in preexisting situations, such as: • Diabetic ketoacidosis • Aspirin overdose • Tricyclic antidepressant overdose • Hyperkalemia	Class I (definitely helpful): • Known preexisting hyperkalemia Class IIa (acceptable, probably helpful): • Known preexisting bicarbonate-responsive acidosis • Overdose of tricyclic antidepressants • Alkalize the urine in drug overdose Class IIb (acceptable, possibly helpful): • If intubated and continued long arrest interval • On return of spontaneous circulation after long arrest interval Class III (not indicated, may be harmful): • Hypoxic lactic acidosis Before considering, try: • Intubation • Hyperventilation • Epinephrine if appropriate • Defibrillation if appropriate	• 1 mEq/kg repeated at 0.5 mEq/kg every 10 minutes thereafter until administration can be guided by blood gases	Not indicated in the routine cardiac arrest, in which the cause of the acidosis is carbon dioxide retention (hypoxic lactic acidosis) Hypernatremia Hyperosmolarity May cause hypokalemia Intracellular acidosis from diffusion of unventilated carbon dioxide across cell membrane

Sodium Bicarbonate

Sodium Nitroprusside

Actions	Indications	Dosage	Precautions
Like all nitrates, sodium nitroprusside is a potent smooth muscle relaxant. It has a vasodilatory effect on both peripheral arteries and veins. This drug decreases both preload and afterload, thereby lowering myocardial oxygen requirement. Decreases pulmonary congestion Pulse rate may elevate when blood pressure decreases. Increases cardiac output, thereby enhancing systolic emptying. Increases left ventricular end-diastolic pressure	• Pump failure • Hypertensive crises	This drug is only given as an IV infusion: • Mix 50–100 mg in 250 mL of NS to give a concentration of 200–400 mcg/mL • Initial dosage range is 0.1–5.0 mcg/kg/min. However, in some more refractory situations, dosages of up to 10 mcg/kg/min may be required.	Observe for thiocyanate toxicity: • Visual blurring • Convulsions • Confusion • Hyperreflexia • Tinnitus Watch for primary problem: hypotension. Used in MIs only when nitroglycerin is refractory Other common side effects are: • Dizziness • Abdominal cramps • Headaches • Nausea and vomiting • Palpitations • Apprehension • Muscle twitching • Chest pain Drug reacts with light.

Thrombolytic Agents

Actions	Indications	Dosage	Precautions
Thrombolytic agents were engineered to break down blood clots. Unfortunately, they are not specific for thrombi in just coronary vessels.	Thrombolytic therapy should be considered in all potential candidates up to 12 hours after onset of pain. The greatest amount of myocardial salvage occurs if thrombolytics are administered within the first 4 hours. If treatment is delayed past 4 hours, the ability to salvage much myocardium is lost. However, even though the amount salvaged is not extensive, thrombolytic therapy is encouraged after 4 hours, to as much as 12 hours after the onset of chest pain.	Four thrombolytic agents are approved by the FDA:	Because these agents break down all blood clots regardless of where they occur, thrombolytics are *absolutely contraindicated* in:
When a clot in a coronary vessel is dissolved, reestablishment of blood flow to involved tissue occurs. This reperfusion can limit the infarct and, depending on the time interval from infarction, may reclaim ischemic tissue.		• APSAC • Streptokinase • Tissue-plasminogen activator (tPA) • Urokinase	• Active internal bleeding • Suspected aortic dissection • Known traumatic CPR • Severe persistent hypertension despite pain relief and initial drugs (>180 mmHg systolic or >110 mmHg diastolic)
By reversing myocardial ischemia, a decrease in ventricular arrythmias may be observed.		Dose is dependent on thrombolytic selected:	• Recent head trauma or known intracranial neoplasm
tPA specifically is FDA approved for treatment of thrombi in acute ischemic stroke		Although both streptokinase and tPA have reduced mortality in acute MI, a front-loaded regimen of tPA showed a clear advantage over streptokinase. This advantage was most pronounced in patients with:	• History of CVA in past 6 months • Pregnancy
	The decision to order thrombolytics is based on a number of variables: the patient's history and age, ECG findings of two or more leads with ST elevation, infarction location, symptom duration, and an estimate of risks versus benefits.	• An infarction time less than 4 hours • An age less than 75 years • Anterior infarcts	There is a long list of *relative contraindications* in the coronary syndrome case study.
	Thrombi in documented cases of acute ischemic stroke	tPA is first FDA-approved therapy for acute ischemic stroke	

Verapamil

Actions	Indications	Dosage	Precautions
Calcium-channel blocker that inhibits calcium's influx across cardiac, skeletal, and smooth muscle. This inhibition causes both negative inotropic and chronotropic effects on the myocardium. Terminates reentrant tachydysrhythmias that pass-through AV node by slowing conduction (atrial fibrillation and flutter) Negative inotropic activity decreases blood pressure Prolongs AV nodal conduction time	• Supraventricular tachydysrhythmias refractory to adenosine administration • Only those wide complex tachydysrhythmias *diagnosed with certainty* to have supraventricular origins. • Atrial fibrillation and flutter with uncontrolled or rapid ventricular responses (>100 beats/minute). Should be withheld in Wolff-Parkinson-White syndrome.	Initial dose: • **2.5 to 5 mg IV slowly over 1–2 minutes** Caution should be exercised and a slower rate of administration should be introduced in the elderly and in patients likely to become hypotensive (consider 3–4 minutes) Second and subsequent doses: • 5–10 mg IV with an interval of 15–30 minutes between successive doses until effect is achieved or a total of 30 mg is reached	Side effects include: • Dizziness • Transient hypotension • Fatigue Contraindicated in patients exhibiting any serious signs or symptoms of: • CHF • AV block • Hypotension • Heart failure • Sinus node dysfunction Contraindicated in atrial fibrillation or flutter masked by Wolff-Parkinson-White syndrome Do not administer IV β-blockers simultaneously with IV verapamil Use cautiously when verapamil therapy must be combined with a history of patient use of β-blockers.

9 Memorization Techniques

This chapter provides a number of diverse tricks to help you remember the large amount of information that constitutes the ACLS protocols, drugs, and drug dosages. Depending on how your brain processes information, some of the following memorization methodology may make retention easier, and some methods may be unhelpful. Do not think that you have to use all of the techniques; just use what works best for you, and ignore the rest! Remember, these techniques work best if you read slowly and follow the instructions.

Each medication and ACLS protocol from the *Advanced Cardiac Life Support* textbook is listed in the following text. After each entry, memorization techniques are provided to help you retain the information. Images are used to assist in memorizing some of the treatment algorithms and drug dosages.

The traditional education system used a textbook-oriented approach to promote student learning. On average, students who enjoyed reading and memorizing the textbook performed well in school. For students who were more visually oriented, however, the textbook often made learning a frustrating experience. These learners found that they could only recall information if they associated the facts with visual images. Because the traditional system did not promote visualized learning strategies, students often struggled to remember the information in the textbook.

Adult learners can usually be grouped into two distinct learning styles:

1. Some learners read the American Heart Association's ACLS textbook from cover to cover, memorize the protocols and associated drug dosages by writing them repetitively, and recite the information with little or no perceived difficulty.
2. Other learners only read what they absolutely have to in the textbook while agonizing over their inability to retain the information. These students dutifully scribble out each protocol over and over again to obtain some semblance of retention. Because stress inhibits memory, these students usually cannot recall all of the information during testing.

In an attempt to assist both styles of learning, mnemonic and visual memory aids are incorporated within this chapter. Note that some of these memory aides may appear confusing or simplistic to you, but they may be helpful for someone else. If an aid does not seem to help you, just proceed to another or make up one of your own.

Right- and Left-Brain Processing

A great deal of research has been done on mapping the right and left hemispheres of the brain. The right half of the brain processes information intuitively and spatially. This half of the brain is usually associated with pictures, intuition, emotions, imagination, humor, spatial concepts, music, color, body movement (dance), creativity, and drama. The left half of the brain, on the other hand, is primarily responsible for processing information in a logical, linear fashion. The left half tends to be linked with verbal skills, logic, and analysis.

People process information using both halves of the brain, but tend to use one side or the other more. In the general population, men tend to process information using the left half more than the right, whereas women are usually right-brain thinkers. This may account for the incredible communication problems that often arise between men and women.

To use the memory aides presented in this chapter, you must determine which side of the brain is dominant during your mental processes. The following scenarios show the difference between right and left brain functions:

- When you visit a museum and go to the dinosaur exhibit, there are hundreds of bones on each wall. Each exhibit has an explanatory placard stating where the bone was found, who found it, what part of the dinosaur it was from, and how old it is (Fig. 9-1). Generally speaking, do you read the placard every time?

If you answered "yes," the necessity of reading the placard is primarily a left-brain function. A right-brain thinker would answer "no." He or she would look at the exhibit and say, "interesting bone," and move on, rarely reading the placard unless specifically interested. Information in right brain thinkers is processed visually. A right-brain thinker would constantly be asking his or her left-brain companion to hurry up during the museum trip.

- Another example might be assembling a piece of furniture (Fig. 9-2). Generally speaking, do you read the complete directions before starting, or only after you get into trouble?

Left-brain thinkers always read the instructions (i.e., verbal skills), whereas right-brain thinkers look at the pictures and make immediate sense of the assembly (i.e., visual skills).

Advertisers know this and employ both right and left clues in their advertisements. Each ad contains a visual portion for the right brain and a verbal component for the left. A cigarette billboard might show a photograph of a smiling woman relaxing on the beach, smoking a cigarette. The tag line below it states, "I smoke for the pleasure of it!" (Fig. 9-3). The visual aspect of a happy person smoking is absorbed by the right brain, and the left half processes the written material that smoking is pleasurable.

Memorization Schemes

This chapter provides both right- and left-brain techniques to assist in memorizing the ACLS protocols and drug dosages.

The memorization techniques employ:

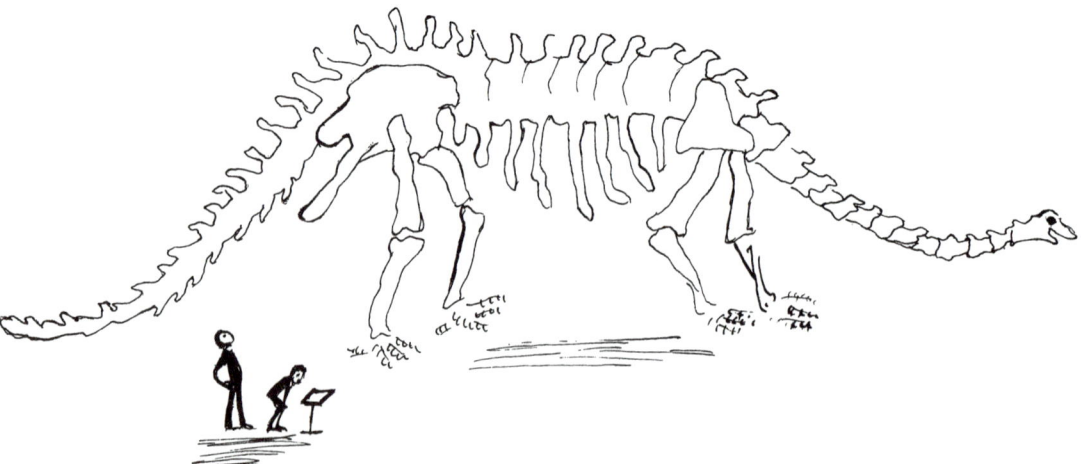

Figure 9-1

Figure 9-2

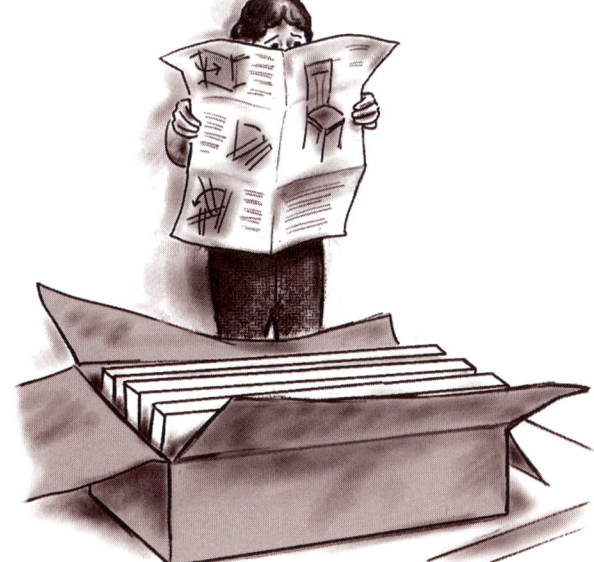

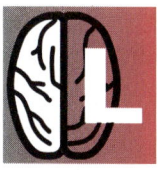
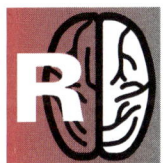

Mnemonics: nonsensical sentences in which the first letters of most words remind you of something to be memorized. "Looks pretty bad but stable" helps the clinician remember the treatment for stable ventricular tachycardia: **l**idocaine, **p**rocainamide, **b**retylium, and **s**ynchronized cardioversion.

Visual images: visualized exactly or chained together. This technique uses visual images made so dynamic, exciting, or bizarre in a ho-hum fashion that they cannot be forgotten. Every image or story conveyed requires you to see an image in your mind—as real and vivid as your imagination can make it. If you just read each description the technique will not work! The visual image must be dynamic, humorous, colorful, exciting, or truly bizarre for the information to be memorable.

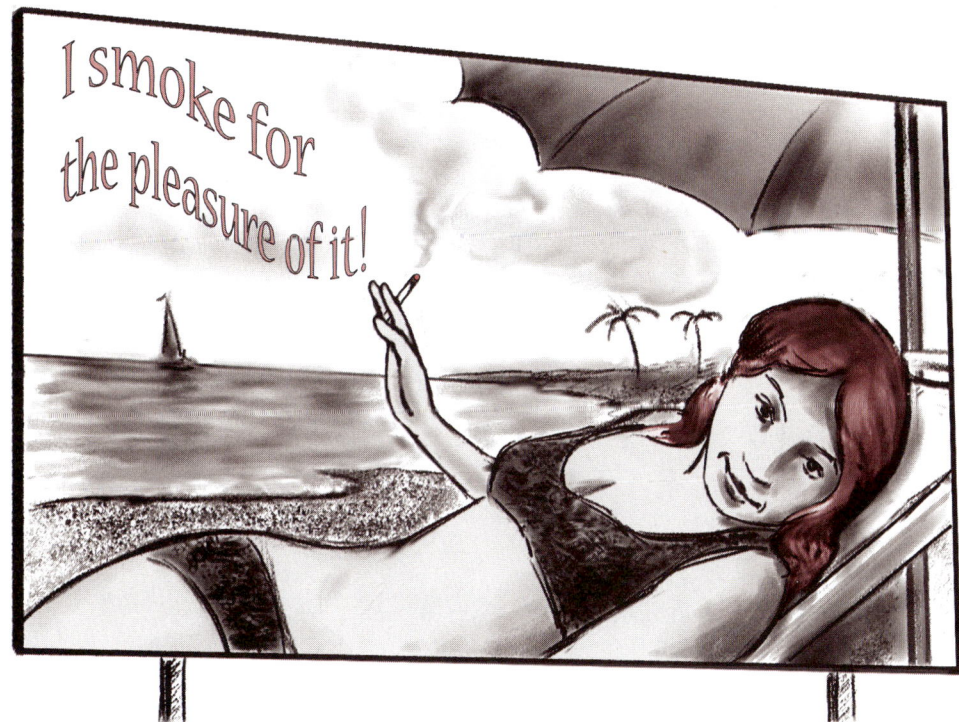

Figure 9-3

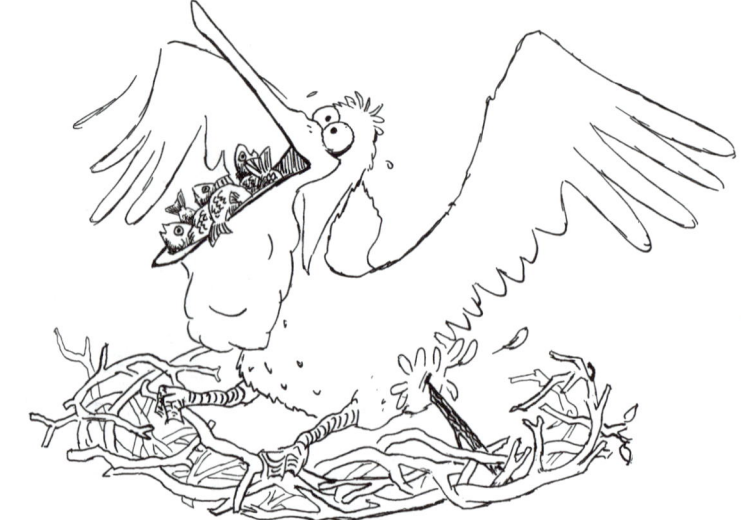

Figure 9-4

For example, if I told you to visualize a pelican sitting on a nest, you may have difficulty. However, if I told you visualize the following description of a pelican, you would probably be able to see it clearly in your mind: the pelican has white gossamer wings that are so bright that they appear to glint in the sun; its floppy pouch is protruding from the bottom of its beak, so stuffed with live fish that the rippling pouch appears to be alive. It is flapping its wings and screeching madly because it is sitting on a nest of twigs arranged so haphazardly that one of the larger branches is poking the pelican so deeply in its rear that one might think it was undergoing an endoscopy (Fig. 9-4).

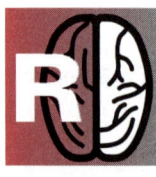
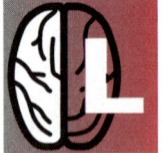

For most people, this image can be recalled easily and effectively. I used visual, auditory, and humor cues to make it memorable. If you can recall this vision easily, those memory aids that employ this technique will be easy; these aids are indicated with a right-brain symbol: If you are a predominantly left-brain thinker, however, you might have found yourself asking questions like, "What is the pelican doing there?" "What sex is it?" "Where did the fish come from?" These questions indicate that right-brained memory aids may cause you frustration. If the images work for you, great! If they do not, try harder to make the image real and dynamic. Put movement, color, and possibly sexual humor into it. If the images are still difficult to recall, drop the technique and use another method, such as repetitive writing—whatever works best for you. I have indicated the memory aids that use left-brain techniques with the left-brain symbol: If both symbols appear, the memory aid would be useful for both right- and left-brain thinkers.

Many drugs and protocols have only one memory aid, usually right-brained. If a left-brain symbol is not present, assume that the only way for a left-brain thinker to memorize it is to write it out repeatedly until it is easily recalled or to use a memorization technique that works for you.

Practice sessions are provided and are set in a different typeface so that they are obvious. Do not skip the practice sessions because they are necessary to force you to make the images clearer and to clue you when you did not make them dynamic enough to retain.

ACLS Drugs

- Adenosine
- Verapamil
- Lidocaine
- Procainamide
- Bretylium
- Atropine
- Epinephrine
- Magnesium sulfate

Adenosine

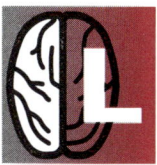 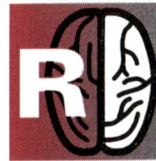

Repeat the drug's name slowly: Ad-din-o-sin. What time does "din-ner" begin in the evening? 6 o'clock. Thus, the first dose of this drug is 6 mg. Now for the second dose. What time do most people equate with biblical "sin," the witching hour?—sin begins at midnight. Therefore, the second dose is 12 mg. The first dose of adenosine is 6 mg, and the second dose is 12 mg. Adenosine can be repeated at 12 mg if the first two doses are refractory.

Verapamil

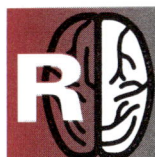

Verapamil: the word sounds like "wrap-a-meal." If you are wrapping up a meal, you must have had leftovers. Leftovers are common when people take their time to eat, usually spreading the meal over 20 to 30 minutes. If you rush, you tend to overeat, and there are no leftovers to wrap up. Therefore, if you are finished eating and food is left over, you must have taken at least 20 to 30 minutes to eat.

Imagine a plate, and spread aluminum foil over it, carefully crimping the edges. Pick it up and look at it carefully. To your astonishment, the foiled-wrapped plate becomes a clock with a mouse on the front. (Due to copyright restrictions a certain well-known mouse cannot be shown. The key here is to visualize the mouse of your choice on the clock.) The mouse is holding his hands to either side, representing the passage of time. The watch, however, no longer bears the traditional time sequence: 1 through 12. The top of the watch bears the number 30—representing that it took that long to eat. Progressing clockwise, the first new digit, 5, appears one quarter of the way around, 10 appears at the bottom halfway through, and the number 20 appears at the three-quarters mark (Fig. 9-5).

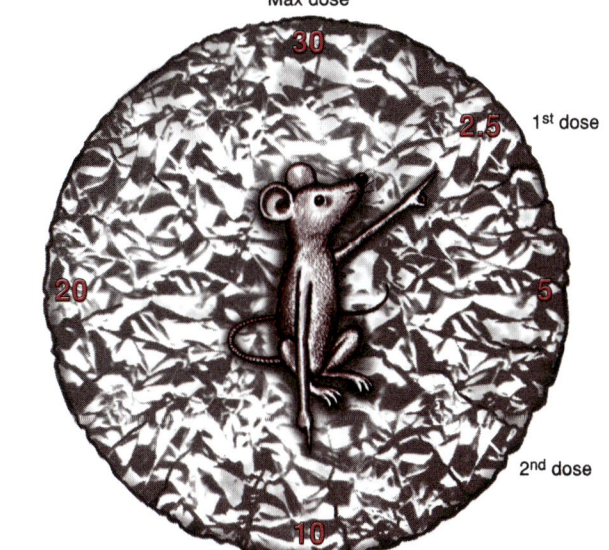

Figure 9-5

Let's Practice

One of the mouse's arms is pointing straight up; what number is there? Good, 30. He is pointing directly down; right, the number here is 10. Now where is 20? Good! His right hand is pointing directly to his right, or if he used his left hand, it would be awkwardly pointing across his body to his right side, about three quarters the way around the clock. What if he moves his hand and progresses clockwise from the top to one quarter the way around the clock? Right, 5. Now let's continue with the description.

Initially, from a vertical position, the mouse moves his hand clockwise halfway to the number 5 mark (one eighth the way around), to about 2.5. He pauses for 2 to 3 seconds and then continues, stopping directly at the number 5 mark. The first dose of this drug is 2.5 to 5 mg. Again, repeat the image. Watch the mouse's hand start at the top, pause halfway to the one quarter mark, and continue to stop at the number 5 mark.

Try to visualize that image before proceeding!

Now the mouse pulls his hand in and hesitates. The hesitation reminds the clinician that there is an interlude of 15 to 30 minutes between successive doses. The mouse then puts the same hand at the number 5 mark and moves it to where it points directly down—the number 10 mark. The second dose is 5 to 10 mg. Once more, he pauses by pulling in his hand, reminding the clinician of the necessary 15- to 30-minute waiting period.

Now the mouse points to the number 10 and drags the pointing finger clockwise from the halfway point, where it eventually becomes vertical, pointing at the number 30—the maximum dose. The patient was given the first and the second dose without effect, so it can be repeated until a maximum dose of 30 mg is reached.

Let's Practice

One of his hands goes clockwise from the top to a stop one eighth the way around, pauses, and stops one quarter the way around.

1. What is the dose? _____

The mouse then points overhead.

2. What is the dose? _____

Yes, I got out of sequence and tried unsuccessfully to fool you.

The mouse's hand points to his left at a right angle to his body and then points toward his shoes. Good, the second dose is 5 to 10 mg. He points overhead: 30. He points to his left at the one-quarter mark and then points down: second dose, 5 to 10 mg.

3. What did the mouse do to help you remember the first dose? _____

Summarizing, the first dose is 2.5 to 5 mg and the second is 5 to 10 mg, waiting at least 15 to 30 minutes between successive doses. The doses can be repeated until a maximum of 30 mg is achieved or side effects become substantial. Remember to "wrap the meal," taking *time* to wrap it right!

Lidocaine

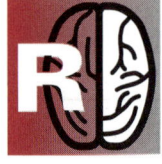

The memorization technique for lidocaine is different. I am going to tell you a story, similar to "Goldilocks and the Three Bears." Try to remember just the gross facts; it will be necessary to repeat them back as close as possible to the original. Each image does not necessarily mean anything; the images are chained together visually to help you imagine them in your mind. When viewed together, these images help you to remember the protocols and the drug dosages. Although this is inherently easy for the right brain, many people who approach this scheme with their left brain (i.e., try to understand it) are frustrated. They think it is nonsense because there is not necessarily a logical connection between one image and another. If you try to understand what each image means (a left-brain process), this system can be difficult and frustrating. Therefore, do not think; just picture the images in your mind.

At the end, I chain each of the individual images together, which results in a sequence to help you recall the dosage of lidocaine, procainamide, and bretylium. Remember, don't be logical, just read the story, keeping in mind that you will have to repeat it to someone else.

THE DOOR

Picture yourself standing on a well-cared-for lawn in a housing subdivision. The lawn feels spongy beneath your feet. The sun is baking the back of your neck, and a breeze is softly blowing through your hair. In a relaxed manner, you are gazing at the front door of a beautiful home. The door is obviously expensive because it is made out of teak. It has a glossy appearance, and you remember that the owner spends an inordinate amount of time waxing it every 2 weeks. Above the door is a stained-glass panel with a rainbow shining out from it and hitting the lawn, where you can almost make out a pot of gold (Fig. 9-6).

Try to visualize the image before proceeding.

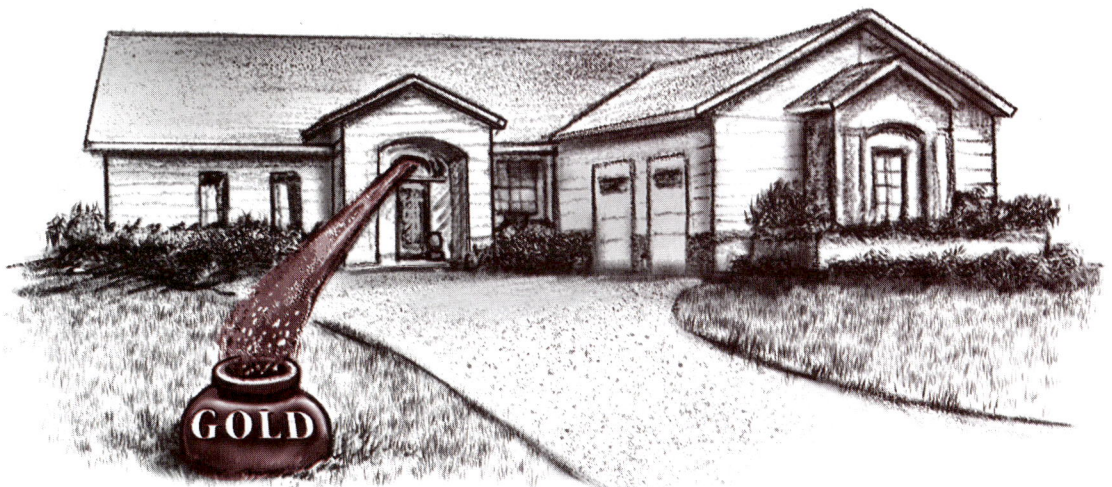

Figure 9-6

Let's Practice

1. What is striking the back of your neck? _____
2. What was the door made of? _____
3. What was shining out from above the door? _____

THE MORTAR

Breaking the peaceful atmosphere, suddenly from behind you comes the sound of a mortar being shot off—schunk! You turn your head and see a teenage boy holding a piece of gray PVC plastic plumbing pipe. The pipe is stuck into the ground at a 45-degree angle, and the boy is dropping Christmas candy canes down the barrel (Fig. 9-7). When the candy canes reach the bottom, they shoot forth with a resounding "schunk!" and strike the beautiful teak door of the home that you were viewing. They hit the door and lie down in front of it.

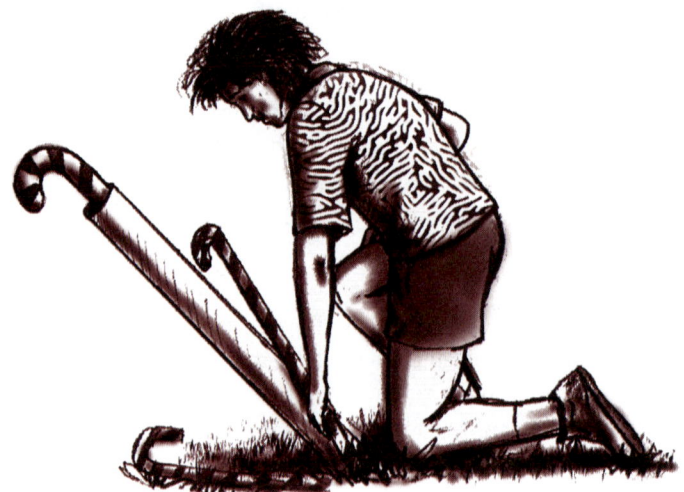

Figure 9-7

Let's Practice

1. What was the boy holding at a 45-degree angle? _____

2. What was shooting out from the barrel? _____

3. What did they do to the teak door? _____

THE CANDY CANES

You walk up to the teak door, being careful not to walk on the scattered candy canes lying in front of the door. You pick up one candy cane in your left hand and turn to your right, spying a cedar keg alongside the door. You can smell the scent of cedar as it wafts up.

Leaning against the keg is a chrome baton. You remember it in high school being thrown above the heads of the crowd by the cheerleaders during homecoming (Fig. 9-8). Picking up the baton in your right hand, you pause, look at the candy cane, look back to the baton, and repeat the process again. Holding the candy cane over the open keg, you purposely strike the candy cane in the middle with the baton, breaking the candy cane in half. You keep returning to the door and pick up candy canes, breaking them in half in the keg, until you have broken a total of three candy canes.

Figure 9-8

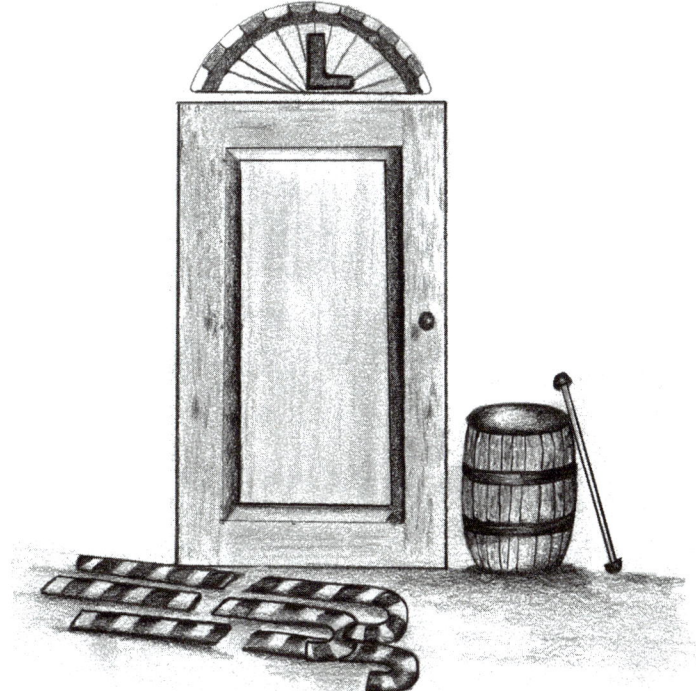

Let's Practice

1. What two objects did you pick up? _____

2. Did you pause and look at both the objects in your hands, or did you immediately break the candy cane in half with the baton? _____

3. How many candy canes did you wind up breaking in half? _____

THE INTERPRETATION

The candy canes strike the door, where they lie down in front of it: Li-dor-caine. The dose of 1 mg is depicted by pausing when holding one candy cane and the baton over the keg. The baton resembles the number 1, while the keg reminds the clinician that lidocaine is administered on a per-kilogram basis. Striking the candy and breaking it in half serves two purposes: illustrating the alternate dose of 1.5 given for more serious situations, and helping the clinician remember that subsequent doses would routinely be half of the first. The act of breaking the candy into halves would be completed when a maximum of three candy canes: 3 mg/kg (per keg) are administered.

Summarizing, lidocaine is given in a dosage of 1 to 1.5 mg/kg, which can be repeated at half doses to a maximum of 3 mg/kg.

Let's Practice

1. What is the maximum dose? How many candy canes? _____

2. What are the subsequent doses for routine situations? _____

3. What are the two initial dosage ranges? _____

4. Are these dosages based on milligrams per minute? _____

Procainamide

THE KEG

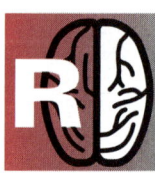

Drop the baton and the pieces of broken candy into the keg, open the beautiful teak door, and enter the house. Enter the first door on your right. Imagine that you enter a room with four gray walls and that the floor is painted a flat black. There are no windows, although there is a skylight overhead. You have just entered from the only door.

Standing upright in the center is a cedar keg. This is the type of barrel that one might use to ship quilts, bedding, screws, or roofing nails (Fig. 9-9). On closer inspection, you can see rusted metal bands strapped around the sides. The smell of cedar fills the room, and you are reminded of the time that you lifted the lid on your grandmother's cedar chest. The scent of home and your grandmother gently relax you. You notice that there are numerous dead moths lying at the base of the keg as you recall that cedar kills moths.

Try to visualize the image before proceeding.

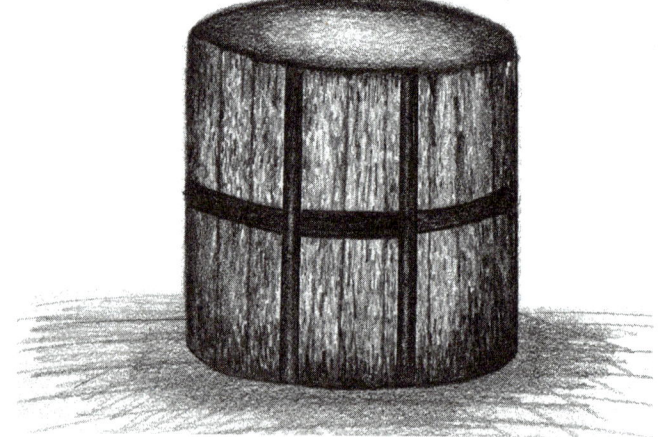

Figure 9-9

Let's Practice

1. What color are the walls?
2. What is the object in the center of the room?
3. How many windows are there?

THE TILL

Sitting on top of the keg is an old-fashioned cash register, commonly referred to as a till. People in small towns would make their own change at the till if the storekeeper was not present. This till is both massive and artistically ornate. If you push any combination of the keys down, the numbers pop up in a glass window located on top. The sides and front are cast iron, painted gold, with intricate scrolling. The name National Cash Register is cast into the back in a flowing script. This till is a beautiful antique that might have been found in any dry goods store at the turn of the century.

Let's Practice

1. What is below the till?
2. What is above the keg?
3. What is the color of the floor?

THE NEST AND THE BIRD

Perched precariously on top of the till is a gigantic nest of twigs. The twigs are arranged so haphazardly that it looks like the nest may fall to the ground with a brisk breeze. On closer inspection, it appears that each of the twigs was taken from a nearby eucalyptus tree because the smell of cough drops is heavy in the air.

Sitting directly in the center of the nest is an enormous pelican. It has immense white gossamer wings that are so bright that they appear to glint in the sun. Its floppy pouch, protruding from the bottom of its beak, is so stuffed with live fish that the rippling pouch appears to be alive. It is beating its wings in a frenzy, screeching madly because one of the larger twigs is poking into its rear. The twig is so deeply embedded that one might have thought the bird was undergoing an endoscopy (Fig. 9-10).

Try to visualize the image before proceeding.

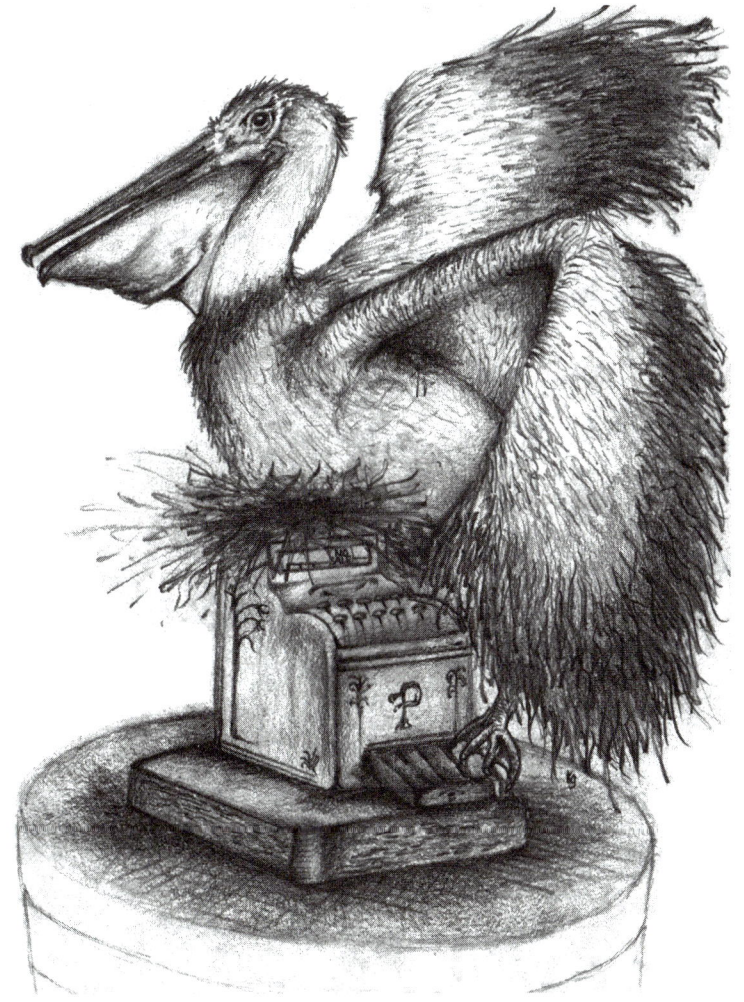

Figure 9-10

Let's Practice

1. What is above the till? _____
2. What is below the nest? _____
3. What is above the nest? _____
4. What is below the till? _____
5. What is on top of the nest? _____
6. What is making the pelican's pouch move? _____

FOOD FOR THE PELICAN

You walk up to the squawking bird and grab its beak in your hands. You pry it open. You then throw two items inside the pelican's pouch: a pack of cigarettes and a watch (Fig. 9-11).

Figure 9-11

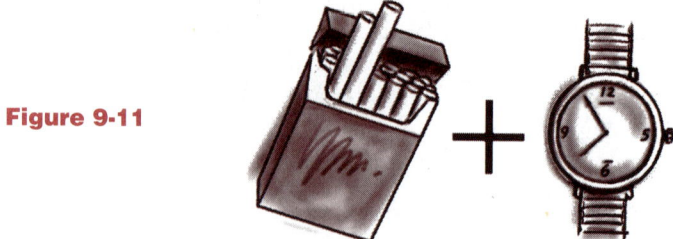

The cellophane wrapper of the cigarette pack crinkles as it slides into the cavernous maw of the pelican. One of the cigarettes falls out of the pack and lands in the mouth of one of the imprisoned fish. This appears strange but appropriate because the condemned are always asked if they wish one last smoke. After the pack of cigarettes you throw in your watch. You regret giving it away, but now you can be assured that the pelican will always know the correct time for dinner. The numbers arranged around the face of the watch sparkle as they cast numerous points of light all over the fish and the interior of the pelican's pouch (Fig. 9-12).

Try to visualize the image before proceeding.

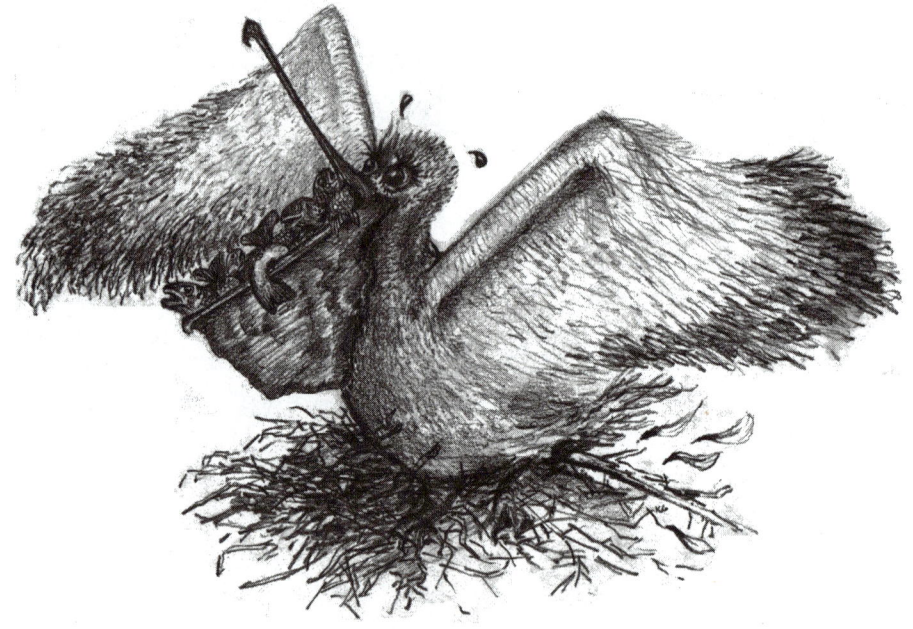

Figure 9-12

Let's Practice

1. What did you put into the pelican's mouth? _____
2. What were the objects you threw in? _____
3. What happened to one of the cigarettes when it fell out of the pack? _____
4. What was interesting about the watch as it fell into the pelican's mouth? _____

THE MAGAZINE

After depositing the pack of cigarettes and your watch, you begin to insult the pelican. You call it names: "son of a sea gull" and the like. It tries to ignore you by standing up, slowly waddling in a clockwise motion until eventually turning its tail feathers toward you. It then leans down, picks up a magazine off the floor, and begins nonchalantly to read it. This infuriates you so much that you grab a mass of tail feathers and spin the pelican around to face you. The magazine's name is now legible, a teenage magazine—*Seventeen* (Fig. 9-13).

Try to visualize the image before proceeding.

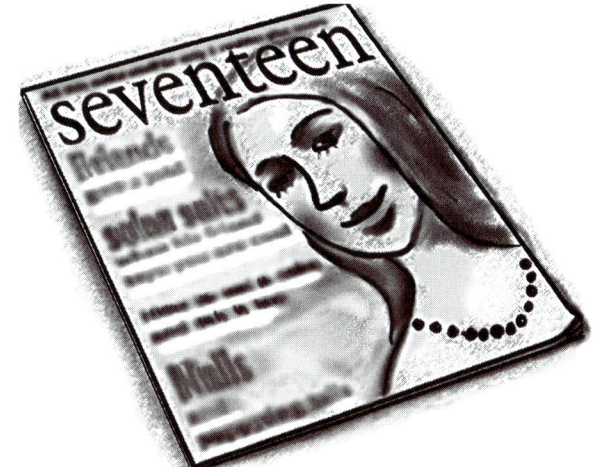

Figure 9-13

Let's Practice

1. Which way did the pelican turn in its effort to ignore you? _____
2. What made you mad? _____
3. What is the title of the magazine? _____

THE INTERPRETATION

The pelican was nesting on the till: Pro-nest-till. The trade name of procainamide is Pronestyl. You put a pack of cigarettes and a watch in its mouth. The visual memory aid for the number 20 is a pack of cigarettes because there are 20 to a pack. There are memory aids for all numbers: 6—a six-gun, 12—a dozen eggs, 3—a three-legged stool, or 5—an open hand. A cigarette pack helps visualize the number 20. The loading dose is 20 mg/min. The watch helps to remind you that this drug is given per *minute,* not per kilogram. Thus, the combination of a pack of cigarettes and a watch reminds you that the dose is 20 mg/min to a maximum dose of what? You got it: 17 mg/kg (keg). The *Seventeen* magazine helps remind you of the maximum dosage, and the keg reminds you that the maximum dose is based on weight, not time.

The higher loading dosage of 30 mg/min has not been covered thus far. The higher dose is only considered in the ventricular fibrillation protocol, in which time is crucial and the drug must be administered more rapidly. Administration at this rapid rate to patients not in ventricular fibrillation may exacerbate an already exaggerated propensity for hypotension.

Let's Practice

1. Starting from the top, name the three top objects. _____
2. What did you put into the pelican's mouth? _____
3. What was the pelican reading? _____

Bretylium

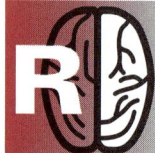

The pelican is sitting in its nest reading *Seventeen* magazine. It upsets you so much that you rip the magazine from its grasp, roll it up tightly, and begin striking the pelican on the head and body; feathers are floating everywhere. Pretty soon, the pelican loses consciousness and falls off the nest in a heap with a resounding thud! The nest, so precariously perched before, falls with the bird and promptly disintegrates on the ground. Now all you have left is a till sitting on top of the keg.

Try to visualize the image before proceeding.

Let's Practice

1. Who took the magazine and rolled it up? _____
2. Where did you strike the pelican? _____
3. Did the nest fall down off of the till? _____
4. What is left at the end? _____

THE FROZEN TILL

The till is getting chilly and beginning to freeze over because the pelican's body heat is no longer available. It is getting so cold, brrr! The till is now frozen solid, and there is a layer of frost on its exterior. The ice is so thick that you can etch your initials with your thumbnail.

To your amazement, from the side of the till sprouts a hand with five fingers wearing a glove. It waves at you with broad strokes. Then another hand grows from the opposite side of the till sporting another five-fingered glove. Both hands are waving madly about trying to get your attention. As the temperature drops, the till tries to keep warm by slapping the sides of its arms. It does this once, twice, three times (Fig. 9-14).

Try to visualize the image before proceeding.

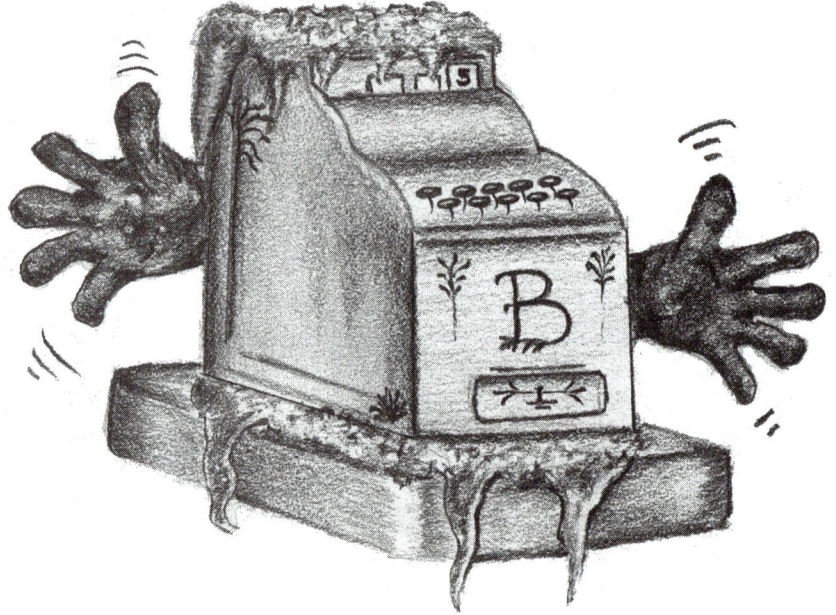

Figure 9-14

Let's Practice

1. How was the pelican removed from its perch? _____
2. Is the nest still there? _____
3. How many hands came out initially? _____
4. How many fingers were on the hand? _____

5. What happened next? _____

6. How many times did the arms slap each other attempting to keep warm? _____

THE INTERPRETATION

The till is getting so cold, brrr . . . -till-ium. Bretylium is the name of the drug. The initial dose of 5 mg/kg was illustrated by the five-fingered hand. The drug is administered on a per-kilogram basis (the keg). The second and subsequent doses are 10 mg/kg—the 10 fingers waving madly at you. The maximum dose of 30 mg/kg is depicted by both hands (10 fingers total) slapping the arms three times. The higher maximum dose of 35 mg/kg depends on whether you start with 5 mg/kg or 10 mg/kg, which is possible in the stable wide complex tachycardia of uncertain type or the documented ventricular tachycardia protocol (the loading dose ranges from 5 to 10 mg/kg).

Atropine, Epinephrine, and Magnesium Sulfate

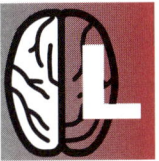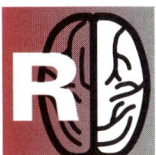

When in doubt about a drug's dosage, say 1. For four out of the eight main ACLS intravenous push drugs, the dose is 1:

- Atropine: 1 mg
- Lidocaine: 1 mg/kg
- Epinephrine: 1 mg
- Magnesium sulfate: 1 g

Another way of remembering these drugs is to drink 1 mug of ale: *a*tropine, *l*idocaine, *e*pinephrine.

To assist in remembering how often to give epinephrine, reverse the capital E in Epinephrine; it becomes a 3. Give this drug every 3 to 5 minutes. Also, when used in an arrest situation, atropine's dosage and time intervals are exactly like epinephrine's: 1 mg every 3 to 5 minutes.

Let's Practice

1. What is the dose of magnesium sulfate? _____

2. What is the dose of epinephrine? _____

3. What is the dose of atropine? _____

4. How often do you give atropine and epinephrine in a cardiac arrest? _____

Easy Ways to Remember Which Drugs Are Given per Kilogram

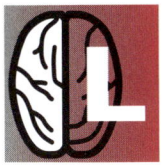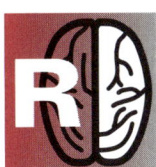

Of the eight main drugs that participants are required to remember, only two are administered as a loading dose on a per-kilogram basis.

- Adenosine: 6 mg
- Verapamil: 2.5 to 5 mg
- **Lidocaine: 1 to 1.5 mg/kg**
- Procainamide: 20 to 30 mg/min
- **Bretylium: 1 mg/kg**
- Epinephrine: 1 mg
- Atropine: 1 mg
- Magnesium sulfate: 1 g

Take the initials of lidocaine and bretylium, l and b, and put them together, lb, the abbreviation for pounds. Lidocaine and bretylium are the only two drugs that deal with weight!

Let's Practice

1. What is the initial dose of bretylium? _____
2. How often should you administer epinephrine? _____
3. What is the second dose of verapamil? _____
4. What is the dose of atropine? _____
5. What is the maximum dose of procainamide (Pronestyl)? _____
6. What is the dose of magnesium sulfate? _____
7. What is the second dose of lidocaine? _____
8. What is the second dose of adenosine? _____

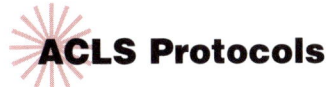

ACLS Protocols

- Respiratory arrest with a pulse (universal algorithm)
- Ventricular fibrillation and pulseless ventricular tachycardia
- Pulseless electrical activity (PEA)
- Asystole
- Acute coronary syndromes
- Bradycardia
- Unstable tachycardias
- Stable tachycardias
- Acute stroke

Each protocol is presented in the subsequent discussion. The entire protocols are featured in the case studies in Chapters 2, 3, and 4. The protocols noted here are heavily abbreviated, concentrating only on making them easy to recall.

Universal Algorithm Protocol

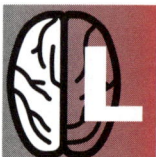 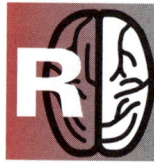

- Assess responsiveness
  - If responsive, observe and treat as indicated
  - If not responsive, continue
- Activate EMS
- Call for a monitor-defibrillator
- Assess breathing
  - If breathing, place in rescue position if no evidence of trauma
  - If not breathing, deliver 2 slow breaths
- Check pulse
  - ■■ **If pulse is present** ■■
    - Secure airway and give oxygen
    - Initiate IV access
    - Monitor pulse rate
    - Check vital signs
    - Obtain history and perform physical
    - Set up 12-lead ECG
    - Assess suspected cause of respiratory arrest
      - Hypotension, shock, acute pulmonary edema (see protocol)
      - Acute MI (see acute coronary syndromes)
      - Acute stroke
      - Arrhythmia
        - Too fast (see tachycardia protocol)
        - Too slow (see bradycardia protocol)
  - ■■ **If pulse absent** ■■

    - Start CPR and check monitor
      - If ventricular fibrillation or pulseless ventricular tachycardia, go to protocol
    - Intubate and confirm tube placement
    - Confirm ventilations
    - Determine rhythm and cause
      - Is there electrical activity?
        - If yes, go to PEA protocol
        - If no, go to asystole protocol

(Reproduced with permission. *Advanced Cardiac Life Support.* Copyright 1997, American Heart Association)

Universal Algorithm Memory Aid

PRIMARY ASSESSMENT

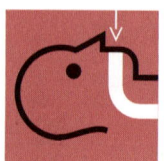 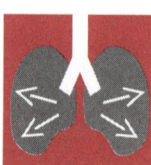 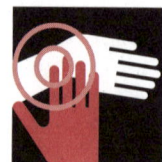 

SECONDARY SURVEY

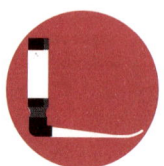 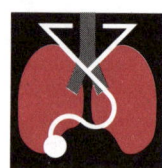 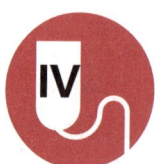 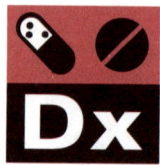

Ventricular Fibrillation and Pulseless Ventricular Tachycardia Protocol

- **Primary assessment**
- CPR, until defibrillator is obtained
- Pulse check
- **Defibrillate** 200 J
- **Defibrillate** 200 to 300 J
- **Defibrillate** 360 J
- Pulse check
- Continue CPR
- **Secondary assessment**
  - Intubate
  - Perform mini-thorax assessment and abbreviated history
  - Assess vital signs and IV access
  - Administer drugs as applicable to diagnosis
- **Epinephrine, 1 mg repeat q 3 to 5 min.** If the standard dose fails, consider other dosage regimens (class IIb: acceptable, possibly helpful):
  - Intermediate: 2 to 5 mg IV q 3 to 5 min
  - Escalating: 1 mg 3 mg 5 mg IV q 3 min
  - High: 0.1 mg/kg IV q 3 to 5 min
- **Defibrillate** at 360 J or a stack of shocks
- **Lidocaine, 1.0 to 1.5 mg/kg** (one dose of 1.5 mg/kg in cardiac arrest is acceptable)
- **Defibrillate** at 360 J or a stack of shocks
- **Lidocaine, 1.0 to 1.5 mg/kg repeated to maximum of 3 mg/kg**
- **Bretylium, 5 mg/kg**
- **Defibrillate** at 360 J or a stack of shocks
- **Bretylium, 10 mg/kg,** repeated at 5-minute intervals to maximum of 35 mg/kg
- **Defibrillate** at 360 J or a stack of shocks

Consider the following medications for their respective indications in refractory ventricular fibrillation or ventricular tachycardia while defibrillating between each dose:

- **Magnesium sulfate, 1 to 2 g,** undiluted IV push
- **Procainamide, 30 mg/min** to maximum of 17 mg/kg
- **Sodium bicarbonate, 1 mEq/kg,** only for specific indications

(Reproduced with permission. *Advanced Cardiac Life Support.* Copyright 1997, American Heart Association)

Ventricular Fibrillation Memory Aid

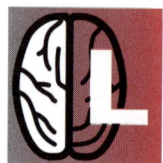 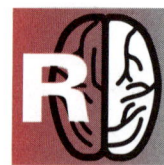

Always
    shock
    shock
    shock
Everybody
    shock
Little
    shock
Big
    shock
Big **B**ig
    shock
Mama
    shock
Papa
    shock
Baby

The mnemonic is chanted from top to bottom. This is only a way of remembering the gross portions of the protocol. It does not give details. You would administer each of the medications, perform cardiopulmonary resuscitation (CPR) for no longer than 30 to 60 seconds to circulate the medication, and check for a pulse before each defibrillation. *Always* reminds you to always **a**ssess—during the primary survey, and after the three defibrillations, during the secondary survey. The first three *shocks* correspond to *defibrillation* at 200, 200 to 300, and 360 joules. *Everybody* signifies **e**pinephrine. The mnemonic assumes that you continue CPR, have started your intravenous line, and have intubated before administering the next shock at 360 joules (or a set of shocks at 200, 200 to 300, and 360 joules). The next word, *little*, stands for **l**idocaine. *Shock* at 360 joules or deliver a set of shocks. The next word, *big*, stands for **b**retylium. Shock at 360 joules or deliver a set of shocks. Then, *Big Big* refers to doubling the dose of **b**retylium and immediately shocking at 360 joules or delivering a set of shocks. *Mama*, *Papa*, and *Baby* refer to considering **m**agnesium sulfate, **p**rocainamide, and **b**icarbonate, shocking every 2 to 3 minutes at a minimum and after and between each dose.

Pulseless Electrical Activity Protocol

- **Primary survey**
- **Absent pulse; continue CPR**
- **Secondary assessment**
  - Intubate
  - Perform mini-thorax assessment and abbreviated history. **Hey, Hey, Hey THAT's EMD!** is a useful mnemonic for remembering the possible etiologies of PEA.
    - ◆ **H**ypovolemia
    - ◆ **H**ypoxia
    - ◆ **H**ypothermia
    - ◆ **T**amponade, Cardiac
    - ◆ **H**yperkalemia
    - ◆ **A**cidosis
    - ◆ **T**ension pneumothorax
    - ◆ **E**mbolism
    - ◆ **M**I
    - ◆ **D**rug overdose
      - **A** Antidepressant Tricyclics
      - **B** Beta Blockers
      - **C** Calcium-Channel Blockers
      - **D** Digoxin
  - Assess vital signs with Doppler and IV access
  - Administer drugs as applicable to diagnosis
- **Epinephrine, 1 mg——repeat q 3 to 5 min.** If the standard dose fails, consider other dosage regimens (class IIb: acceptable, possibly helpful):
  - Intermediate: 2 to 5 mg IV q 3 to 5 min
  - Escalating: 1 mg 3 mg 5 mg IV q 3 min
  - High: 0.1 mg/kg IV q 3 to 5 min
- **Consider sodium bicarbonate.** Administer if patient has preexisting hyperkalemia or has any other specific indications.
- **If absolute or relative bradycardia, give atropine 1 mg,** repeat q 3 to 5 min to 0.04 mg/kg.

(Reproduced with permission. *Advanced Cardiac Life Support.* Copyright 1997, American Heart Association)

Pulseless Electrical Activity Helpful Memory Aid

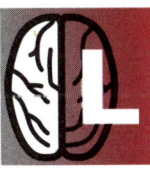
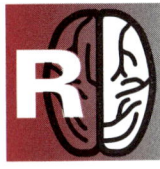

- **P**ossibilities (etiologies)
- **E**pinephrine (nonspecific; makes CPR more effective)
- **A**tropine (if bradycardic)

Pulseless electrical activity is a collection of syndromes in which an apparently normal electrocardiogram (ECG) presents with no accompanying pulse. The rhythm displayed may be sinus, idioventricular, or any rhythm that does not present as asystole, ventricular fibrillation, or ventricular tachycardia. Most etiologies represent problems with generating an acceptable cardiac output. The mnemonic stresses assessment. P refers to checking for **p**ossible etiologies of the arrest. If a specific treatable cause is determined, employ the treatment immediately (e.g., hypovolemia—fluids, or pericardial tamponade—pericardiocentesis). While investigating and treating any suspect etiologies, administer E, **e**pinephrine. Epinephrine improves the efficiency of CPR, which is poor at best. If the rhythm is bradycardic, suspect vagal domination and administer A, **a**tropine.

Asystole Protocol

- **Primary survey**
- Absent pulse; continue CPR
- **Secondary assessment**
  - Intubate
  - Perform mini-thorax assessment and abbreviated history. **Ho, Ho, Ho, Accidents Do Happen** is a useful mnemonic for remembering the possible etiologies of asystole.
    - **H**ypoxia
    - **H**ypothermia
    - **H**ypokalemia
    - Preexisting **A**cidosis
    - **D**rug overdose
    - **H**yperkalemia
  - Assess vital signs and IV access
  - Administer drugs as applicable to diagnosis
- **Confirm** in more than one lead
- **Consider transcutaneous pacing** (perform early with simultaneous drug therapy)
- **Epinephrine, 1 mg repeat q 3 to 5 min.** If the standard dose fails, consider other dosage regimens (class IIb: acceptable, possibly helpful):
  - Intermediate: 2 to 5 mg IV q 3 to 5 min
  - Escalating: 1 mg 3 mg 5 mg IV q 3 min
  - High: 0.1 mg/kg IV q 3 to 5 min
- **Consider sodium bicarbonate.** Administer if patient has preexisting hyperkalemia or any other specific indications.
- **Atropine, 1 mg, repeat q 3 to 5 min to 0.04 mg/kg.** (Consider shorter dosing levels in cardiac arrest.)
- **Consider termination of efforts.**

(Reproduced with permission. *Advanced Cardiac Life Support.* Copyright 1997, American Heart Association)

Asystole Memory Aid

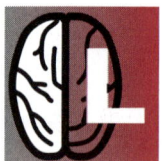 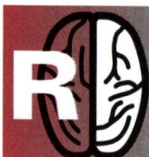

Consider application of a transcutaneous pacemaker (TCP).

- **P**ossibilities (etiologies)
- **E**pinephrine (nonspecific makes CPR more effective)
- **A**tropine (to rule out vagal domination)

This is the exact same treatment as for PEA, with the addition of a TCP!

Acute Coronary Syndrome Protocol

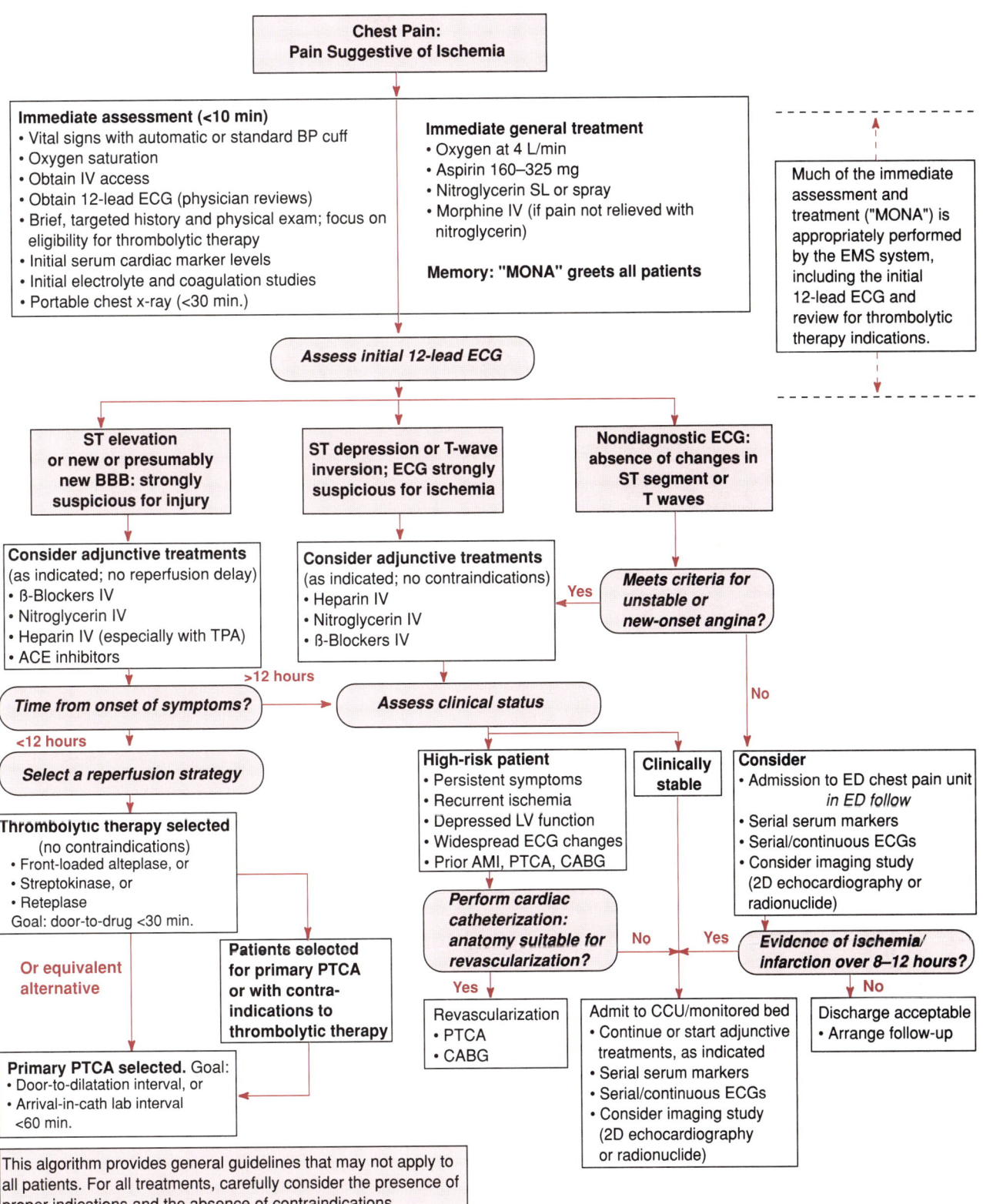

(Reproduced with permission. *Advanced Cardiac Life Support*. Copyright 1997, American Heart Association)

Acute Coronary Syndromes Memory Aid

There is no need to memorize this protocol. I have only included it for completeness.

Bradycardia Protocol

- Assess patient with primary and secondary survey
- Attach monitoring devices
- Perform targeted history & physical
- Administer oxygen
- Initiate IV. Do not delay transcutaneous pacemaker (TCP) while IV is secured if patient has serious symptoms.

If signs and symptoms are serious

(Do not delay application of a TCP while waiting for atropine to work)

- **Atropine, 0.5 to 1.0 mg q 3 to 5 min to 0.04 mg/kg**
  (Consider shorter dosing intervals in severe situations. Watch carefully in second-degree type II or third-degree)
- **TCP (if available)**
- **Dopamine drip, 5 to 20 mcg/kg/min**
- **Epinephrine drip, 2 to 10 mcg/min**
- **Isoproterenol drip**
  Use only with caution! At low doses, isoproterenol is class IIb (possibly helpful). At higher dosages, it is class III (harmful).

If NOT serious

Diagnose rhythm

- If second-degree type II or third-degree AV block, administer transvenous pacemaker
- If not, monitor patient

(Reproduced with permission. *Advanced Cardiac Life Support.* Copyright 1997, American Heart Association)

Bradycardia Protocol Memory Aids

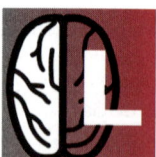

Check out an easy way to memorize drip concentrations in the Flash Cards in the Appendix.

One way to remember the bradycardia protocol is as follows:

At
this
Pace
the
Dope
needs
Epi
Immediately

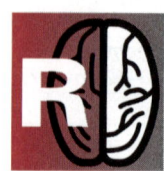

At stands for **a**tropine, *pace* for **p**acemaker, *dope* for **d**opamine, *epi* for **e**pinephrine, and *immediately* for **I**suprel.

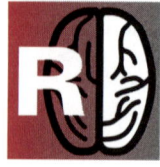

Another memory aid for bradycardia uses visual images. Take your time and make each image easily recallable. When you try to remember what to do when a rhythm goes too slow, think of a turtle. I use a turtle image in this section to help you recall each of the treatments for the bradycardia protocol.

THE TURTLE

Picture a Galápagos land turtle in your mind's eye (Fig. 9-15). The shell is hard and oval, with bumps protruding all over it. It is colored forest green and covered with a patchwork quilt of squares, each containing a maze-like design. Each of the shell designs is like a fingerprint, unique to that turtle. The myriad of designs also helps recall the fact that bradycardia comes in many forms: sinus, junctional, second-degree blocks, and third-degree blocks. Every turtle has but one shell, however, and all the different forms are treated with but one protocol.

Its four legs and head project out past the edge of the domed shell, which flares out at the base. If you think of the turtle as a clock, the head protrudes at 12 o'clock, while the front legs stick out at 10 o'clock and 2 o'clock, respectively. The rear legs are at 4 o'clock and 8 o'clock. Before we proceed, picture numbers at each of these areas. The head is number 1, and proceeding clockwise, the right front leg is number 2, right rear leg is number 3, left rear leg is number 4, and left front leg is number 5.

Close your eyes and visualize the turtle.

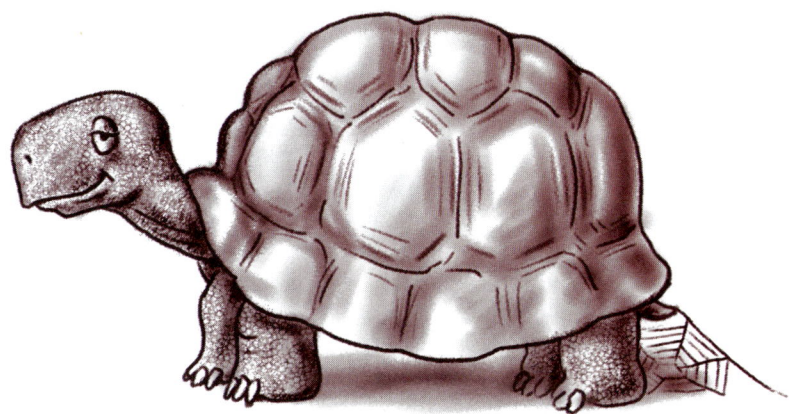

Figure 9-15

Let's Practice

1. What body part is number 3? _____
2. What body part is number 5? _____
3. What body part is number 1? _____
4. What body part is number 2? _____
5. What body part is number 4? _____

If you cannot visualize them, try harder, but do not continue until it becomes easy. I am going to give you some visual images for each of the limbs. Later, when you see them in your mind, it will become easy to recall all of the drugs in order.

A TROPHY

In the popular childhood fairy tale, "The Tortoise and the Hare," the turtle surprisingly beats the rabbit and wins the race. Although the turtle is a slow-moving animal, he is able to win "a trophy" because the overconfident rabbit decides to take a nap during the race. Visualize the turtle with a trophy on his head (Fig. 9-16). This image can help you to remember the first drug in the bradycardia sequence: atropine. "A trophy in" the race sounds like the beginning of the drug, atropine. Although the two do not sound exactly alike, the image of a trophy on the turtle's head will remind you of the drug atropine.

Try to visualize the image before proceeding.

Figure 9-16

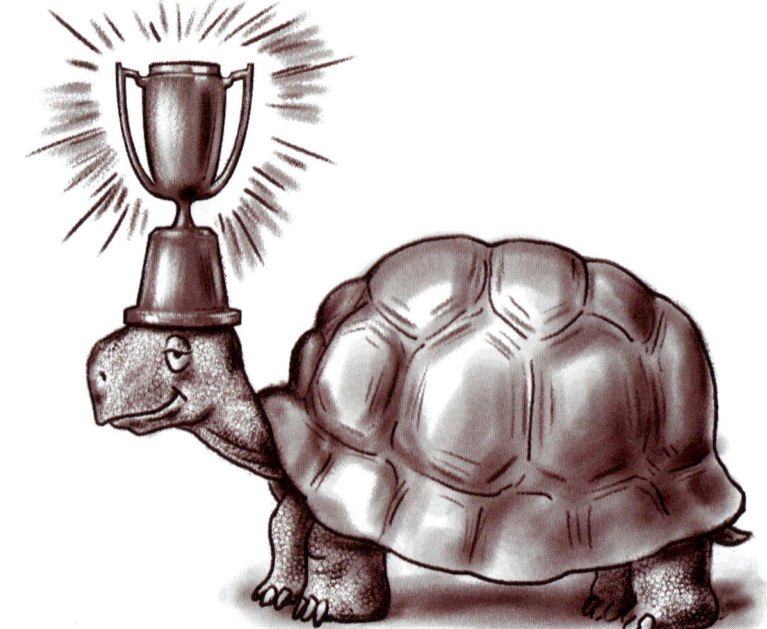

Let's Practice

1. What body part is number 2?　　_____
2. What is on top of number 1?　　_____
3. What body part is number 3?　　_____
4. What is on the turtle's head?　　_____

SETTING THE PACE

Move clockwise to number 2, the right front leg. Strapped to the turtle's right front leg is a huge grandfather clock (Fig. 9-17). The face of the clock features the phases of the moon, and the pendulum bounces around with every movement of the turtle's leg. The hard rosewood exterior is smooth and heavily waxed.

The turtle is dragging the clock along as it strides forward. Every time the turtle jerkily moves his leg for another stride, the clock crashes down and bongs! Imagine this turtle with this massive time-piece strapped to its leg striking chimes with each forward motion. The clock reminds you to set the pace: an external pacemaker, or TCP.

Try to visualize the image before proceeding.

Figure 9-17

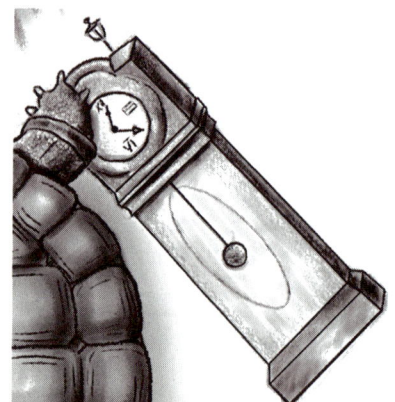

Let's Practice

1. What form of treatment is on number 2? _____
2. What form of treatment is on number 1? _____
3. What body part is number 5? _____
4. What body part is number 4? _____

THE DOPE ADDICT

Move to the number 3 position, the right rear leg. The turtle has had a drug problem for most of his life. He furtively looks around and removes his thin turtle leather belt from around his waist and wraps it around his right front leg. He sticks the end of the belt in his mouth to put tension around the limb, causing the leg veins to stand out. The veins are in intricate patterns, appearing red and blue with green streaks throughout. With his free right front paw, he picks up a hypodermic syringe and fills it with a milky white substance, probably heroin. The turtle then tries to stick the needle into a vein. He is having difficulty because his legs do not sport opposing thumbs. He keeps stabbing at the veins, trying to inject the substance. Each time that he is off the mark, he lets forth a bellow of agonized pain. The white, dope-filled syringe plunges up and down, blood spurting with each stab. The acrid odor of blood fills your nostrils as the turtle's howls fill your ears. At the end of his patience, the turtle lifts the syringe over his head and thrusts it deep into his leg. It enters the bone with a sickening "crunch." The syringe quivers perpendicular to the skin as it slowly oscillates back and forth. You can see the milky white fluid rippling at the meniscus (Fig. 9-18). The **dope-filled** syringe is meant to provide the visual link to the next drug in the sequence, dopamine.

Try to visualize the image before proceeding.

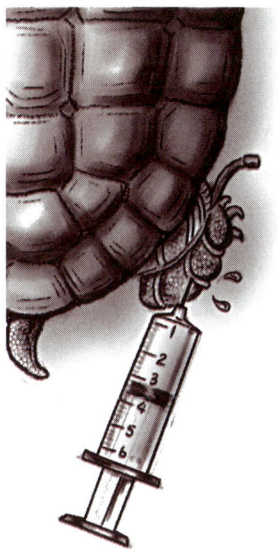

Figure 9-18

Let's Practice

1. Visualize the right back leg; what is the form of treatment? _____
2. What form of treatment is on the right front leg? _____
3. What form of treatment is on the head? _____
4. What form of treatment is on number 2? _____
5. What form of treatment is on number 1? _____
6. What form of treatment is on number 3? _____

THE A IS DRILLING

Now progress to number 4, the left rear leg. Picture the capital letter **A** with arms coming out of its sides. It is colored pink with blue polka dots, sporting track shoes with spikes. It is skipping up and down the leg, puncturing the turtle's skin, each step resulting in a bellow. The A jumps down and picks up a drill—like the ones used to drill holes through wood. It crawls back up on top of the leg and starts moving the drill all over the leg, drilling into the muscle, bone, and sinew. The turtle is screeching in pain. There are big chunks of turtle meat being ripped off, accompanied by showers of blood as the A is drilling (Fig. 9-19). "A drilling" sounds like adrenaline. Adrenaline is also known as the generic drug epinephrine. If you wish to say adrenaline instead of epinephrine, feel free.

Try to visualize the image before proceeding.

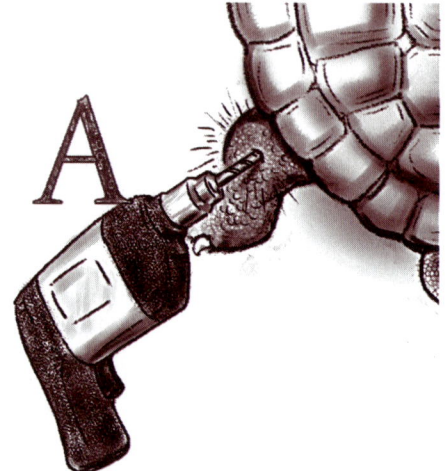

Figure 9-19

Let's Practice

1. Visualize the left back leg; what is the form of treatment? _____
2. What form of treatment is on number 2? _____
3. What form of treatment is on number 1? _____
4. What form of treatment is on number 3? _____
5. What form of treatment is on number 2? _____
6. What form of treatment is on number 4? _____

FROZEN SHAMPOO

Move to number 5, the left front leg. Strapped to the ankle of the left front leg is a massive block of ice. This is the same block that the iceman would leave in your refrigerator every day in 1890s America. The ice has been there for so long that frostbite, along with extensive tissue damage, has occurred. The skin near the toes is blackened and has curled back, revealing stark white bone. Because the area is deadened due to the cold, the turtle is unaware of the problem and blithely trudges through life. If you examine the interior of the ice block, there appears to be an object: a bottle of Prell shampoo (Fig. 9-20). Putting them both together: ice-u-prell. Isuprel (isoproterenol) is the last treatment in this protocol.

Try to visualize the image before proceeding.

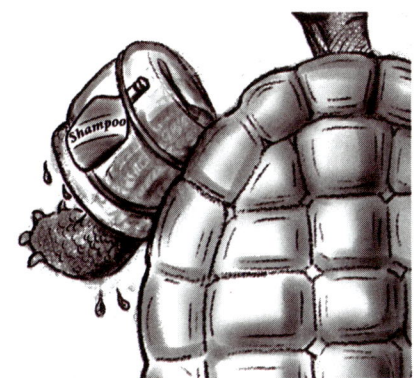

Figure 9-20

Let's Practice

1. What form of treatment is on number 4? _____
2. What form of treatment is on number 2? _____
3. What form of treatment is on number 5? _____
4. What form of treatment is on number 1? _____
5. What form of treatment is on number 2? _____
6. What form of treatment is on number 3? _____

(Figure 9-21 presents the image of the whole turtle.)

With this method, memorizing the bradycardia protocol is easy. However, don't think of it just one time. Repetition is the mother of memory. Rethink the images in your mind a couple of times per day until the test. Soon, you'll wonder if you could ever forget it.

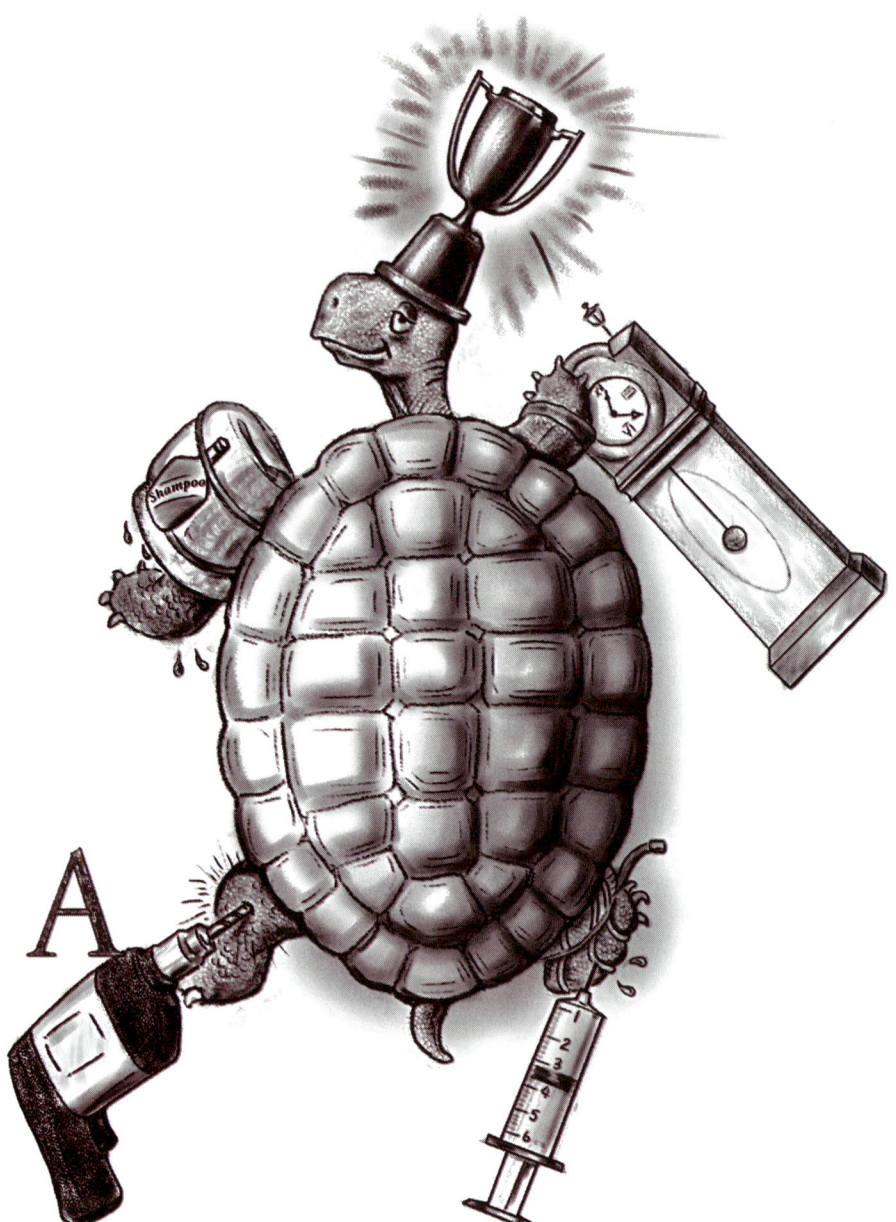

Figure 9-21

Chapter 9 Memorization Techniques 273

Tachycardia Protocols

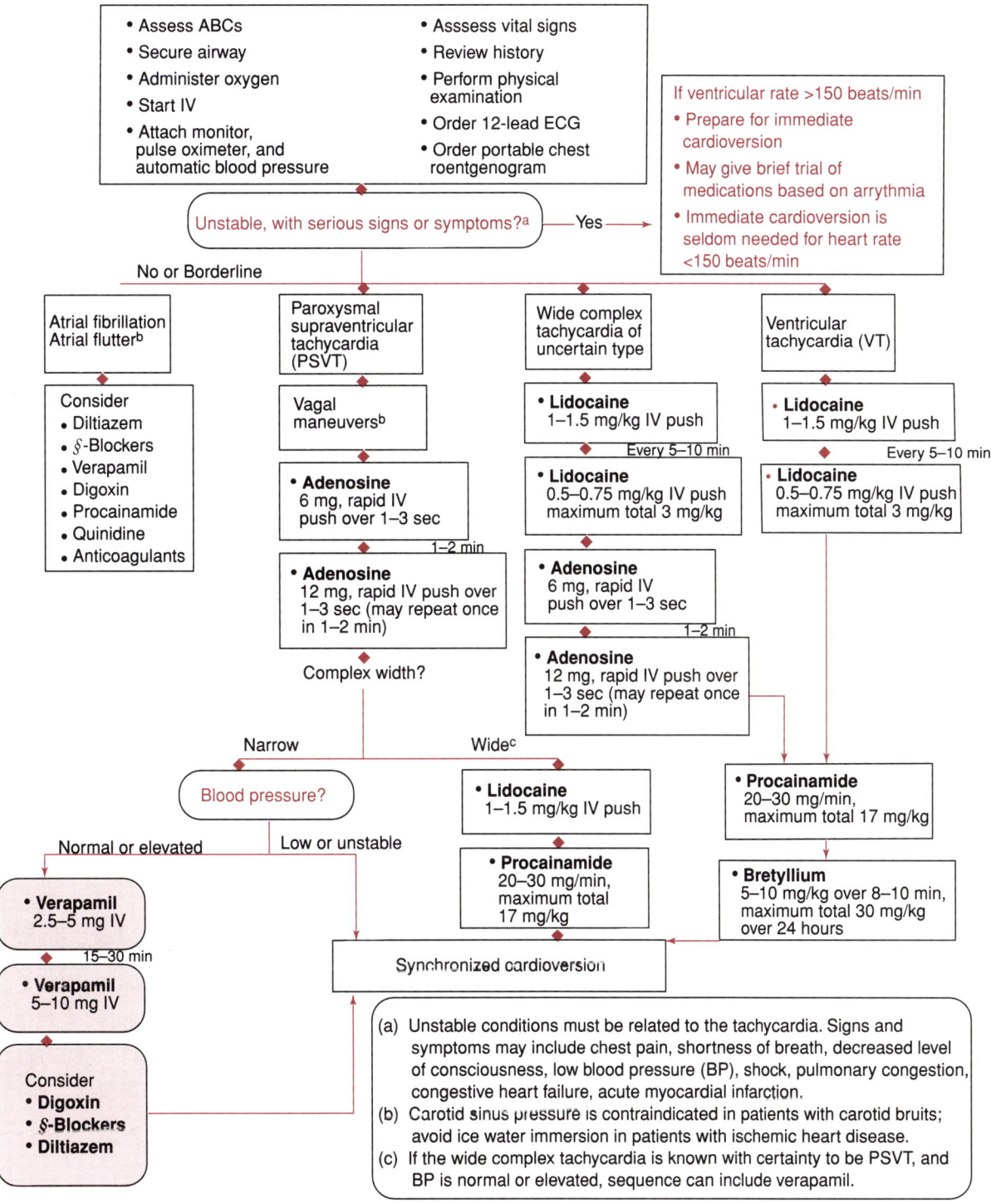

(Reproduced with permission. *Advanced Cardiac Life Support.* Copyright 1997, American Heart Association)

274 Unit 2 *Learning Adjuncts*

Tachycardia Memory Aid

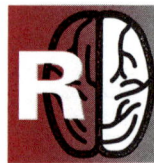

Because this protocol is the most intricate, I have developed visual images that will make it easy to memorize. If you have ventricular fibrillation on the monitor, go to the ventricular fibrillation protocol. If you have a pulseless rhythm with an ECG, go to the PEA protocol. If you have a bradycardic rhythm, consider the turtle. If the rhythm is an excessive noncompensatory tachycardia (narrow complex, more than 170, or wide complex, more than 100, and not atrial fibrillation or flutter), this memory aid using a car will help you recall the appropriate treatment for any given noncompensatory tachycardia.

Visualize yourself in the driver's seat of your car. In front of you is your steering wheel, and the dashboard spreads out all the way to the right. In the center of the dashboard is the car radio, and on the far side, near the passenger door, is the glove box (Fig. 9-22).

STABLE TACHYCARDIAS: THE SPEEDOMETER

The seat feels familiar as you scrunch your rear around and sit straight up. Your steering wheel is smooth and cool as your hands caress its exterior. You glance to your rear-view mirror as you secure your seatbelt. As you lower your gaze to see through the steering wheel, the speedometer becomes visible. It has a red needle that tracks back and forth from 0 to 100 miles/hour.

Try to visualize the image before proceeding.

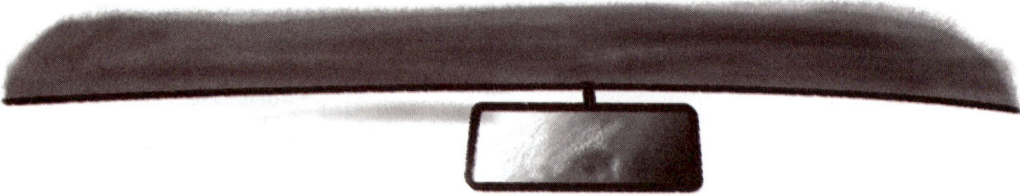

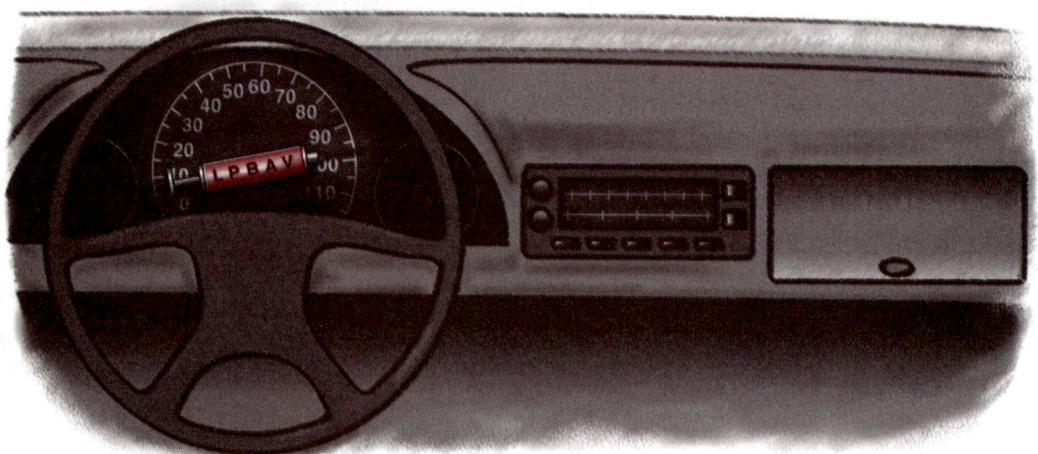

Figure 9-22

Let's Practice

1. What do you think about when you see an noncompensatory tachycardia?

2. What is the item set into the dashboard nearest the passenger door?

3. What item is centered in the dashboard? _____

4. What tracks back and forth from 0 to 100 miles/hour in the speedometer? _____

To your amazement, the red speedometer needle transforms itself into an antique syringe, similar to a blood gas hypodermic (Fig. 9-23). As you peer to examine it, you note that it has a removable needle that has to be resharpened and autoclaved after each use. The glass exterior is frosted, making it appear like the outside of a cold drink, whereas the numbers representing milliliters are skillfully etched along one side. The plunger has a metal ring, where you insert your thumb, and your index and middle fingers slide into rings along the sides of the barrel. As you pull back your thumb, the glass plunger scrapes against the inside glass bore with a sound similar to scratching a blackboard, sending a chill down your spine.

Try to visualize the image before proceeding.

The inside of the syringe is bubbling and swirling with colors, such as lemon yellows, violets, blues, purples, and aquas. The syringe glows with an eerie light as the various colors whirl and pulsate, creating intricate patterns much like those of a kaleidoscope. As you gaze at the colors, you make a mental note that the first letter of each color corresponds to a drug: **l**emon yellow, **l**idocaine; **v**iolet, **v**erapamil; **b**lue, **b**retylium; **p**urple, **p**rocainamide; and **a**qua, **a**denosine.

The first letter of speedometer is **s**, **s**table. Hence, we will put all of our stable tachycardias into the speedometer and treat them with drugs. It does not matter which of the noncompensatory tachycardias that you encounter; if they are stable, look for their drug-oriented treatment in the speedometer.

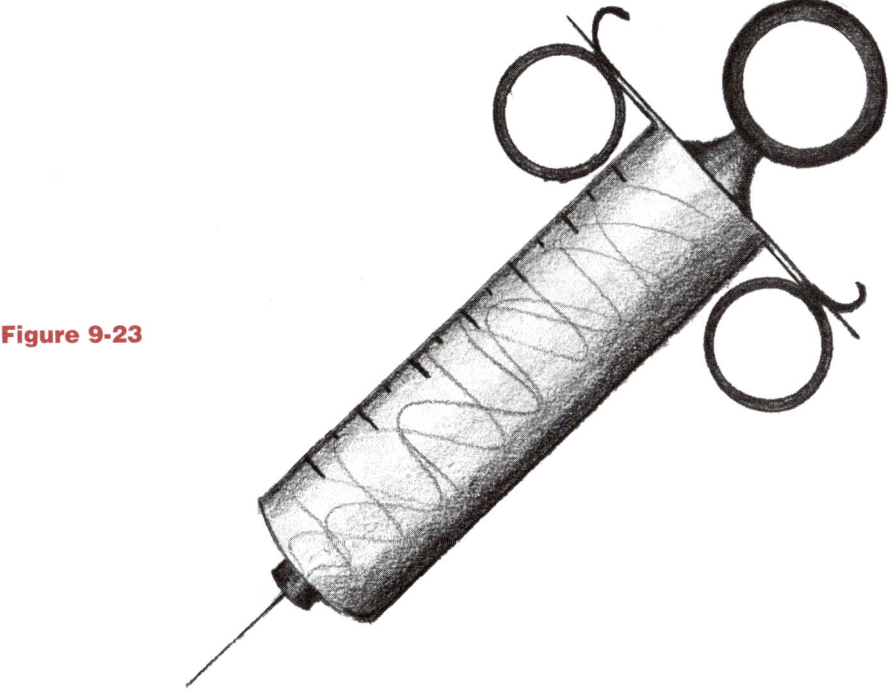

Figure 9-23

Let's Practice

1. What color was procainamide? _____

2. What was blue? _____

3. What color was verapamil? _____

4. Do you recall aqua? _____

5. What did the speedometer needle become? _____

6. Can *all* tachycardias be treated in the speedometer? _____

Try to visualize the image before proceeding.

At the tip of the needle, a solitary drop of medication forms, coruscating with brilliance. As if in slow motion, it falls and strikes the base of the speedometer. The colors liberated by the collision are so bright that you momentarily shield your eyes. When the spots before your eyes become manageable, you notice that the speedometer has become a round 1950s television screen. Portrayed on the screen is the interior of a patient's room. Your vantage point is as if you were standing in the doorway.

THE MONITORS: THE PROTOCOLS

As you gaze in astonishment at the speedometer screen, you see a male patient standing in front of a hospital bed. Above his head are three large television monitors (Fig. 9-24).

- On your left (nearest the driver's door), the monitor is flashing *Obvious SVT*. The color of the text alternates from aqua to violet, holds, and repeats the sequence.
- On the middle monitor, directly above his head, a giant **question mark** (wide complex tachycardia of uncertain type) flashes. Its color scheme starts off with lemon, changes to aqua, dissolves to purple, and then ends with blue. The sequence continues to repeat itself.
- The monitor on the far right (nearest the car radio) sports the text *Documented V-tach*. The text's color scheme starts with lemon like the middle monitor, changes to purple, and ends with blue.

The flashing colors are distracting but they seem, to scream out a message to you. As you observe more closely, a pattern begins to emerge. The question mark monitor and the Documented V-tach monitor both start with the same color: lemon yellow. With the exception of aqua (present in the question mark monitor but not in the Documented V-tach monitor), both continue to turn from purple to blue. There is no doubt about it. The middle monitor has one color that differs in the sequence—aqua—inserted between lemon yellow and purple.

"Aha!" you say to yourself, the colors on the monitors are telling me which drugs to give and their administration order. The only difference between the drug protocols of the question mark and Documented V-tach is aqua: adenosine.

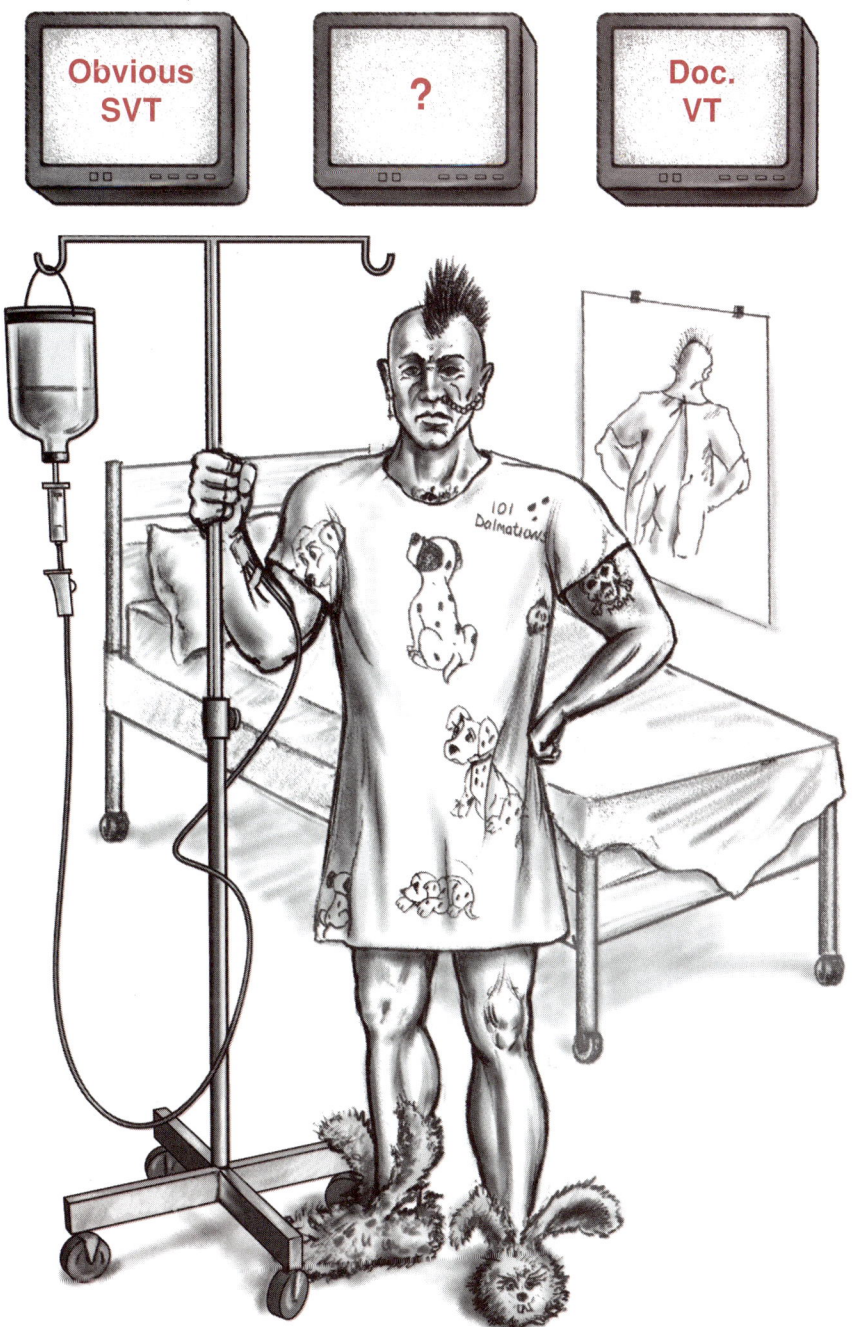

Figure 9-24

Let's Practice

1. The monitor over the patient's head is what? _____
2. The one to your right (closest to the car radio) is what? _____
3. The one in the middle is what? _____
4. The overhead monitor on your left (closest to the driver's door) is what? _____
5. The monitor on your right (closest to the car radio) is what? _____

The bed appears to have been slept in for many days without a change in linen because the sheets appear filthy and in disarray. The patient is standing upright, not lying down or sitting up, in front of the bed and appears about 22 years of age. He is wearing a pair of fluorescent pink "bunny" slippers with huge ears that end at his knees. He sports a hospital gown patterned with a dalmatians motif. From a mirror at the sink behind him, the gown does not reach all the way behind, leaving his rear fully exposed, his gluteal crack painfully obvious. His skin is a pasty white except for both of his arms and his neck, which are a deep bronze. He has an intravenous line attached to his right arm. On both arms, he has tattoos. On the right just above the elbow is written: "Kill them all and let God sort them out." On the left arm is a picture of a skull and crossbones with "Mom" stenciled beneath. Moving up to his face, you note that he has a bright silver ring in his left nostril. The ring is attached by a small chain to his left earlobe. He has a mohawk down the center of his otherwise bald skull. The mohawk is dyed lemon yellow, purple, blue, aqua, and violet.

Let's Practice

1. What was interesting about the patient's hair?
2. What was the patient wearing on his feet?
3. What was attached to the patient's arm?
4. Name either of the tattoos on the patient's arms.
5. What is reflected in the mirror?

The patient is alert and his jet-black eyes lock onto yours. He can see you through the steering wheel. He can read your name tag, so he knows who you are if you should hurt him. He bellows with a throaty yell, "Hurt me and you'll regret it. I'll rip off your head and shove it down your throat!" With that statement, he snarls, turns his head, and spits on the floor.

Visualize the image before proceeding.

You make a decision to stay at least an intravenous tube length away from him at all times. Never touch him; give him any treatments through his intravenous line. Although scary, this man is stable cardiovascularly. If his cardiac rhythm appears on any of the monitor screens, only consider drug therapy. You should never approach him with the defibrillator paddles; that would be a lethal mistake!

The first letter of speedometer is **s**, as in **s**table. Speedometer people are stable: drugs only, no overly aggressive therapy. Summarize the speedometer to yourself: "If the patient is cardiovascularly stable, I will only consider drug therapy." He'll fall out of the speedometer onto the dashboard if he becomes unstable, because only *stable* patients are treated in the speedometer.

Let's Practice

1. The patient is unstable (T or F)?
2. The s in speedometer stands for scary (T or F)?
3. If the patient become unstable, intravenous therapy should become more aggressive (T or F)?

Visualize the image before proceeding.

OBVIOUS SVT MONITOR

The patient then looks at you and screams with a voice that can only be described as Neanderthal, "Watch me and learn!" On both sides of the patient, below each of the TV monitors, are three wooden planks resembling signs. The patient points to each and tells you what is written on them. The planks are located at the level of his head, the level of his chest, and the level of his thighs on both sides of his body. He then points to the monitor on the above left and looks at you. You respond: "Obvious SVT."

Vagal Maneuvers. Underneath the obvious SVT monitor, the placard at the level of the patient's head has the following burned into the wood: vagal maneuvers. The text has been burned black with a blow torch but has been outlined in white paint. The white outline appears to glow and ripple across the entire title.

The patient then forms his fingers into a victory sign in front of the wooden placard (Fig. 9-25). "Tell me quickly what this stands for or I'll take your first born!" Having experienced the joys of raising a teenager, you start to reply, "Take him, I can make another!" but at the last moment you see the answer burned into the wooden placard behind his fingers and shout out: "Vagal maneuvers!" You now note that every time he makes the peace sign in front of this wooden sign, you should respond with vagal maneuvers.

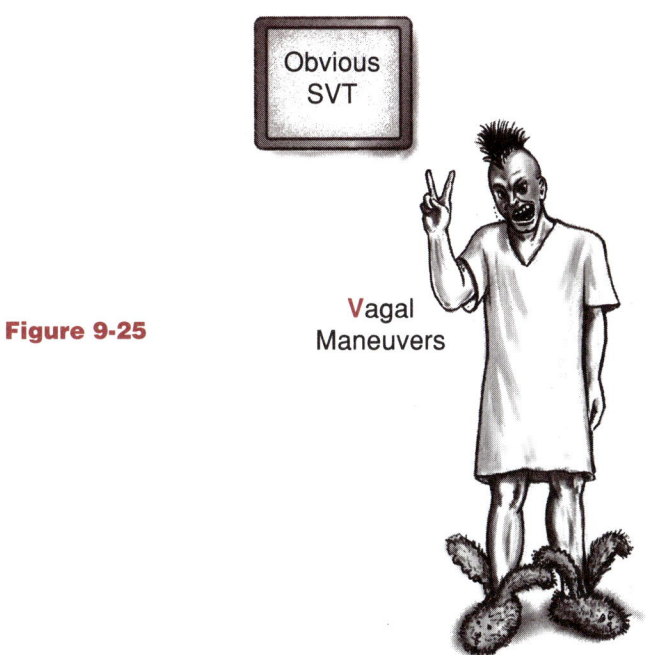

Figure 9-25

Let's Practice

1. The overhead monitor over the patient's head is _____

2. The overhead monitor closest to the car radio is _____

3. When the patient makes a victory sign just below the Obvious SVT monitor, it means _____

4. The overhead monitor closest to the driver's door is _____

5. When the patient makes a victory sign just below the monitor closest to car door, it means _____

Adenosine. Still staying directly under the Obvious SVT monitor and the vagal maneuvers placard, the patient then makes a letter A with his fingers over the next wooden placard—the one level with his chest (Fig. 9-26). Yes, he is trying to convey the next treatment—adenosine! In fact, when he moves his fingers slightly, you can make out the word *adenosine* painted on the sign. On closer examination, the bright aqua paint used to write adenosine appears to move. As you get closer to it, it appears to be a three-dimensional ocean. The waves move back and forth across each letter in the word. You can see starfish along the edge of each letter. Dolphins jump back and forth from the a to the e. Then something hurtles from the depths and jumps out at you, and it appears to be all teeth. You violently push away from the placard and regain your poise.

Visualize the image before proceeding.

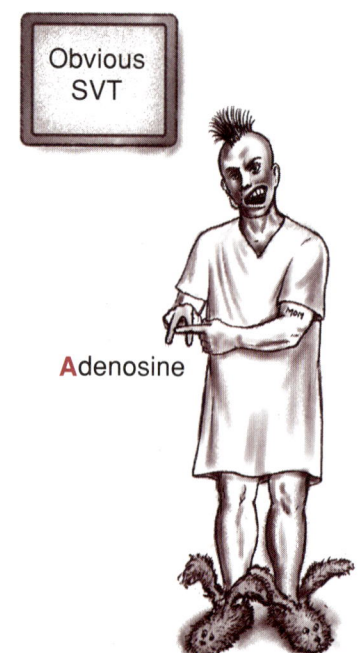

Figure 9-26

Let's Practice

1. When the patient makes a victory sign just below the Obvious SVT monitor, it means _____

2. The overhead monitor closest to the car radio is _____

3. When the patient makes an A, even with his **a**xilla just below the vagal maneuver placard in line with the Obvious SVT monitor, it means _____

4. The overhead monitor closest to the driver's door is _____

5. When the patient makes a victory sign just below the monitor closest to car door, it means _____

6. The placard just below vagal maneuvers is _____

Verapamil. The patient then makes another victory sign over the bottom wooden placard at the level of his thighs just below the adenosine sign (Fig. 9-27). You know it is the next drug in the SVT protocol, *assuming that the QRS complex is still narrow*, but you cannot remember what it is. Sweat breaks out on your forehead as his gaze locks with yours. He mumbles under his breath just loud enough for you to hear, "Tell me or I will make a seven-course meal of you!" Grasping at straws, the word *meal* reverberates in your brain. Verapamil sounds like "wrap-a-meal." Then, trying to summon what is left of your demeanor, you disdainfully say, "Verapamil!" "Good!" he says. The word verapamil instantly appears on the bottom placard. "Verapamil" has been written on the placard in violet. The word is so bright that it appears to glow with an unearthly hue. The glowing violet color hurts your eyes. It looks like a neon sign at its brightest setting.
Visualize the image before proceeding.

Chapter 9 *Memorization Techniques* 281

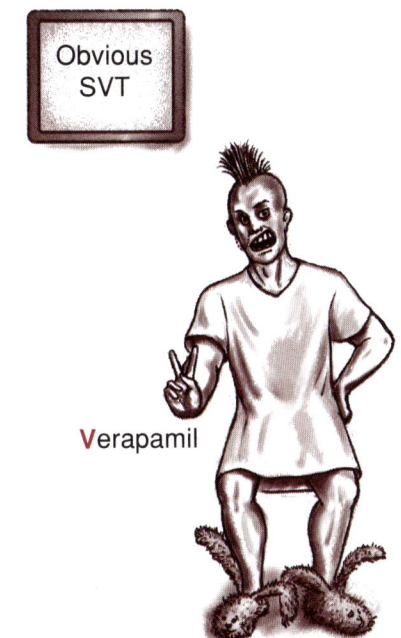

Figure 9-27

Let's Practice

All of the following are directly beneath the monitor closest to the driver's door:

1. The patient points to the monitor itself. _____ ?
2. He makes a peace sign over the top placard. _____ ?
3. He makes an A even with his axilla. _____ ?
4. He makes a victory sign at the level of his thighs. _____ ?
5. Again, victory sign, top placard. _____ ?
6. Victory sign, bottom placard. _____ ?
7. An A on the middle placard. _____ ?
8. Middle placard with an A. _____ ?
9. Victory sign, top. _____ ?
10. Victory sign, bottom. _____ ?
11. Middle placard with an A. _____ ?
12. Victory sign, bottom. _____ ?
13. And finally, victory sign, top. _____ ?

DOCUMENTED V-TACH MONITOR

Now the patient points to the overhead monitor on his left (your right—the one closest to the car radio). Documented V-tach is flashing on the monitor in the following colored sequence: lemon yellow, purple, and blue: lidocaine, procainamide, and bretylium.

The patient lunges through the speedometer and tries to grab your shirt, but you quickly lean back, making his gesture futile. He glares into your eyes and yells, "The same thing here!" There are three placards in exactly the same position as in the Obvious SVT monitor. The top placard under the Documented V-tach monitor is lidocaine, the middle placard is procainamide, and the bottom placard, about mid-thigh, is bretylium (Fig. 9-29). "Don't try to run, I know where you live." He then becomes less threatening by receding back and visibly relaxing. All these ventricular antiarrhythmics are given as initial boluses and, when successful, as a drip. The drips are piggybacked onto the main line. We will refer to them as little **p**iggy **b**acks: **l**idocaine, **p**rocainamide, and **b**retylium (Fig. 9-28).

Lidocaine. You then notice that, magically, the top placard has *lidocaine* printed in bright lemon yellow. On closer examination, the word is made up of individual lemons lined up to make each letter. You push on the top lemon in the letter L, and it squirts back at you and hits the patient on his eyelid. How convenient, the **lid**ocaine is at the same level as the patient's eye**lid**. The smell of lemons pervades the air as saliva collects under your tongue.

Visualize the image before proceeding.

Let's Practice

1. The lidocaine placard is below the monitor closest to the car radio and even with the _____

2. Each letter in lidocaine is made up of arranged _____

3. What is the placard on the opposite side of the patient at the same level as lidocaine? _____

Figure 9-28

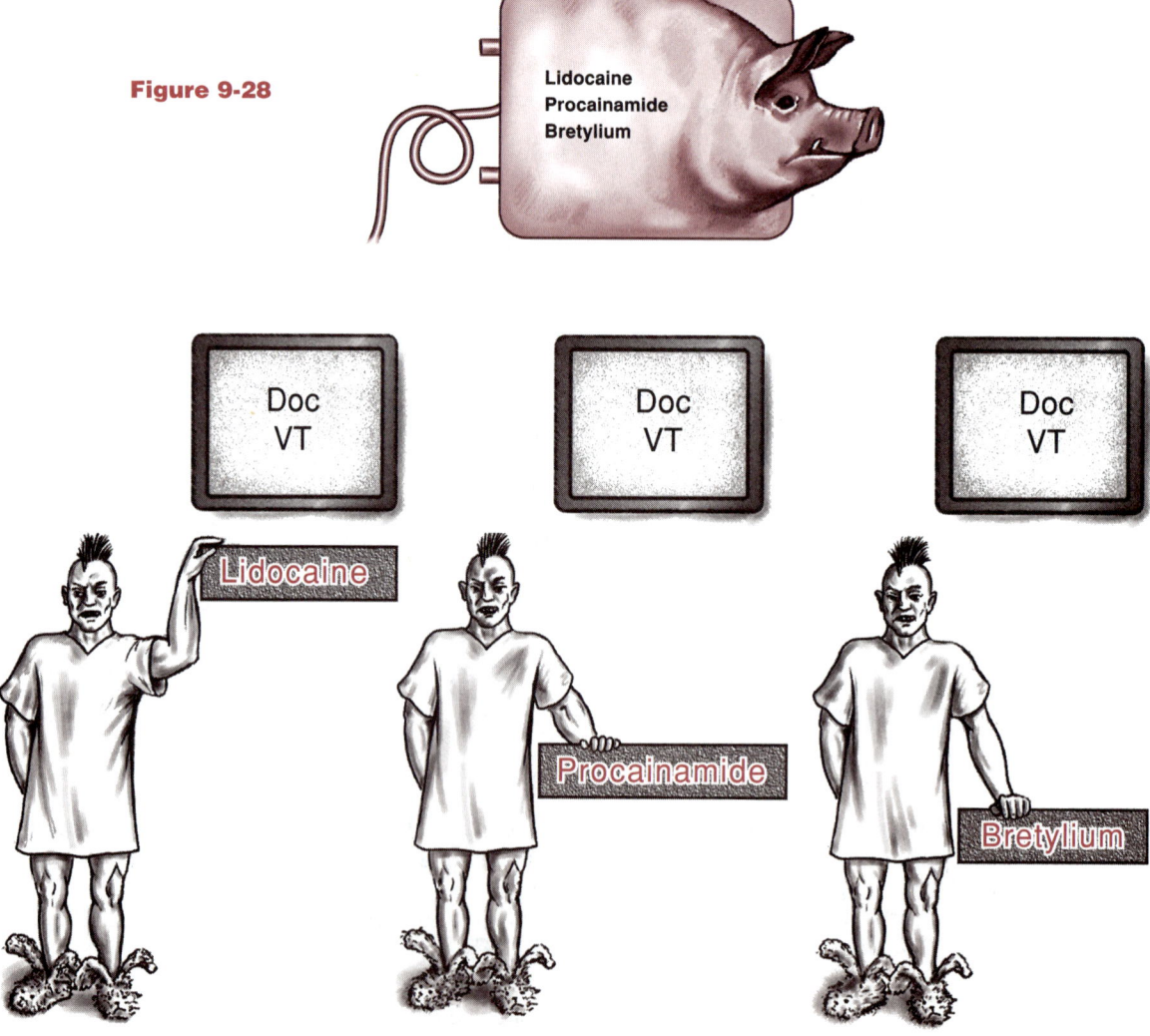

Figure 9-29

Procainamide. Underneath the Documented V-tach monitor, bathed in a hue of royal purple and situated at the level of the patient's **p**ants beneath lidocaine, is the wooden placard that says *procainamide*. As you examine the placard closely, you note that what you took for purple paint is not paint at all. Each letter of procainamide has been cut from a king's robe. The fur is luxurious to the touch as you slowly stroke it, but it must have been a poor dye job because some of the purple comes off on your hands. Notwithstanding, the texture and feel of the royal purple fur remind you of procainamide.

Visualize the image before proceeding.

Let's Practice

1. The drug beneath the lidocaine placard with the monitor closest to the car radio is _____
2. The color associated with procainamide is _____
3. Where is procainamide situated on the patient under the Documented V-tach monitor? _____

Bretylium. When the other therapies prove refractory, you turn your attention to the third wooden placard located at the level of the patient's thighs beneath procainamide. As you get closer, the word *bretylium* is made out painted in a brilliant blue. The paint color reminds you of the hue of the sky at dusk.

As you stare at the word *bretylium,* you begin to see twinkling stars scattered throughout each of the letters. Blazing comets shoot between the b and the m with increasing rapidity. Pretty soon, all of the lights shooting out from the placard make it resemble a fireworks display.

Visualize the image before proceeding.

Let's Practice

1. Under the Documented V-tach monitor, he points to the placard even with his pants? _____
2. He then points to the sign just beneath this monitor? _____
3. Then he tries to trick you by using his other hand. The patient points to what placard just under the Obvious SVT monitor (don't be taken in by switching protocols)? _____
4. He then points to the placard at the bottom of the Documented V-tach monitor? _____
5. The placard at mid-level beneath the Obvious SVT is _____
6. What is the bottom placard of the Documented V-tach monitor? _____
7. What is the top placard beneath the Obvious SVT monitor? _____
8. What is the top placard beneath the Documented V-tach monitor? _____

THE QUESTION MARK MONITOR

Now move your eyes to the middle monitor above the patient's head. The sequencing colors cascading from the question mark are lemon yellow, aqua, purple, and blue, repeating continually. The colors repeat in the same sequence as documented ventricular tachycardia, except for aqua, which flashes between lemon yellow and purple. Adenosine (aqua) is in the question mark protocol but not in Documented V-tach.

The patient points to the middle monitor (the question mark): "I don't know what this means—could you explain it to me?" You roll your eyes but gather your thoughts so you can explain it in layman terms. The question mark stands for wide complex tachycardia of uncertain type.

The explanation:

- *Usually,* any pacemaker cell that originates from the atria (supraventricularly) is conducted down the bundle branches, resulting in a narrow QRS complex. Thus, SVTs usually exhibit narrow QRS complexes.
- *Usually,* any cells in the ventricles that depolarize spontaneously take a backward pathway toward the atria. This retrograde pathway, depending on how low in the ventricle the beat arises, usually results in a wide QRS complex. Thus, ventricular tachycardia usually presents with a wide QRS complex.
- In some instances, however, a tachycardic, supraventricular pacemaker cell may initiate a pathway that doesn't employ the standard route, resulting in a wide QRS complex. This peculiarity is referred to as *aberrant conduction*. Because the pacemaker was initiated in the atria, the tachycardic rhythm is referred to as *SVT with aberrant conduction*.

Anytime that you are viewing what appears to be ventricular tachycardia, don't be fooled; it could be SVT with aberrant conduction. Both look *exactly* alike in lead II. Even with a 12-lead ECG, it is extremely difficult to tell the difference between these two rhythms. Any wide complex tachycardia is ventricular in origin in only 80% of cases; in the remaining 20% of cases, it is supraventricular with aberrant conduction. Both rhythms look so similar that they are difficult for most clinicians to differentiate without the assistance of a cardiologist.

If an immediate consult is not possible, do not hesitate—use the question mark protocol (i.e., wide complex tachycardia of uncertain type).

Helpful Hints

- Some clinicians think that ventricular tachycardia is inherently more symptomatic than SVT with aberrant conduction and that it is easy to differentiate between them clinically. This is *incorrect*. It is possible for some ventricular tachycardias to be asymptomatic; whereas some supraventricular tachycardias (with or without aberrancy) may be cardiovascularly devastating. *Don't use clinical criteria to differentiate between the two.*
- Ventricular antiarrhythmic drugs do not work on supraventricular pacemakers, and vice versa. The question mark (wide complex tachycardia of unknown origin) protocol allows for this idiosyncrasy by sequencing medications for both.

The patient thanks you for the information while emitting a deep, resonating belch. He again points to the monitor above his head—question mark. You now understand that this means any wide complex tachycardia that you are not absolutely certain is ventricular tachycardia. If a wide complex tachycardia appears on the monitor, and there is no cardiologist to consult, no specific history on the patient, and a 12-lead ECG is not definitive, treat with the wide complex tachycardia of uncertain type protocol.

In the question mark protocol, you do not know for certain if the presenting rhythm is ventricular or supraventricular. The origin is important because ventricular pacemakers do not respond to supraventricular drugs, and vice versa. Because there is an 80% chance that any wide complex tachycardia is ventricular in origin, the first treatment of choice in the question mark protocol is lidocaine, the same first drug as in the documented ventricular tachycardia protocol.

Lidocaine. The patient reaches over to the placard directly under the documented ventricular tachycardia monitor and slides it to a spot directly underneath the question mark monitor, centering it to a point in the middle of his face. The placard has **lidocaine** painted on it in lemon-yellow letters. The sign is obscuring the patient's jaundiced, yellow eyes. When he points to the placard that covers his face, remember the color of the eyes—lemon yellow—lidocaine (Fig. 9-30).

Visualize the image before proceeding.

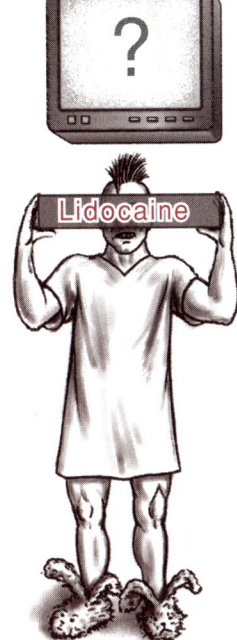

Figure 9-30

Let's Practice

1. The drug beneath the question mark monitor covering the patient's eyes is _____

2. The therapy that is at the level of the patient's thighs under the Documented V-tach monitor is _____

3. The first drug of choice in either the Documented V-tach or the wide complex tachycardia of unknown origin protocol is _____

Adenosine, Procainamide, Bretylium. If the rhythm is refractory to lidocaine, you might conclude that the rhythm does not have a ventricular pacemaker. Thus, you consider the possibility that the pacemaker might be supraventricular but conduct aberrantly, making the QRS complex appear wide.

The patient grabs the adenosine placard from the middle slot under the Obvious SVT monitor and slides it directly across to position it beneath the lidocaine directly across his chest. If the adenosine works, the rhythm has a supraventricular origin. If the adenosine is unsuccessful, it is more likely that the rhythm was ventricular but just did not respond to lidocaine. If the rhythm is refractory, procainamide is slid underneath adenosine. If procainamide proves ineffective, bretylium would be considered and placed below the procainamide. The procainamide placard is hooked on the patient at the level of the pants (if he was wearing some): **p**ants reminds you of **p**rocainamide. Bretylium is pasted at about mid-thigh, about the level of his **b**uttocks. Now the placards beneath the question mark monitor read: lidocaine, adenosine, procainamide, and finally, bretylium (Fig. 9-31).

Visualize the image before proceeding.

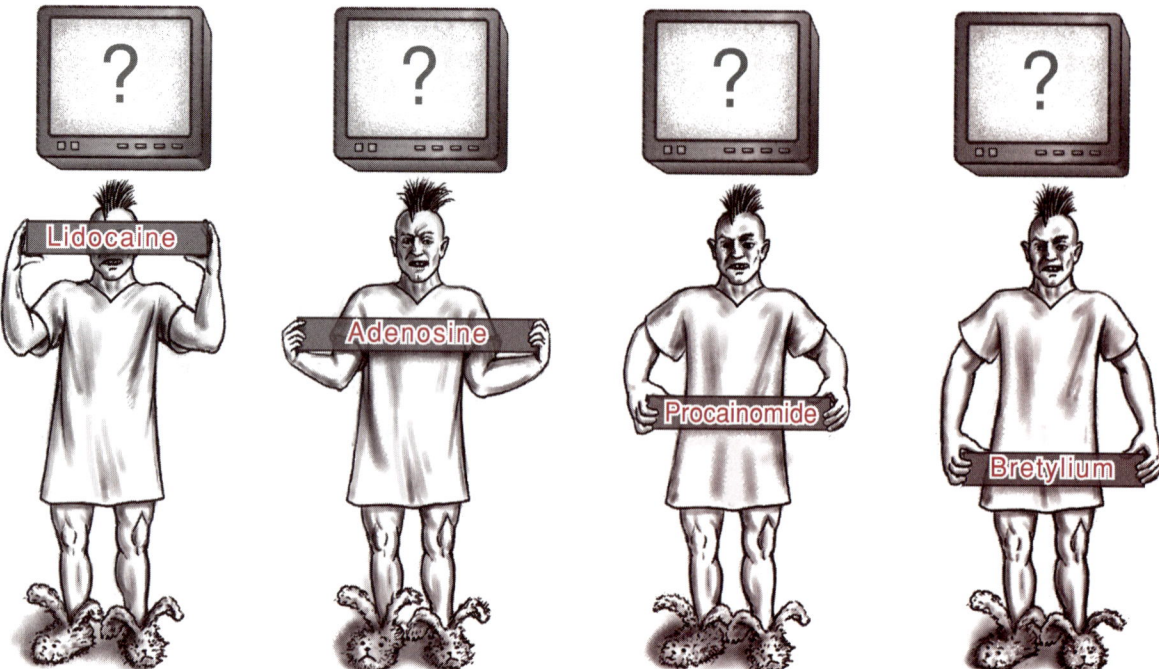

Figure 9-31

Let's Practice

1. Under the documented ventricular tachycardia monitor, the patient points to what placard even with his pants? _____

2. He then points to what sign just beneath the Obvious SVT monitor? _____

3. Then he tries to trick you by using his other hand. He points to what placard just under the question mark monitor covering his face? _____

4. He then points to what placard at the bottom of the Documented V-tach monitor? _____

5. What placard is placed mid-axillary beneath Obvious SVT? _____

6. What is the second placard beneath the question mark monitor even with the patient's chest? _____

7. What is the bottom placard beneath the Obvious SVT monitor? _____

8. What placard is at the level of the patient's pants under the Documented V-tach monitor? _____

The patient looks at you with those implacable jet-black eyes and says, "Always treat me with drugs because I am stable. Always treat patients who look like me with drugs *unless* they lose consciousness, have chest pain, become hypotensive, or exhibit symptoms of pulmonary edema."

You thank him for his time, slam the door in his face, and relax back in the driver's seat.

UNSTABLE TACHYCARDIAS: THE CAR RADIO

After the harrowing discourse with the patient in the speedometer, you are glad to get away, and you allow your eyes to roam across the dashboard. They center over the car radio in the middle. To your annoyance, lying there with his head pointing toward the steering wheel and his feet toward the passenger door is the same bizarre patient who was in the speedometer (Fig. 9-32).

Although this patient appears unconscious, in general, unstable tachycardic patients may present as either:

- Unconscious
- Going unconscious
- Alert but exhibiting signs and symptoms of cardiovascular compromise (i.e., hypotension, chest pain, or pulmonary edema)

You know that the patient on the car radio is alive without touching him because his tachycardic heart beat resonates from the radio speakers: "lub-dub, lub-dub, lub-dub." This patient is unconscious, and his ruby-red tongue is hanging out of his mouth so far that it becomes the red indicator on the radio dial. His eyes are rolled so far back in their sockets that only the sclera are visible. Spittle is dripping along the corner of his mouth, and he is making a snoring sound. The top of his multicolored mohawk haircut is listing toward the right. The reflection from the windshield reveals that his rear is still uncovered.

Visualize the image before proceeding.

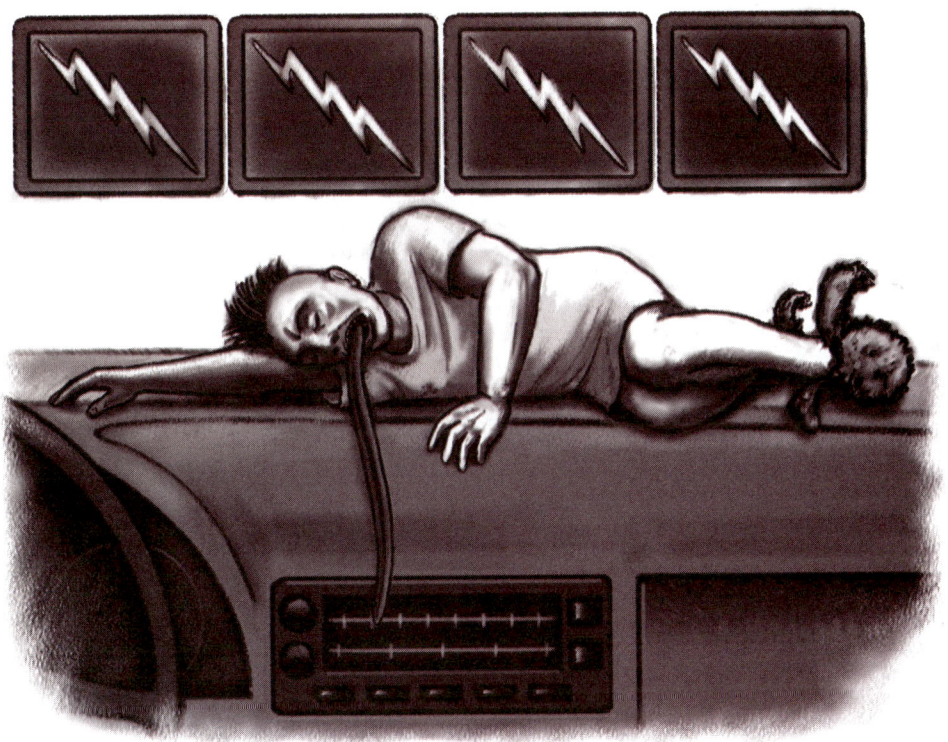

Figure 9-32

Let's Practice

1. Is the patient lying on the dashboard pointed toward the steering wheel or the passenger door? _____
2. Is the patient always unconscious when on the car radio? _____

This patient is no longer considered stable, thus no longer in the speedometer. He is now unstable. An unstable patient is not solely treated with drugs because his cardiovascular system is quickly deteriorating. Concurrent drug therapy is acceptable but should not delay or take the place of more immediate therapy—cardioversion. During cardioversion, the time required to wait for a drug's effect is unacceptable; therefore, if you administer any antiarrhythmics, give them quickly while the machine is charging or between the shocks.

Unstable patients may present with chest pain, pulmonary edema, shortness of breath, or altered level of consciousness. Even an apparently stable "speedometer" patient *who has any of these symptoms* should be considered *unstable* and moved onto the car radio. For example, if the patient in the speedometer suddenly experiences chest pain or pulmonary edema, even though the blood pressure and other vital signs are acceptable, he is considered unstable and moved to the car radio. The chest pain or pulmonary edema is a symptom of a too rapid heart rate.

If the patient is alert enough to know what is going on, sedate him. A hypnotic, such as Versed or Valium, can institute the proper mood. If you do not have the time to sedate, warn the patient that the procedure may be painful, and then shock.

The patient is lying on top of the car radio. Repeat the words "car radio." Again, say it faster. Again, faster. You want to car-radio-vert (cardiovert) the patient. Because this person is alive, synchronized cardioversion, not defibrillation, is the preferred treatment of choice. The machine can synchronize on the R wave, keeping far away from the vulnerable area of the T wave. If your monitor-defibrillator does not have the capability to synchronize or is having trouble synchronizing, *do not hesitate to turn off the synchronizer and immediately defibrillate.*

It does not make any difference which of the monitors above the patient exhibits the rhythm, "car-radio-version" is the treatment of choice. The patient could be in ventricular tachycardia, SVT, or atrial fibrillation or flutter; it makes no difference. Treating any unstable tachycardia, in which the *heart rate is the cause* of the instability, is as simple as 1—2—3. These are the joule settings times 100, which can progress up to 360 joules. Some rhythms, SVT or atrial fibrillation or flutter, may use lower settings, but they are not as easy to remember.

If the patient is stable, treat him with drugs in the speedometer. If he is found lying on the radio or falls out of the speedometer onto the radio, car-radio-vert him 1—2—3. A brief trial of medications, such as rapidly acting adenosine or lidocaine, may be given while preparing for cardioversion. A routine medication trial, however, is not meant to be part of the standard protocol for unstable tachycardias.

Let's Practice

1. Adenosine and lidocaine have a higher priority than cardioversion in an unstable tachycardia. True or false? _____

2. Defibrillation is the same as synchronized cardioversion except that defibrillation takes place at a higher joule setting. True or false? _____

3. A routine trial of medications of antiarrhythmics is part of the standard protocol for all unstable tachycardias. True or false? _____

PULSELESS VENTRICULAR TACHYCARDIA: THE GLOVE BOX

Now move your eyes all the way to the right of the dashboard and visualize the glove box. Its dark exterior and lock makes it look similar to a casket. When you open it up, your bizarre patient, recently deceased, rolls out (Fig. 9-33). This patient looks dead. His pasty white skin tone is in stark contrast to his dilated jet-black eyes. He has no pulse. In this situation, because pulseless ventricular tachycardia is treated like ventricular fibrillation, the patient is defibrillated at once.

A way of remembering this: if the patient is alive, always attempt to synchronize. If the patient is dead, defibrillate. Both *dead* and *defibrillate* start with the letter **d**. You start with 200 joules rather than 100 joules for cardioversion because you have to raise them from the dead!

Visualize the image before proceeding.

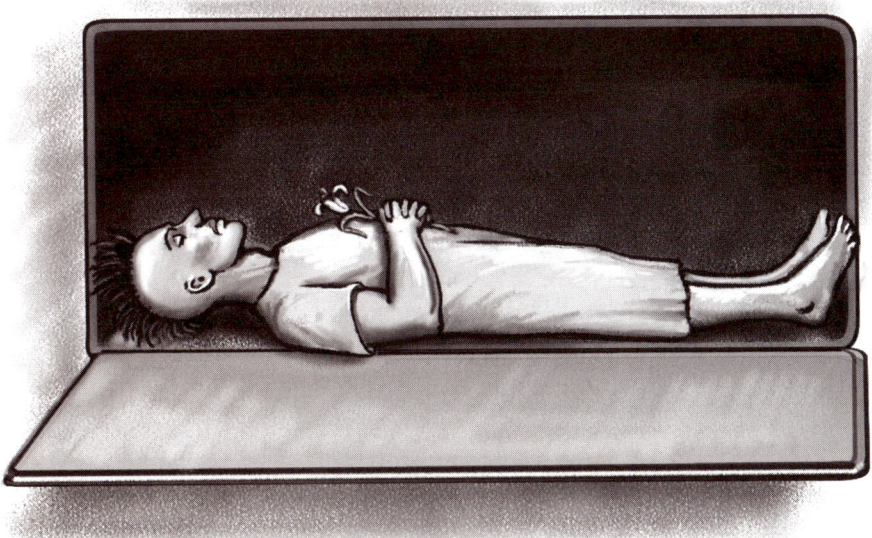

Figure 9-33

Let's Practice

1. What is the difference between the car radio and the glove box? _____
2. Is a patient in the glove box deemed unstable? _____
3. Is the glove box the ventricular fibrillation protocol _____?

(See Figure 9-34 for a review of the tachycardia dashboard.)

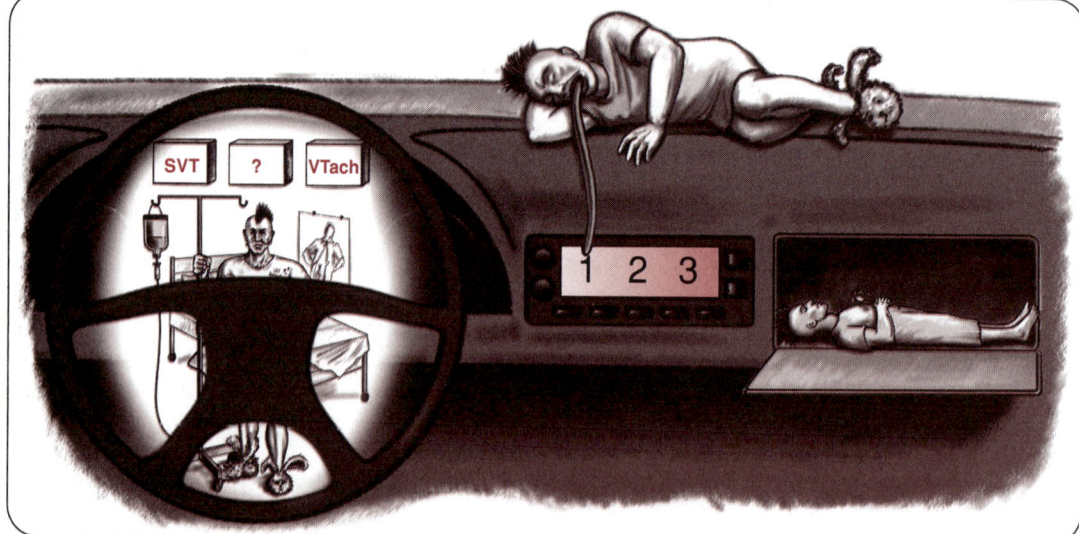

Figure 9-34

Tachycardia Summary

In summary, *with the exception of atrial fibrillation and atrial flutter,* if your patient develops either a wide complex tachycardia (more than 100) or a narrow complex tachycardia (more than 170), mentally sit in your car. Gather assessment data and decide what the patient looks like.

- If he is conscious and alert with no symptoms of cardiovascular compromise, treat him as a speedometer and give the drug treatment appropriate to the rhythm.
- If he is unconscious, going unconscious, or cardiovascularly compromised, treat him on the car radio—cardiovert him.
- If he exhibits a pulseless ventricular tachycardia, treat him in the glove box—defibrillate.
- Remember that it is necessary to recognize atrial fibrillation and flutter before contemplating standard therapy because they usually present with much slower rates than 170 beats/minute and have different drug protocols in the speedometer. However, unstable atrial fibrillation and atrial flutters are treated with synchronized cardioversion.

Emphasizing decisions on stability, as long as you approach all tachycardias by sitting in the car *before* treating them, you will deal with them appropriately.

Chapter 9 Memorization Techniques

Acute Stroke: Acute Ischemic Stroke and Hemorrhagic Stroke

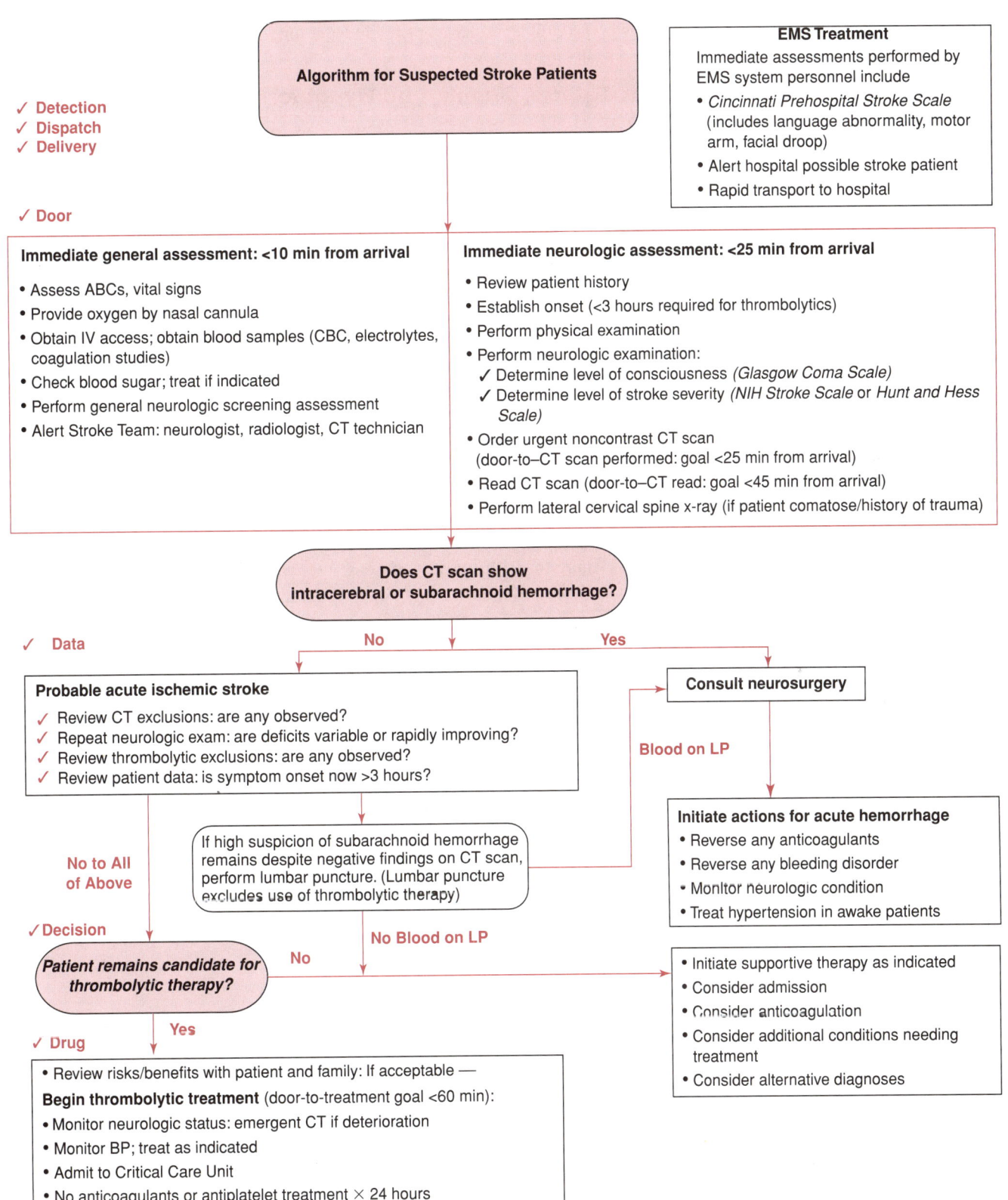

(Reproduced with permission. *Advanced Cardiac Life Support*. Copyright 1997, American Heart Association)

Acute Stroke Memory Aid

There is no need to memorize this protocol. I have only included it for completeness.

Acute Pulmonary Edema, Heart Failure, Shock, and Hypothermia

These protocols are not part of a generic ACLS course. They are included in certain customized courses for specific clinicians. This book includes all but hypothermia as part of the unstable tachycardia protocol (rate–volume–pump). Hypothermia is discussed as part of case studies 2 and 3: ventricular fibrillation and pulseless ventricular tachycardia.

Let's Practice

1. What is the second therapy in the bradycardia protocol? _____
2. What are the main components of PEA? _____
3. What is the second antiarrhythmic in the ventricular fibrillation protocol? _____
4. What is the difference between the asystole and PEA protocols? _____
5. What is the third therapy in the stable SVT protocol? _____
6. What is the treatment of choice for any unstable wide complex tachycardia (more than 100) or unstable narrow complex tachycardia (more than 170)? _____
7. What is the fourth drug in the bradycardia protocol? _____
8. What is the second drug in the stable ventricular tachycardia protocol? _____
9. What is the first drug in either the wide complex tachycardia of unknown origin or the ventricular tachycardia protocol? _____
10. Which is the only drug to differ between the wide complex tachycardia of unknown origin and the ventricular tachycardia protocols? _____

Answers

Chapter 2

Answers to Respiratory Interim Evaluation

1. (b) It is often hampered by a poor seal. A BVM is a sophisticated piece of equipment, providing up to 100% oxygen. If improperly applied, it may cause more problems than it solves. It can be used to ventilate a cardiac arrest or just assist the respirations of a patient displaying respiratory compromise.

2. (a) 1, 3, and 4. A BVM should include a self-expanding bag, a transparent face mask, and a nonrebreathing valve. To ensure 100% oxygenation, the flow should be at least 12 to 15 liters/minute.

3. (b) False. An OPA is not long enough to reach the vocal cords.

4. (c) 1. The only selection that is considered part of the primary survey is suctioning the airway. All other selections should be accomplished during the secondary survey. The primary survey is reserved for what is absolutely necessary to keep the patient alive—no extras. This does not imply, however, that treatment cannot be ordered simultaneously. The assessment mnemonic is used to help the clinician structure the appropriate priorities.

5. (a) True. An NPA is pliable and soft and may kink, causing blockage. When an OPA or NPA is employed, make certain that the patient's airway is patent.

6. (a) True. Previously used to make intubation easier, cricoid pressure is now advocated when ventilating nonintubated patients. Direct pressure on the cricoid cartilage collapses the esophagus, stopping air from entering the stomach.

7. (d) 1, 2, and 3. Intubation diminishes the chance of aspiration by protecting the airway. If intravenous routes are delayed or unavailable, atropine, lidocaine, and epinephrine can be given through the ET tube. In no way does intubation abrogate a supplemental oxygen source.

8. (b) 2, 3, and 4. Intubating a patient allows a clinician to ventilate with less effort while reducing the risk of aspiration. Nevertheless, pushing the tube past the level of the carina can result in unilateral inflation. To allow for the inevitable period of apnea, a patient should be ventilated by other means before intubating.

9. (d) 1 and 2. Attempts at tracheal intubation may result in both laryngeal trauma and esophageal intubation. The other selections represent pathologies that are too deep for an ET tube to be involved.

10. (b) 2, 3, and 4. Because the patient may become hypoxic, ET suction should be preceded by increased ventilation. Suctioning should be limited, however, to 10 to 15 seconds while withdrawing the catheter.

11. (d) 3 and 4. The curved blade is designed to fit in the vallecula, whereas the straight blade lifts up the epiglottis. Use of either blade is entirely dependent on the clinician's preference.

12. (a) Patient supine, neck flexed, and head extended. This positioning is commonly called the *sniffing position*. None of the other answers provides positions in which the vocal cords can be visualized.

13. (b) Intubated the esophagus. Even though pressed against the carina, breath sounds will still be heard because the base of the tube has another hole on the side. The other two selections generate breath sounds somewhere in the lungs. Assuming no chest trauma, absent bilateral breath sounds usually represent esophageal intubation.

14. (b) False. For a short period after an arrest, it is possible for a patient to exhibit breathing movements but no concurrent pulse. Likewise, it is possible for a patient to be apneic but have a pulse, but only for a brief period of time. Do not assume anything during the primary survey—verify each step.

15. (a) Esophageal intubation. If the esophagus is intubated, there will be no breath sounds—right or left. The other selections represent situations in which breath sounds will be absent on the right.

16. (d) Oxygen face mask with reservoir. Both the nasal cannula and oxygen face mask deliver between 20% and 60% oxygen. Although the amounts of oxygen are not large, a Venti mask is usually used only when exact oxygen concentrations are required.

17. (b) False. Clearing the airway by suctioning is part of the primary survey, but trying to find an oxygen bottle is not. Stopping to put a person on 100% oxygen without progressing to assessing circulation (i.e., checking for a pulse) is inappropriate. Oxygen employment is necessary, but not during the 15-second primary survey.

18. (c) 2, 3, and 4. Verifying bilateral lung fields is part of advanced airway assessment and should be verified before progressing to the next portion of the survey—beware blinders. The clinician should think of beware blinders as a reminder to perform a quick thorax examination. Things to look for include rales, rhonchi, wheezing, chest symmetry, jugular distention, tracheal deviation, and signs of trauma. In addition, it serves to remind the clinician to check pertinent history (e.g., alcoholism, diabetes). Do not think of beware blinders as part of just verifying lung sounds. Use it to remind you to think about the cause and impacting symptoms of the emergency.

19. (c) Peripheral arm vein. The other selections could be used but are not the most accessible or suitable as the *initial* vein during CPR.

20. (b) Medial. Progressing from lateral to medial, the mnemonic NAV—*nerve, artery,* and *vein*—is an easy way to remember them. The femoral vein is medial to the femoral artery.

21. (b) 1 and 2. Lactated Ringer's and normal saline are the solutions of choice in cardiac arrest. D-5-W and 5% Dextrose in half-normal saline are not isotonic. Use of nonisotonic solutions results in fluid shifts in the vascular compartment. Multiple bags of dextrose in an arrest may result in hyperglycemia in some predisposed patients, resulting in a poor neurologic outcome.

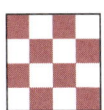

ANSWERS TO RESPIRATORY CROSSWORD PUZZLE

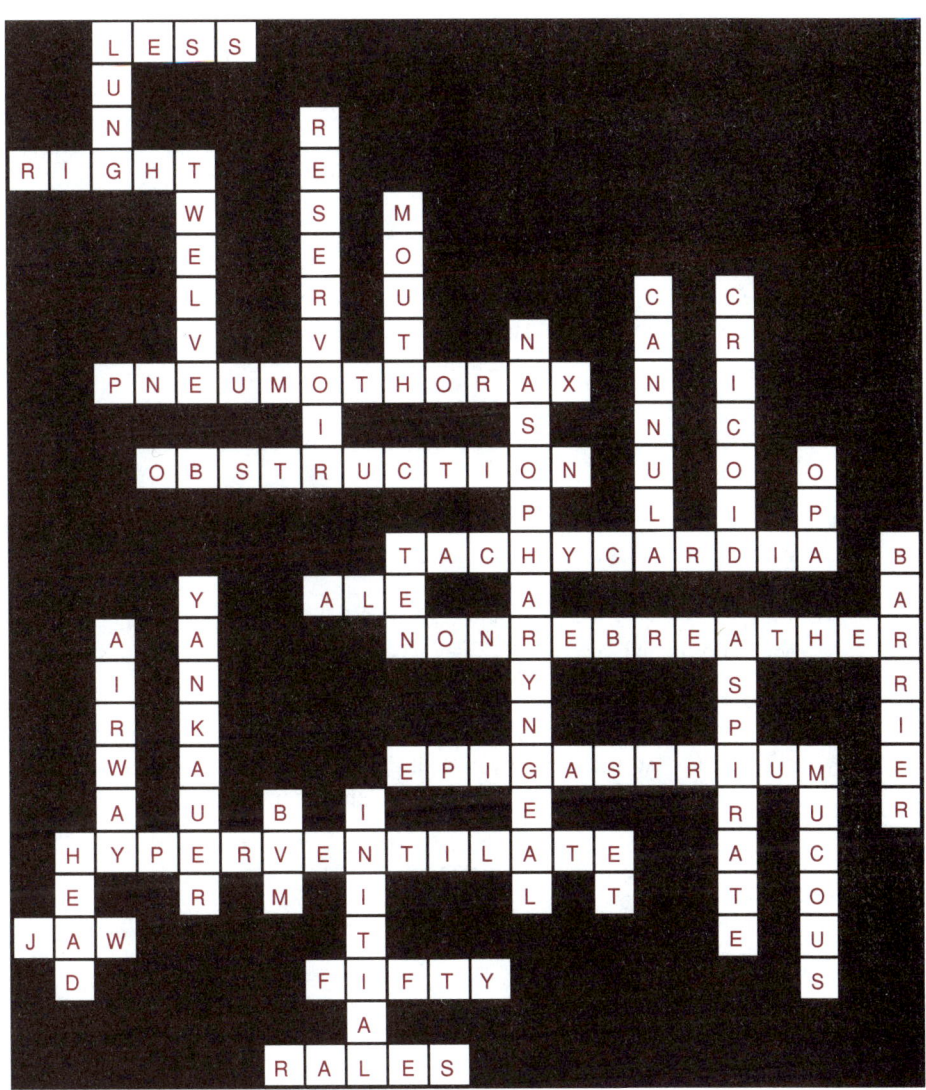

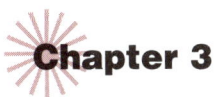

Chapter 3

Answers to Ventricular Fibrillation and Pulseless Ventricular Tachycardia Interim Evaluation

1. (c) 1, 2, and 3. Magnesium sulfate, sodium bicarbonate, and procainamide are part of the refractory ventricular fibrillation and pulseless ventricular tachycardia protocol. The clinician should consider these medications early in the protocol. Morphine sulfate and propranolol may be used in specific portions of the myocardial infarction (MI) protocol but are not part of the cardiac arrest protocol.

2. (b) False. Although most protocols appear to progress from top to bottom, that is not the case. When a clinician suspects an etiology of an emergency, it should be treated promptly. In this scenario, if nutritional deficit was suspected, the chance of hypomagnesemia would be high, and therefore this condition should be treated as soon as it is suspected, directly after epinephrine.

3. (a) An immediate unsynchronized countershock, up to three times if necessary. After A, B, and C comes D for defibrillation. Nothing is more critical than timely defibrillation in the ventricular fibrillation protocol. The other drugs listed are important, but not as crucial as immediate defibrillation. Answer (d) is best performed during the secondary survey, not the primary.

4. (d) Immediate defibrillation. During a witnessed arrest of either ventricular fibrillation or pulseless ventricular tachycardia, and when a monitor-defibrillator is available, you would not start CPR initially but immediately defibrillate. Synchronized cardioversion is only appropriate for unstable ventricular tachycardia, not pulseless ventricular tachycardia. Lidocaine should not be given in preference for immediate defibrillation.

5. (c) 360 joules. An initial stack of unsynchronized shocks (defibrillations) should be given at 200, 200 to 300, and 360 joules. Because the patient had been shocked at 250 joules, the next shock would have been 360 joules.

6. (a) Vasoconstriction. Epinephrine has a variety of adrenergic effects on the body. Among these are beta effects: increased automaticity, positive inotropic effects, and positive chronotropic effects. The alpha effects of epinephrine, however, are the primary reason it is administered during a cardiac arrest. It makes CPR more effective by increasing the blood supply to the brain and the left ventricle by vasoconstriction of peripheral vessels.

7. (b) The key strategy in the treatment of ventricular fibrillation is timely defibrillation. Although CPR, epinephrine, and intubation are necessary in the cardiac arrest scenario, the key strategy is: the faster and more often you defibrillate, the more high-energy phosphates are available to allow the heart to contract once the problem is corrected.

8. (c) Lying on the ground with no one touching the patient. If the answers from (a), (b), and (d) were being performed and motion detected, the AED's analyze cycle would be interrupted.

9. (a) True. Sernum-to-apex placement requires less patient manipulation to expose the pad locations.

10. (a) AED. The AED will have the most far-reaching impact for most of the population because it will bring larger numbers of people closer to defibrillation access. Although external pacemaker capability, surgically implanted defibrillators, and cryotherapy have an impact, each is not necessarily the most far-reaching for most of the population.

11. (d) All of the above. Sodium bicarbonate therapy may produce metabolic alkalosis, should always be guided by blood gases and pH when available, and is considered harmful in a hypoxic-related acidosis. If you suspect a preexisting bicarbonate-responsive situation (i.e., hyperkalemia or aspirin overdose) during a cardiac arrest, you should administer sodium bicarbonate early in the protocol.

12. (d) 2 to 2.5 times the intravenous dosage diluted to a total of 10 mL. Answers (a) and (b) have incorrect dosages. Answer (c), 2.5 mL of 1:1000 dilution, is too small a volume to distribute throughout the lung.

13. (b) 1, 2, and 3. In ventricular fibrillation, lidocaine may be given as an initial bolus of 1.5 mg/kg and repeated at the same dosage to a maximum dose of 3 mg/kg. It may also be given as a single bolus of 1.5 mg/kg, but then moving to the first dose of bretylium. Lidocaine may cause seizures in doses above 3 mg/kg. In addition, lidocaine is contraindicated in idioventricular rhythms without mechanical pacemakers because it stops ventricular ectopic activity.

14. (b) Excessive length of administration time. Ventricular fibrillation is remarkably time dependent, and therefore the longer it takes to administer a drug, the less is the chance of success. Given in ventricular fibrillation at 30 mg/minute, it would take 40 to 60 minutes to administer procainamide to the total dose for a 100-kg patient. In addition, procainamide decreases automaticity, elevates the ventricular fibrillation threshold, and when the cardiovascular system is restored, may cause hypotension.

15. (d) An initial 5 mg/kg bolus followed by a 10 mg/kg bolus every 5 minutes to a total of 30 to 35 mg/kg. The other answers did not reflect the correct dosage scheme.

16. (d) 1 to 2 g diluted to 10 mL given as an intravenous push. This drug can be given as an intravenous push during a cardiac arrest. The other selections either dilute it excessively or give an incorrect dosage.

17. (c) Check the ECG leads. If the patient has a pulse, the monitor must be faulty—ventricular fibrillation does not deliver a pulse.

18. (b) 2 and 3. Epinephrine and oxygen are the only class I drugs noted. Magnesium sulfate and procainamide are both class IIa—probably helpful but not definitely helpful.

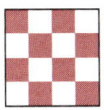

ANSWERS TO VENTRICULAR FIBRILLATION AND PULSELESS VENTRICULAR TACHYCARDIA CROSSWORD PUZZLE

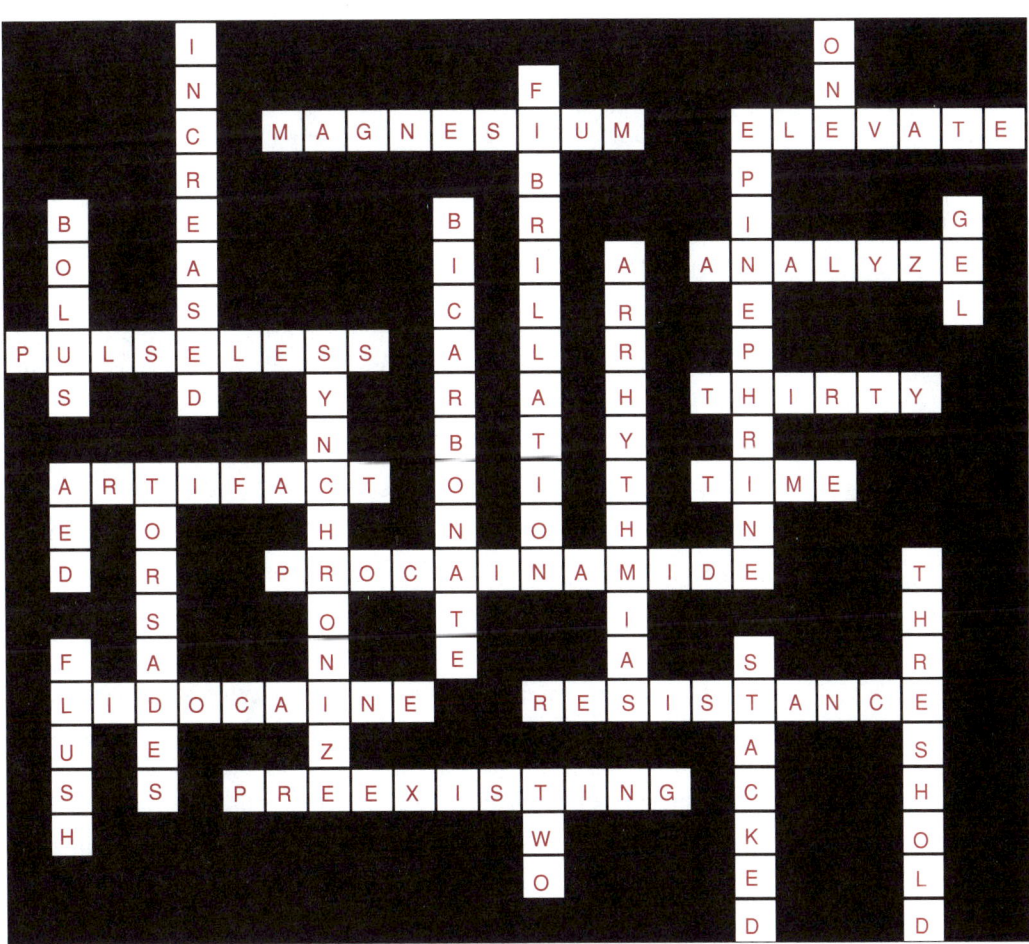

Answers to Pulseless Electrical Activity Interim Evaluation

1. (b) False. Ventilation and oxygenation are not the same. Hyperventilation primarily only affects the $Paco_2$, the Pao_2 is affected by inspired oxygen. Because hypoxia represents an oxygen deficit, hyperventilation without adequate oxygenation does not quickly correct underlying hypoxia. In treating PEA, speed in correcting the hypoxia is paramount, thus oxygen is a requirement.

2. (d) Hypovolemia. Although (a), (b), and (c) are all etiologies of PEA, only hypovolemia qualifies as the *most* common while matching the symptoms noted.

3. (a) 1, 2, and 3. Lidocaine is not an intervention in PEA. Interventions include: a rapid fluid challenge, an abbreviated patient assessment, and epinephrine to make CPR more effective.

4. (d) Ruptured diaphragm. The remaining selections are documented causes of PEA; however, ruptured diaphragm is not.

5. (b) Perform a pericardiocentesis. Because they are in cardiac arrest, patients in PEA have no time to have a chest radiograph or cardiac catheterization. Although helpful in certain drug-overdose situations, a TCP is not routinely employed because PEA already has electrical activity—it just lacks sufficient cardiac output to generate a pulse. If you suspect cardiac tamponade, rule out the possibility quickly with a pericardiocentesis; you cannot make the situation any worse.

6. (a) Normal treatment for acute hyperkalemia consists of trying to force potassium back inside the cell by immediately administering calcium chloride along with a combination of glucose, sodium bicarbonate, and insulin. Although some of the other distracters have calcium chloride and bicarbonate, they contain other choices inappropriate for hyperkalemia.

7. (a) Perform a brief patient assessment considering possible causes. The key strategy of PEA is to find an etiology and treat it. PEA is not shocked, given fluid challenges of D-5-W, or given calcium-channel blockers. A heart rate of 130 beats/minute does not qualify as a rate treatable with verapamil. The rate is more indicative of a compensatory tachycardia due to a fluid-deficit hypovolemia, the most common cause of PEA.

8. (b) Institute a TCP. Although helpful in certain drug-overdose situations, a TCP is not *routinely* part of the protocol for PEA because the rhythm already has an endogenous pacemaker—it just is not delivering an adequate cardiac output. The remaining selections are appropriate during the PEA protocol.

9. (d) All of the above. Acidosis in a routine cardiac arrest should be treated with increased ventilation until perfusion has been restored. An acidosis, in which carbon dioxide retention is the etiology, is not routinely treated with sodium bicarbonate.

10. (d) 2 to 2.5 times the intravenous dosage in 10 ml of NS. The endotracheal dosage of atropine is documented differently in two portions of the ACLS textbook. In Chapter 1: Essentials of ACLS, it is listed along with others as 2 to 2.5 times the intravenous dosage. In the Pharmacology I chapter, it is listed as 1 to 2 mg diluted in 10 mL of NS. Therefore, it is a safe bet that it can be given as low as 1 mg and as much as 2.5 mg diluted in 10 mL of NS. Selections (a) and (b) are obviously incorrect, but answer (c) appears correct until the dilution amount is noted.

11. (a) True. Atropine, the antidote for vagal domination, is indicated for both a relative or absolute bradycardia if the etiology of the PEA involves the vagus nerve.

12. (b) Warm blankets. Severe hypothermia is treated with warm intravenous fluids, warm humidified oxygen, peritoneal lavage, and warm enemas—anything but warm blankets. Peripheral warming with blankets causes vasodilation of the extremities carrying cold, lactic acid–rich blood back to the core, which could cause ventricular fibrillation. The problem in PEA is the time necessary to rewarm a patient while performing basic life support.

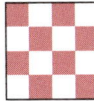

ANSWERS TO PULSELESS ELECTRICAL ACTIVITY CROSSWORD PUZZLE

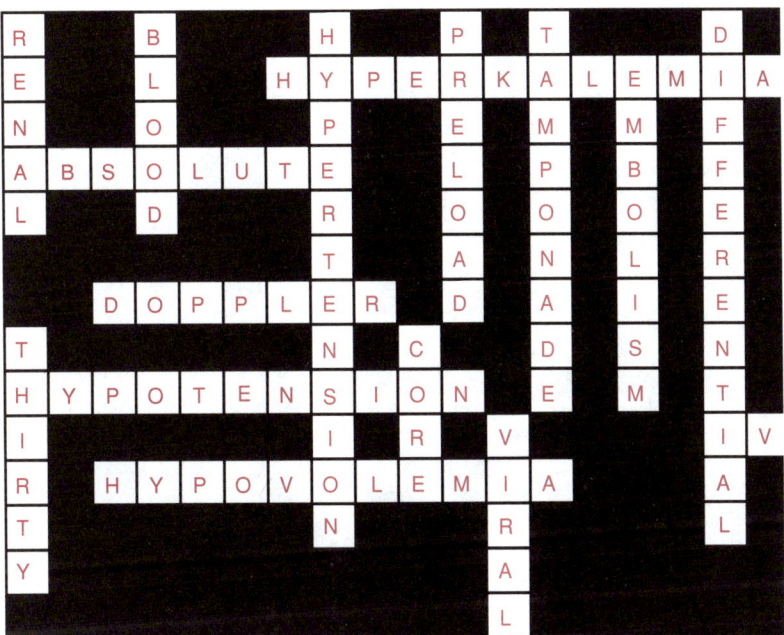

Answers to Asystole Interim Evaluation

1. (d) The presenting rhythm might be ventricular fibrillation. The asystole protocol does not contain defibrillation—a critical component of ventricular fibrillation. Therefore, it is important to make the distinction early when immediate defibrillation might be successful. The chaotic depolarization waves of ventricular fibrillation may be moving at 90 degrees to the lead that you are viewing, thereby making the activity invisible in that lead. Therefore, quickly verify the asystolic rhythm from another angle. The remaining three answers were just distracters, containing no medical validity.

2. (b) False. Most people think that atropine makes the heart go faster; however, this is not specifically correct. Atropine reduces vagal domination, allowing the sympathetic system to dominate, thereby increasing heart rate. It makes the heart rate accelerate indirectly. Atropine only reduces parasympathetic tone; therefore, if it is administered without effect, you can rule out the vagus nerve as the etiology of the bradycardia.

3. (b) Digitalis toxicity. Digitalis toxicity is more frequent in patients with hypokalemia. The other three answers are all situations of increased, not decreased, potassium level.

300 Unit 2 Learning Adjuncts

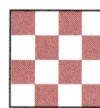

ANSWERS TO ASYSTOLE CROSSWORD PUZZLE

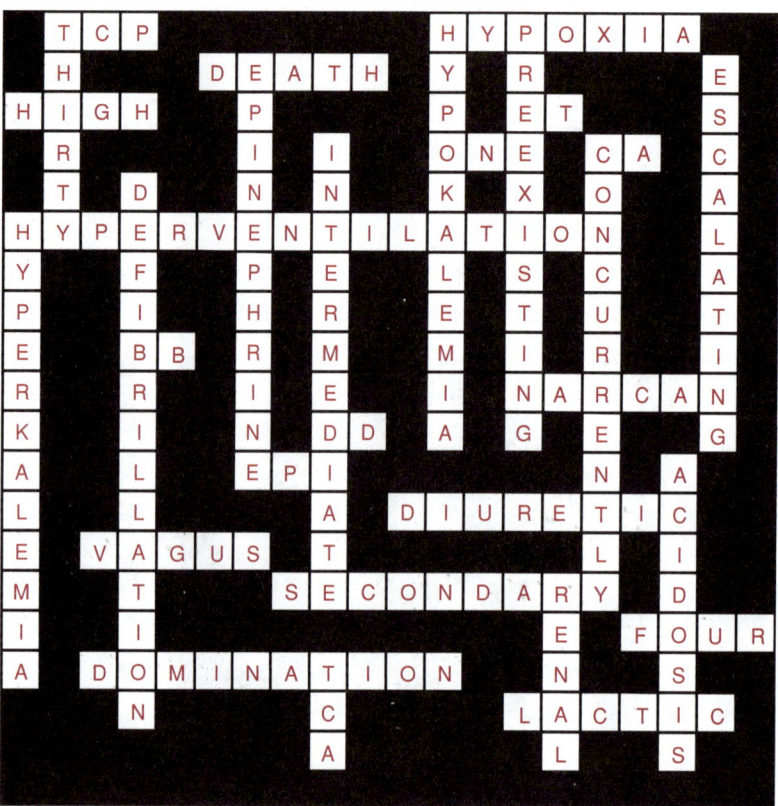

Chapter 4

Answers to Acute Myocardial Infarction Interim Evaluation

1. (b) False. A normal ECG does not exclude the diagnosis of MI. A significant group of infarctions do not have any initial changes in the ECG, only showing up much later or not at all.

2. (d) 1 and 4. All patients with chest pain should be monitored for cardiac arrhythmias and given supplemental oxygen. Giving oral β-blockers prophylactically is inappropriate. If β-blockers are used, they should be given intravenously and only if the patient is neither hypotensive nor bradycardic. Isoproterenol is only given in bradycardia when nothing else is successful.

3. (b) Morphine sulfate. Morphine sulfate is routinely given for relief of chest pain and associated apprehension. Furosemide is given in the presence of congestive heart failure, not mentioned here. Atropine is not administered because the patient's pulse is 98 beats/minute. Procainamide is not given prophylactically and is given only when a ventricular ectopic rhythm is refractory to lidocaine.

4. (c) 50%. The percentage of acute MI deaths outside the hospital is about 50%, usually occurring within the first hour after the onset of symptoms.

5. (d) All of the above. All of these selections will have a substantial impact on survival from prehospital cardiac arrest.

6. (a) True. Aspirin can achieve the same decrease in mortality as streptokinase if administered within 24 hours. For this reason, the AHA encourages aspirin administration in the prehospital sector in all patients exhibiting chest pains with no specific allergies or contraindications.

7. (a) Most occur during heavy physical exercise. MIs can occur at any time, unlike angina, which may be precipitated by heavy physical exercise. Although they may appear improbable, (b) and (c) are true. In addition, 66% (most) of all patients who have MIs die before reaching the hospital.

8. (a) True. Diagnosis of an MI is based on changes in the ECG, changes in the cardiac enzymes, and a patient history. In some instances, it may take time for the first two to show any changes; so initially, diagnosis of a suspected MI should be primarily based on the patient's physical examination and pertinent history.

9. (b) False. Lidocaine is no longer administered prophylactically to a patient with chest pain. Routinely treating premature ventricular contractions is discouraged unless they are significant (i.e., runs of ventricular tachycardia).

10. (d) None of the above. All three selections represent etiologies in which magnesium sulfate may prove useful. Magnesium may be used in the first 24 hours after MI, in the obstetrical and gynecologic sector for eclampsia, and is the pharmaceutical of choice for treating torsades de pointes.

11. (d) 3. β-Blockers, such as propranolol, directly depress the pumping function (negative inotropic effect). Neither atropine, lidocaine, nor isoproterenol decreases the pumping function of cardiac muscle. Both atropine and isoproterenol are positive chronotropes and, like lidocaine, have no negative inotropic effects.

12. (c) Narrow complex tachydysrhythmias refractory to adenosine and verapamil. Propranolol would not be given to further slow a ventricular rate of 80 beats/minute, even when there is an underlying rhythm of atrial fibrillation. Propranolol is contraindicated in compensatory tachycardias, such as congestive heart failure, and in complete heart blocks.

13. (a) True. Sublingual nitroglycerin is the treatment of choice for ischemic cardiac pain. In the past, sublingual nitroglycerin was used to rule out the presence of an MI. If the patient responded to the nitroglycerin, an infarction was ruled out. However, it is inappropriate to use nitroglycerin as the sole basis of ruling out an MI because there are a number of noncardiac etiologies that respond to nitroglycerin (e.g., esophageal pain).

14. (b) 1, 2, and 3. Nitroglycerin is commonly given sublingually. It may be useful in relieving pain in an acute MI and is known to produce hypotension. If necessary, sublingual nitroglycerin should be repeated every 5 minutes.

302 Unit 2 Learning Adjuncts

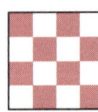

ANSWERS TO ACUTE MYOCARDIAL INFARCTION CROSSWORD PUZZLE

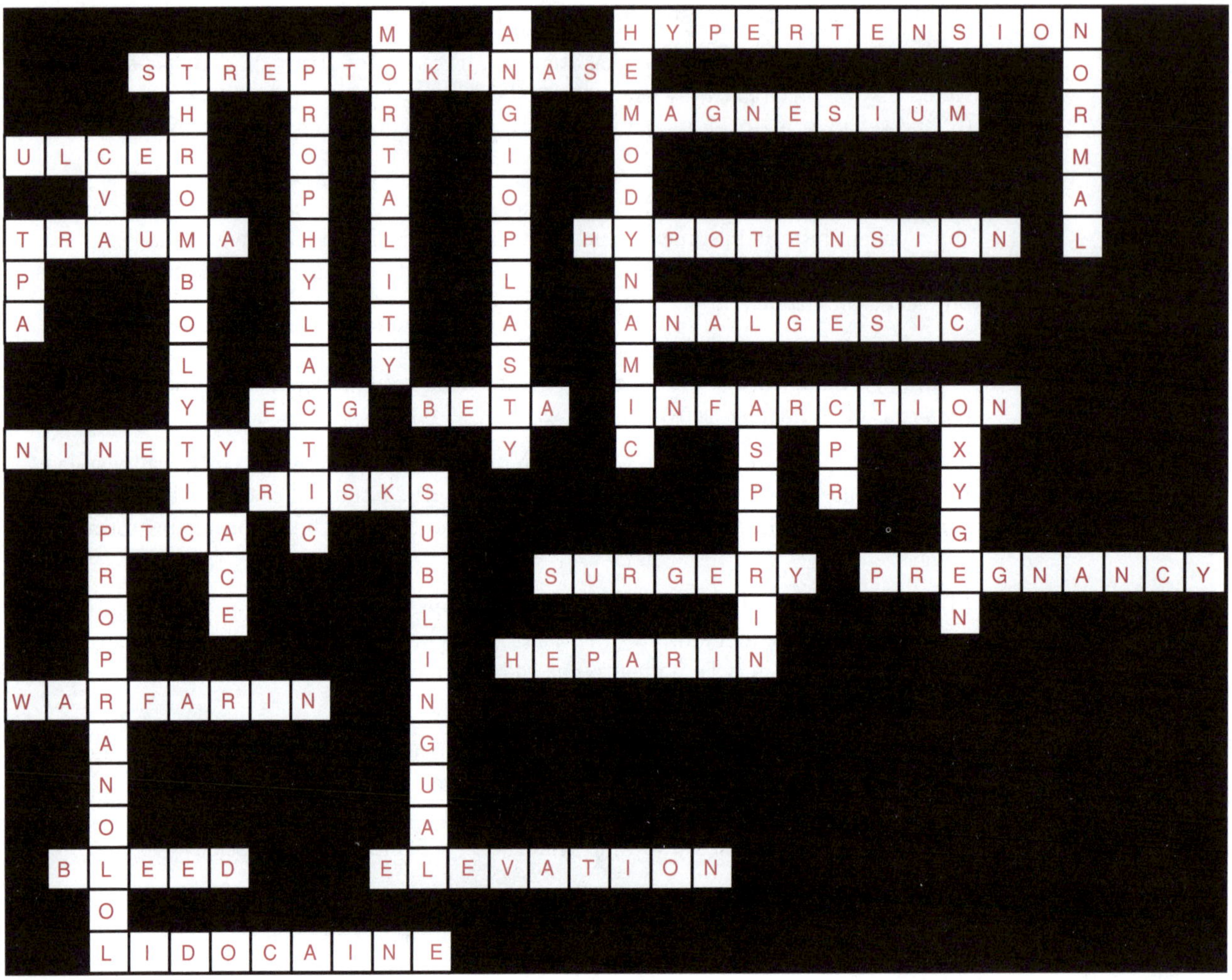

Chapter 5

Answers to Bradycardia Interim Evaluation

1. (c) 2, 5, 1, 3, and 4. All treatments begin with improving oxygenation and then selecting the most benign of the noted drugs—atropine—followed quickly by a pacemaker, dopamine, and an epinephrine drip. The other selections are incorrect because they either did not start with oxygen or the pacemaker was employed too late.

2. (b) Chronotropic. Although epinephrine evidences all of the effects noted, when used as an intravenous drip in the bradycardia protocol, it is used to increase the heart rate.

3. (a) 1 and 3. A sinus tachycardia of 130 beats/minute is consistent with a possible fluid deficit. Although most bradycardias are treated with the bradycardia protocol, right ventricular MIs may present as special cases. Poor contractility due to an MI may decrease preload; therefore, a cautious fluid challenge may improve the situation. Selection 2 is incorrect because fluid

deficits are usually associated with tachycardias, not bradycardias. Selection 4, an SVT, has a rate of 190 beats/minute, consistent with a possible rogue pacemaker cell gone awry. Fluid would not be appropriate; stopping the pacemaker abnormality through drug therapy or immediate cardioversion would be appropriate.

4. (d) Any form of hemodynamically significant bradycardia. Selections (a), (b), and (c) are not indications for a TCP. A sinus rhythm with a first-degree block is not bradycardic per se and is rarely treated. With the exception of overdrive pacing for torsades des pointes, ventricular tachycardia is not paced. Except for some drug overdoses, pulseless electrical activity would not profit from a TCP because it is usually a cardiac output problem.

5. (b) Sex of the patient. Although patient size, pad location, and pericardial effusion are all conditions that might interfere with TCP capture, the patient's sex has no effect on whether a TCP will capture.

6. (b) 3 to 10 mcg/kg/min. Dopamine is entirely dose dependent, and at low dosages of 1 to 2 mcg/kg/min, it stimulates the dopaminergic receptors, keeping the kidneys open and mesentery vasodilated. At rates above 11 mcg/kg/min, only β- and α-adrenergic receptors are stimulated, not the dopaminergic ones; hence, the kidneys no longer diurese. Selection (b) is correct because this dosage keeps the kidneys perfusing while increasing stimulation to the β-adrenergic receptors (heart and lung). Stimulation of β-adrenergic receptors increases cardiac contractility, resulting in blood pressure elevation.

7. (a) True. In rare instances, atropine may cause hypotension in certain infranodal blocks—second-degree, type II AV block or complete heart block. Atropine suppresses vagal stimulation, allowing the atria to accelerate. The AV node responds to the rapid atrial depolarization by slowing conduction, hence exacerbating the poor to nonexistent conduction caused by blocks below it. The end result is an even more decreased ventricular rate and hypotension.

8. (b) Atropine. Although PVCs in a hemodynamically significant bradycardia may cause the clinician to pause, they are usually viewed as a symptom of a reduced heart rate. Suppressing them with lidocaine would further exacerbate the failing rate. Treatment should consist of increasing the heart rate, and the PVCs should terminate on their own. β-Blockers, such as propranolol, are inappropriate because they would further reduce the heart rate. Bradycardias are not treated with cardioversion.

9. (b) 1 and 4. Isoproterenol, a hazardous intervention, is only administered with extreme caution and then only if necessary. It causes increased oxygen consumption, which may increase muscle death in an MI. The drug is only administered in low doses by intravenous drip.

10. (a) True. Normally discouraged, lidocaine may be used to treat significant ectopic beats in a bradycardic patient who is being paced. The pacemaker ensures that the rate does not decrease while ectopic beats are suppressed.

11. (d) 1 and 5. Isoproterenol, administered at 2 to 10 mcg/min, increases myocardial irritability and potential for arrhythmias. It is a pure β-adrenergic receptor with no α-adrenergic receptor qualities stimulating forceful contractions while increasing the heart rate. Because the drug is potentially harmful, it is only considered when all other interventions are deemed ineffective.

12. (c) 1 and 2. At 7 mcg/kg/min, dopamine stimulates both dopaminergic and β-adrenergic receptors, resulting in both increased contractility and mesenteric vasodilation. At rates above 10 mcg/kg/min, however, dopamine stops stimulating the dopaminergic receptors, which results in mesenteric vasoconstriction. α-Adrenergic receptors are not stimulated at this dosage.

13. (a) True. It is *always* necessary to verify that the QRS complexes generated by a pacemaker generate a pulse.

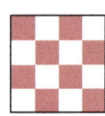

ANSWERS TO BRADYCARDIA CROSSWORD PUZZLE

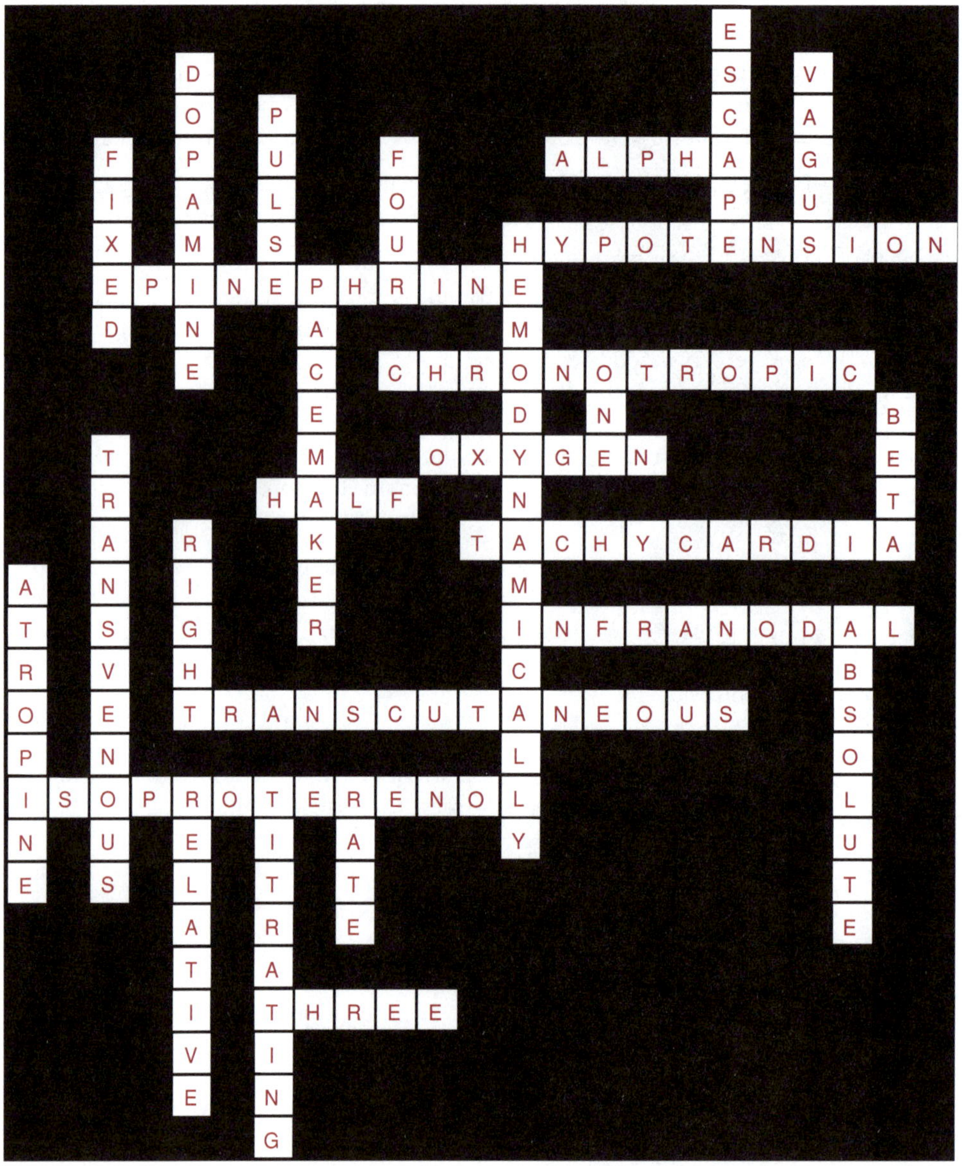

Answers to Unstable Tachycardia Interim Evaluation

1. (a) 4 and 5. Cardioversion is not the treatment of choice for rhythms: (1) when the rate is less than 100 (controlled atrial fibrillation), (2) that have no R wave to synchronize on (standstill), or (3) that represent a compensatory tachycardia (sinus tachycardia). Cardioversion is the treatment of choice in unstable SVT, unstable atrial fibrillation or flutter, and unstable ventricular tachycardia.

2. (b) False. Although helpful, the patient's level of consciousness is not the sole factor used to determine stability. A conscious and coherent patient who has crushing chest pain or pulmonary edema concurrent with ventricular tachycardia, even though alert, is deemed cardiovascularly unstable. Treatment would consist of prompt sedation and immediate cardioversion. Rhythm-specific medications may be administered so long as they do not interfere with the cardioversion sequence.

3. (d) Proceed immediately with an unsynchronized countershock. If during the act of cardioversion a patient develops ventricular fibrillation, pulselessness should be verified and the patient immediately defibrillated (unsynchronized countershock). Most defibrillators automatically turn off the synchronizer after each shock; however, in older defibrillators, the switch must be physically turned off before proceeding with defibrillation. Lidocaine and CPR should not be used initially to treat ventricular fibrillation.

4. (b) False. When discerning stability, concentrate on the symptoms, not the rhythm. The origin of the tachycardia does not make any difference when the patient is deemed unstable because rate-driven tachycardias are all treated the same, with cardioversion. Origin only makes a difference after the patient is considered stable because each rhythm requires its own drug protocol.

5. (a) Administer oxygen by bag-valve-mask and immediately cardiovert with 50 to 100 joules. The patient is apneic, but not pulseless; thus, CPR is not necessary. The patient requires both ventilation and immediate cardioversion. Adenosine or lidocaine may be given quickly, but they are not as high a priority as cardioversion. Adenosine would be appropriate if you thought that the origin of the tachycardia was supraventricular; however, lidocaine is probably more logical because wide complex tachycardias have an 80% chance of being ventricular.

6. (d) Sedation and synchronized countershock. Although the patient appears stable, the presence of crushing chest pain relegates him to the unstable protocol: sedation and synchronized countershock. In this scenario, the chest pain is caused by the tachycardia. Stop the rapid rhythm, and the chest pain should desist. Although part of individual stable tachycardia protocols, vagal maneuvers, lidocaine, and adenosine, unless performed or administered while charging the machine, are not priorities in the unstable protocol.

306 Unit 2 Learning Adjuncts

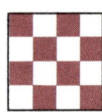

ANSWERS TO UNSTABLE TACHYCARDIA CROSSWORD PUZZLE

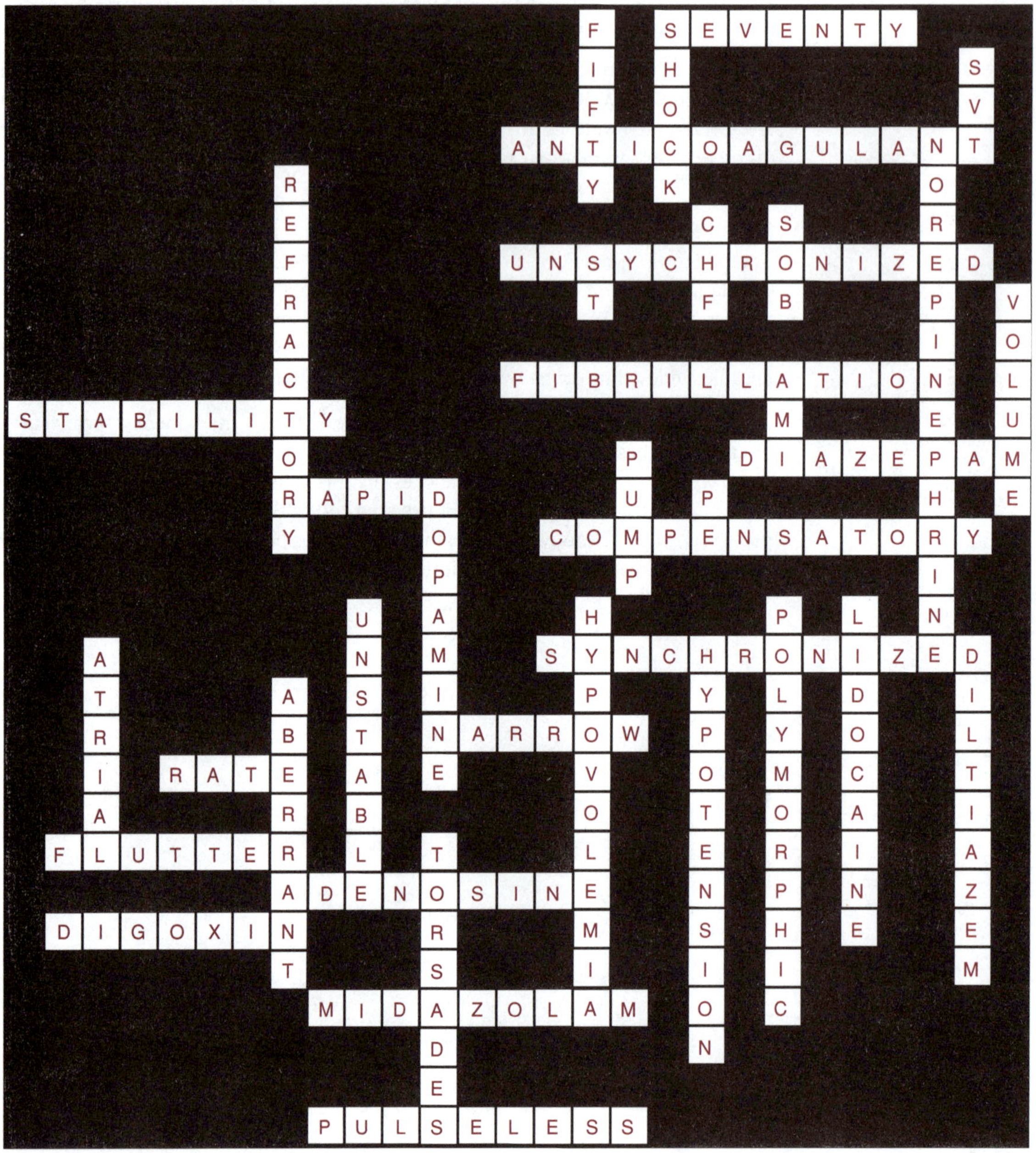

[Crossword puzzle solution with the following answers visible: SEVENTY, FIFTY, SHOCK, SVT, ANTICOAGULANT, STORE, REFRACTORY, UNSYNCHRONIZED, PIE, VOLUME, FIBRILLATION, STABILITY, DIAZEPAM, RAPID, DOPAMINE, COMPENSATORY, UNSTABLE, NARROW, SYNCHRONIZED, ATRIA, RATE, BARREL, FLUTTER, ADENOSINE, DIGOXIN, MIDAZOLAM, PULSELESS, LIDOCAINE, DILTIAZEM, and others]

Answers to Stable Tachycardia Interim Evaluation

1. (c) Administer 6 mg of adenosine. Based on only one lead, any wide complex tachycardia is most likely originating from the ventricles; thus, lidocaine is administered first. After lidocaine, adenosine is employed to rule out a supraventricular origin. Bretylium, owing to its multiple side effects, is only indicated after the rhythm is refractory to procainamide. Cardioversion is employed when the patient becomes unstable, which is not the case in this scenario. Verapamil is contraindicated in any wide complex tachycardia.

2. (d) 1, 2, and 4. Verapamil is one of the drugs of choice for atrial fibrillation or flutter but should not be given in the case of a wide QRS complex. Because atrial fibrillation and flutter do not use a reentry mechanism, adenosine has no significant effect. Adenosine does have a short half-life, so tachycardias can recur easily. Nevertheless, apparently stable patients (acceptable vital signs) with signs of cardiovascular compromise (chest pain or pulmonary edema) are not considered stable and should be immediately treated with the unstable protocol (cardioversion).

3. (c) 75 to 112 mg followed by an infusion of 2 to 4 mg/min. Other selections differ in the correct dosages per weight or drip rates of the infusion.

4. (a) Examining the heart rate. When examining a patient with hypotension of unknown cause, you should consider rate–volume–pump, in that order (with the exception of atrial fibrillation and flutter). Never consider volume or pump until you have ruled out the possibility of a heart rate problem. If the heart rate is less than 60 beats/minute, consider the bradycardia protocol (exception: some right ventricular infarcts). If the rate is faster than 60 beats/minute, the hypotension may be due to either a volume deficit or an ectopic pacemaker cell accelerating the heart to rapid rates. Never treat the patient as having pump failure before considering rate or a volume deficit. Likewise, initiating a fluid challenge without considering the situation as a possible rate problem would be inappropriate for most bradycardias. The last selection is incorrect because it is difficult for an adult to lose an amount of blood in the cranium sufficient to cause hypotension.

5. (c) 2. Lidocaine elevates the ventricular fibrillation threshold. In addition, it is the drug of choice for ventricular or unknown wide complex, not supraventricular, arrhythmias.

6. (b) False. Adenosine works well on SVTs that employ a reentry mechanism at the AV node. Because the depolarization sequences of atrial fibrillation and atrial flutter simply pass through the AV node, they do not respond well to adenosine.

7. (b) False. Eighty percent of all wide complex tachycardias have a ventricular origin. The remaining 20% have a supraventricular origin but are widened by aberrant conduction.

8. (b) Consider vagal maneuvers. The question describes a patient in stable SVT; therefore, cardioversion is initially inappropriate. Adenosine given initially, and verapamil given if adenosine is refractory, would be an acceptable procedure if the SVT does not respond to the vagal stimulation.

9. (c) 2 and 3. Common reactions are nausea and vomiting and postural hypotension. Both respiratory depression and metabolic acidosis were simply distracters—not side effects of bretylium.

10. (b) 3, 4, and 5. Calcium chloride is no longer an integral part of the ACLS protocols. However, it is an essential part of the treatment of hyperkalemia, hypocalcemia, and calcium-channel blocker overdoses. The first two answers in the question are indications for magnesium sulfate, not calcium.

11. (c) 2 and 3. Both a generic SVT and atrial tachycardia (usually synonymous with SVT) are reentry mechanism tachycardias and therefore would respond to adenosine. Because atrial fibrillation and flutter do not employ this mechanism, however, they would not respond to adenosine. Ventricular tachycardia does not originate in the AV node, so it is unaffected by adenosine.

12. (c) 2.5 to 5 mg infused slowly over 1 to 3 minutes. The other selections are incorrect because of the dosage or the manner of administration. Verapamil is famous for its hypotensive side effects, so administer it slowly.

13. (a) True. Unless you are highly skilled in 12-lead ECG interpretation, it is difficult to differentiate SVT with aberrant conduction from ventricular tachycardia. It is definitely impracticable to do so in only one lead. The differences are moot if the patient is unstable

because all unstable cases are treated with synchronized cardioversion. If the patient is stable, both wide complex tachycardic protocols begin with lidocaine, and they only differ by the addition of adenosine if the clinician is uncertain about the cardiac origin.

14. (b) 2 and 3. The heart rate in acute hypovolemia rarely increases to more than 160 beats/minute. The heart rates for CHF and SVT are appropriate.

15. (d) 1 and 2. Hypotension and a prolonged administration time are common problems when administering procainamide. Procainamide increases Q-T intervals and should be discontinued if the QRS complex widens by more than 50% of the pretreatment width. Heart rate and hypertension were distracters and have no medical validity.

16. (b) False. Verapamil is one of the drugs of choice for atrial fibrillation. The narrow ECG signature of atrial fibrillation becomes wide by the Wolff-Parkinson-White syndrome. In response to the verapamil, this syndrome can cause the ventricular rate to accelerate, precipitating ventricular fibrillation. Verapamil should not be given to any kind of wide complex tachycardia because it may be masking Wolff-Parkinson-White syndrome.

17. (a) True. When employed for stable, refractory ventricular tachycardia, bretylium has an initial sympathomimetic effect—the heart rate and the blood pressure begin to rise. After 20 minutes, the catecholamine stores are exhausted, and the blood pressure and pulse drop precipitously.

18. (a) True. Adenosine depresses the AV node, briefly stopping reentry tachycardias.

19. (b) False. Contrary to common belief, patients with ventricular tachycardia do not necessarily show any greater or lesser signs of cardiac compromise than patients with SVT. A patient with ventricular tachycardia might be completely symptomless, as opposed to an elderly patient exhibiting unconsciousness from SVT. Therefore, do not differentiate between forms of tachycardias based solely on the presenting signs and symptoms.

20. (a) Ice-cold water in the outer ear. Carotid massage, intraocular pressure, and rectal stimulation stimulate the vagus nerve. Although ice-cold water on the face induces vagal domination, ice-cold water in the outer ear does not.

21. (b) Terminates those tachyarrhythmias in which reentry is through the AV node. Adenosine, known for its incredibly short half-life, does not stimulate any adrenergic receptors (α-adrenergic, β-adrenergic, or dopaminergic).

22. (a) True. The prior use of digitalis does not appear to contraindicate the use of calcium-channel blockers.

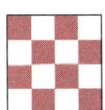

ANSWERS TO STABLE TACHYCARDIA CROSSWORD PUZZLE

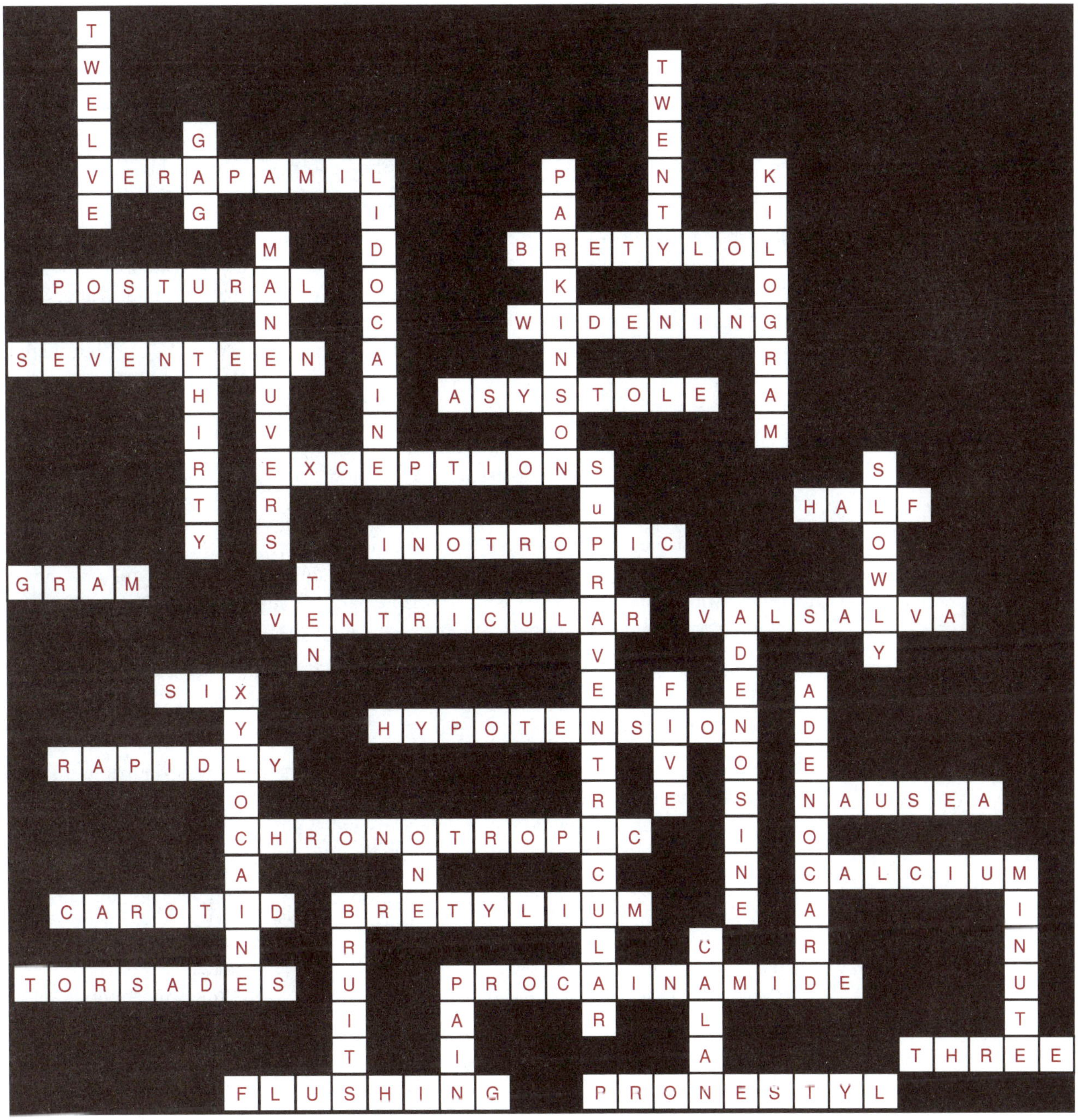

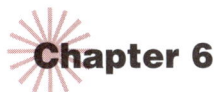

Chapter 6

Answers to Stroke Interim Evaluation

1. (b) False. Any suspected stroke patient presenting with hypotension should be scrutinized for other causes of hypotension besides stroke. An adult cannot lose enough blood in the cranial vault to cause hypotension.

2. (b) 2, 3, and 5. Intravenous lifelines for stroke patients should be isotonic (normal saline [0.9] and lactated Ringer's solution). Both D-5-W and 0.45 saline (half normal saline) are hypotonic, which may contribute to edema and increase ICP.

3. (b) Subarachnoid hemorrhage. Sudden onset of excruciating headache, nausea, vomiting, and photophobia are seen commonly in both migraine headaches and subarachnoid hemorrhage. Nuchal rigidity, a common sign of subarachnoid hemorrhage, may help differentiate them, but it may not show up for several hours or may be missed in a comatose victim. These two are not always easy to differentiate.

4. (b) False. Intubation can stimulate the gag reflex, which can increase ICP. Therefore, although a clear airway is required, intubation should not be performed routinely but rather only when **required** to maintain a clear airway.

5. (d) Recent lumbar puncture. Thrombolytics cannot be administered if the patient has undergone recent arterial blood gases at an *uncompressible* anatomic site, lumbar punctures, or central line introduction. Thrombolytics can be administered up to 180 minutes after onset of symptoms; a reliable time of onset of symptoms must be established; and patients younger than 18 years are considered unacceptable candidates for thrombolytic therapy, but there is no maximal age limit.

6. (d) TIAs have similar signs and symptoms but resolve quickly. Thrombolytics are not used for known TIAs because they resolve on their own; acute ischemic stroke can occur in person who has not had TIAs; and TIAs present with symptoms similar to, not harsher than, stroke symptoms, but because the occlusion resolves spontaneously, the patient recovers swiftly.

7. (d) Focal neurologic deficits are more pronounced in ischemic strokes than in subarachnoid hemorrhage. Patients with hemorrhagic strokes tend to deteriorate quicker and look more ill than those with acute ischemic strokes; and nausea and vomiting, although present in ischemic strokes, tends to be more pronounced in hemorrhagic strokes.

8. (d) Hypotension. Headache, focal weakness, and aphasia all are common in either category of stroke, but hypotension is not common. Always search for an alternate cause when encountering hypotension in the stroke setting.

9. (b) Vertigo. The other three symptoms can be described in patients with both anterior and posterior territory strokes. Because the vertebrobasilar arterial system is responsible for perfusing the brain stem, however, abnormal signs and symptoms involving balance and coordination most likely arise from damage there.

10. (b) False. Although stroke is categorized by origin (occlusive or hemorrhagic), the subsets of hemorrhagic stroke are SAH and ICH.

11. (c) Age. Although male gender, older age, and the presence of heart disease all are contributing factors to an increased risk of stroke, older age is the single most important factor contributing to stroke worldwide.

12. (a) Hypertension. Hypertension is the most common cause of stroke worldwide. Although high red blood cell count is a risk factor, it is not a cause. Stress and migraines are not valid causes of ICH.

13. (d) Discharge. I introduced Discharge as the final phase of stroke treatment. Hazinski's steps were Detection, Dispatch, Delivery, Door, Data, Decision, and Drug Therapy. I thought that Discharge was missing from the continuum.

14. (b) Pupil response. The Cincinnati Prehospital Stroke Scale was designed to be quick and easy. The scale evaluates only obvious traits of a stroke victim: facial droop, arm drift, and speech patterns. Pupil response is more difficult to document properly in the prehospital realm.

15. (c) 3 hours. Thrombolytics cannot be administered after 3 hours (180 minutes).

16. (d) Facial droop. The Glasgow Coma Scale is used to evaluate initial and subsequent levels of consciousness. Facial droop is part of the Cincinnati Prehospital Stroke Scale, which is a one-time test used to determine if the patient is a possible stroke victim. Eye opening and verbal and motor response are the only areas evaluated in this scale.

17. (a) A positive doll's eye reflex. A negative (absent) doll's eye reflex is suggestive of brain-stem involvement, which occurs when the eyes do not rotate in their sockets when the head is rotated.

18. (b) A magnetic resonance imaging scan is a quick and effective means for differentiating hemorrhagic stroke from acute ischemic stroke. The other selections were correct. Lumbar punctures are a contraindication to the use of thrombolytics; diazepam is commonly employed to control reoccurring seizures; and people taking aspirin, although an antiplatelet-aggregating drug, can still be given thrombolytics.

19. (a) True. Treatment of hypertension in the acute stroke setting should be based on the type of stroke presenting (hemorrhagic or ischemic) and whether the patient is a candidate for thrombolytics. Stroke patients commonly develop elevated blood pressures as a sequelae of stroke. If the hypertension exceeds acceptable bounds (systolic pressure of more than 185 mmHg or diastolic pressure of more than 110 mmHg) *and the patient is a thrombolytic candidate*, the AHA has established guidelines for treatment. Hypertension increases the risk of bleeding and must be treated aggressively in thrombolytic therapy candidates.

20. (b) False. Short-term anticonvulsants may be used initially to control recurring seizures, but some clinicians prefer to use long-term anticonvulsants initially. The short-term anticonvulsant may be repeated, but anticonvulsants such as phenytoin should be employed afterward on a long-term basis.

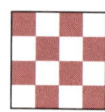

ANSWERS TO STROKE CROSSWORD PUZZLE

Comprehensive Posttest

Posttest Answers

1. (d) Removes the necessity for proper head and jaw positioning in the unconscious patient. This is the only incorrect statement. An OPA is only used for unconscious patients because it can cause gagging and vomiting in patients with higher levels of consciousness. Along with a

slight head tilt, it is placed in the oropharynx to keep the tongue from blocking the airway. It may be used in conjunction with an ET tube to protect the ET tube should the patient awake and bite down on the tube.

2. (b) False. Ventricular fibrillation represents uncoordinated contraction of myocardial muscle; hence, it delivers no pulse or cardiac output.

3. PEA. Any cardiac arrest rhythm not identified as ventricular fibrillation, asystole, or ventricular tachycardia should be treated as PEA. The ECG in this strip is a sinus rhythm—without a pulse—PEA. The suspected cause appears to be a drug overdose of verapamil. Therefore, in addition to the routine medication protocol for PEA, consider administering the antidote—calcium chloride.

4. (b) False. The statement has no medical validity. True EMD indicates a problem with electrical activity without contraction. Although it resembles true EMD, pseudo-EMD reflects a problem with cardiac output. The heart, for some reason (medical or traumatic), is unable to create sufficient cardiac output to generate a pulse.

5. (c) 2, 3, and 4. Routine cardiac arrests are not treated with sodium bicarbonate unless the cause of the acidosis is a preexisting bicarbonate-responsive situation, such as diabetic ketoacidosis (DKA), aspirin overdose, hyperkalemia, or TCA overdose. Increased anaerobic metabolism produces increased carbon dioxide (a respiratory problem), which is the cause of acidosis in a routine arrest.

6. Acute coronary syndrome. The scenario describes symptoms typical of an MI. Because lead II is the usual monitoring lead, the ST elevation in this lead marks the inferior aspect of the heart as the likely candidate for damage. The key strategy is to make the patient comfortable with analgesics while considering the following therapies if not contraindicated: oxygen, aspirin, β-blockers, and nitroglycerin given intravenously, all while quickly gathering data to make a decision about whether the patient could best be treated with thrombolytics or angioplasty. Time is the crucial factor because myocardial tissue dies within 1 to 4 hours.

7. (a) True. Fifty percent of persons who develop an acute MI die before reaching a hospital. The majority who die have VF as the primary dysrhythmia.

8. (a) 1 mg in 250 to 500 mL of NS or D-5-W at 2 to 10 mcg/min. The other answers are incorrect owing to either the rate of administration, dilution, or both.

9. Stable ventricular tachycardia. The 45-year-old woman described in this scenario appears stable without any overt signs or symptoms of cardiovascular compromise. If present, these would include, but are not limited to, a depressed level of consciousness, hypotension, chest pain, or difficulty breathing. The rhythm displayed looks like ventricular tachycardia but has a 20% chance of being SVT with aberrant conduction. The cardiology consult cinches the diagnosis as ventricular. Ventricular antiarrhythmics would be appropriate—synchronized cardioversion would not be necessary unless the patient began to evidence signs of instability.

10. (c) Synchronized cardioversion at 50 to 100 joules. The patient has become hypotensive, but her pulse rate and rhythm remain unchanged. The cardiac rate is making her unstable, so synchronized cardioversion should be employed. An additional dose of adenosine while charging the machine is both reasonable and acceptable. If the rhythm were a wide complex tachycardia of unknown origin, lidocaine could be given while preparing for cardioversion. Verapamil is contraindicated in hypotension. A precordial thump is not performed in SVT.

11. (a) True. Adenosine only works on supraventricular ectopic pacemakers, not ventricular ones. This behavior makes this drug an ideal mechanism for differentiating between true ventricular tachycardia and SVT with aberrant conduction (wide complex tachycardia of uncertain type).

12. Unstable tachycardia. The patient's compromised status, as noted by unconsciousness, diaphoresis, and hypotension, denotes that the *unstable* tachycardia algorithm should be chosen. Although antiarrhythmics are allowed during the unstable tachycardia sequence, they should not interfere with immediate synchronized cardioversion. It is not necessary to establish pacemaker origin, since all are treated alike when they become unstable.

13. (a) Administer lidocaine, 1.0 to 1.5 mg/kg. The first drug of choice in stable ventricular tachycardia is lidocaine. Both procainamide and cardioversion are not employed initially for stable ventricular tachycardic situations. Adenosine is only used if the tachycardia is a suspected SVT. Because a 12-lead ECG confirmed ventricular tachycardia, it was not necessary to employ the wide complex tachycardia of uncertain type protocol.

14. (d) An endotracheal tube. When a patient is unable to control his own airway, the clinician must act. If the patient is unlikely to wake up in the near future (i.e., deeply unconscious or cardiac arrest patient), you should select the best airway—an endotracheal tube. An OPA and an NPA are helpful but are not the best. The nasogastric tube has nothing to do with airways.

15. Pulseless ventricular tachycardia. The scenario describes an obvious wide complex tachycardic pulseless patient—treat it just like ventricular fibrillation.

16. (a) 1 and 4. Ventricular fibrillation can easily be mimicked by artifact on a monitor and should be treated with early defibrillation. Because ventricular fibrillation does not have a coordinated contraction, it cannot have any possibility of a cardiac output.

17. (a) Finding an appropriate cause and treating it. The other choices have no medical validity.

18. Stable wide complex tachycardia of uncertain type. Because the pulse is tachycardic with a wide QRS complex, the rhythm is identified as either ventricular tachycardia or SVT with aberrant conduction. The patient is not suffering from acute cardiopulmonary distress, so a stable protocol is selected. A 12-lead ECG was not available to differentiate between the the two rhythms; thus, the clinician should select the stable wide complex tachycardia of unknown origin protocol because it encompasses treatment modalities for both.

19. (b) Parasympathetic. This is the main reason that routine defibrillation is not part of the asystole protocol. Vagal stimulation makes the myocardium even more refractory to normal therapy. Defibrillation does not cause adrenergic stimulation. Selections (c) and (d) have no medical validity since they are words I invented.

20. (b) False. A pulse oximeter is not necessarily an accurate representation of a patient's PaO_2, especially during peripheral vasoconstriction. Research evidence shows that a slight increase in the patient's PaO_2 is associated with limiting the ultimate size of an infarct; thus, oxygen should not be withheld, even with a normal pulse oximeter reading.

21. The patient is in respiratory arrest, and there is no specific respiratory arrest algorithm for this situation other than the universal algorithm. Perform a primary survey. Start by making sure that the airway is open. A head-tilt and chin-lift maneuver is acceptable if there is no history of trauma. After the airway has been secured, check for any rudimentary breathing attempts. Because the patient is apneic, immediately perform positive-pressure ventilation using a BVM, mouth-to-mask, or barrier device. When the patient is being adequately ventilated, continue with the survey. From the scenario, the respiratory arrest appears to be the only problem. A ventilator should be considered until the patient regains control of her own breathing.

22. (a) True. A TCP is only a temporary therapy until a more definitive transvenous pacemaker can be implanted.

23. (d) Synchronized cardioversion at 50 to 100 joules. Because the patient is obviously unstable, synchronized cardioversion should be employed. The rhythm was a wide complex tachycardia, however, so lidocaine, and then adenosine, can be administered if given while preparing for cardioversion. Verapamil is contraindicated in hypotension.

24. Unstable tachycardia. The patient's compromised status, as noted by crushing chest pain, denotes that the unstable tachycardia algorithm should be chosen. Even though the patient's vital signs make him appear stable, the chest pain changes that status. In this situation, the chest pain is not a symptom of an MI; rather, it is the result of ischemia caused by the excessive tachycardia. The clinician should employ synchronized cardioversion to stop the ectopic pacemaker. This should slow the rate, and the chest pain should resolve by itself. Although antiarrhythmics are allowed during the unstable tachycardia sequence, they should not interfere with immediate synchronized cardioversion. It would be appropriate to rule out an MI after the tachycardia has been terminated.

25. (a) PVCs. Common side effects of adenosine are chest pain, a brief period of asystole, and facial flushing. Ventricular irritability is not a common side effect.

26. (c) Lidocaine, 1.0 to 1.5 mg/kg. The patient is presenting with significant ventricular irritability. After an initial loading dose (1.0 to 1.5 mg/kg), a lidocaine infusion should be established, *but not before* the loading dose. Another dose given by intravenous push—half that of the initial dose—should be administered within 10 minutes to allow enough time for the therapeutic blood level to be maintained. Neither atropine nor β-blockers (propranolol) are indicated because the pulse is 90 to 95 beats/minute.

27. Stable SVT. The rate of this narrow complex tachycardia is 180 beats/minute, much higher than a compensatory tachycardia (e.g., hypovolemia, CHF). A narrow QRS complex and an excessively rapid pulse indicate that this patient should be treated with the SVT protocol. Because she is alert and coherent, her vital signs appear stable, and she denies chest pain or breathing difficulty, the patient should be treated with the stable protocol.

28. (c) 1 and 3. BVM devices are difficult for one person to apply effectively and so should only be used by trained clinicians. If a reservoir is used and 12 to 15 L/min of oxygen are added, BVM devices deliver close to 100% oxygen. Because the lungs contain a greater tidal volume than a relatively small BVM, mouth-to-mask resuscitation provides a greater amount of ventilation.

29. (c) Ventricular fibrillation. Ventricular fibrillation is the most common arrhythmia in the first 60 seconds of an arrest. Although interesting, none of the other selections are the most common.

30. PEA. Any cardiac arrest rhythm not identified as ventricular fibrillation, asystole, or ventricular tachycardia should be treated as PEA. The rhythm presenting is sinus tachycardia. The scenario does not provide any clues to the cause of this particular PEA. Because the most common cause of PEA is hypovolemia, however, a fluid challenge would be appropriate while investigating other treatable causes.

31. (c) Renal failure. Although the others are signs, symptoms, or pertinent history of pulmonary embolism, renal failure is not.

32. Stable tachycardia (atrial fibrillation). The rhythm's rate of 150 beats/minute and its gross R-R wave irregularity, combined with a narrow QRS complex, indicate a diagnosis of atrial fibrillation with a rapid ventricular response. Even though the rhythm's rate of 150 beats/minute is consistent with a *compensatory* rate, both atrial fibrillation and flutter are exceptions to the rate–volume–pump rule. They have to be recognized as exceptions before treatment can commence. If the patient is deemed *stable*, these two arrhythmias are treated with drugs that block the AV node. If the patient has been diagnosed as *unstable*, synchronized cardioversion is appropriate. The patient's status appears stable because chest pain, hypotension, and pulmonary edema are not present. Therefore, the stable tachycardia algorithm should be chosen. The clinician is encouraged to consider any of the following medications for their value in treating this condition: diltiazem, β-blockers, verapamil, and digoxin. Procainamide and quinidine should be considered after the rhythm has been converted. The clinician is cautioned to maintain a high index of suspicion that atrial fibrillation or flutter may be a symptom of an underlying MI.

33. (c) 1, 2, 3 and 4. Epinephrine does cause the effects in the first four selections. However, its purpose during a cardiac arrest is to increase blood supply to the brain and the left ventricle. It accomplishes these effects through the primary stimulation of α-adrenergic receptors (vasoconstriction) rather than β-adrenergic (positive inotropic and chronotropic) receptors. Epinephrine does not increase parasympathetic tone.

34. Stable ventricular tachycardia. The patient described in this scenario appears stable without any overt signs or symptoms of cardiovascular compromise. If present, these would include but are not limited to a depressed level of consciousness, hypotension, chest pain, or difficulty breathing. The rhythm displayed looks like ventricular tachycardia but has a 20% chance of being SVT with aberrant conduction. The 12-lead ECG verifies the ventricular pacemaker. Ventricular antiarrhythmics would be appropriate.

35. (c) Half NS. In the past, D-5-W was the exclusive intravenous lifeline for cardiac patients because salt solutions were thought to potentiate pulmonary edema. NS and lactated Ringer's solution are now routinely given for all lifelines because NS, aside from other benefits, was not found to cause fluid shifts. Half NS, a hypotonic solution, causes fluid to leave the vascular container where it enters cells causing edema; thus, it is not routinely indicated in suspected cardiac arrest. Since this is not a cardiac arrest, D-5-W could be used.

36. (b) Transvenous pacemaker. Although selections (a), (c), and (d) are helpful intermediaries, the definitive therapy is a transvenous pacemaker.

37. Ventricular fibrillation. This patient is in obvious ventricular fibrillation. The key here is to obtain a defibrillator as quickly as possible. Remember that if you do not deliver an initial shock quickly, the amount of high-energy phosphates dwindles rapidly. If you are alone and the defibrillator is close at hand (available within 2 minutes), you should leave the patient and bring it back and deliver the shock, rather than waiting for it to be brought to you. Timely defibrillation is the key strategy.

38. (a) 2 and 4. At dosages above 10 mcg/kg/min, β-adrenergic (heart and lung) and α-adrenergic (vasoconstriction) receptors are stimulated. Dopaminergic (renal and mesentery) receptors are not stimulated at this dosage level, leading to renal arteriole vasoconstriction and mesenteric vasoconstriction. Respiratory depression has no medical validity in dopamine administration.

39. (b) False. Stability of a tachycardia should be primarily based on the patient's symptoms—not cardiac origin. If a patient is unstable, the origin of the pacemaker cell is inconsequential because the treatment is the same: synchronized cardioversion.

40. Unstable tachycardia. The patient's compromised status, as noted by crushing chest pain, denotes that the unstable tachycardia algorithm should be chosen. Even though the patient's vital signs make him appear stable, the chest pain alters that status. In this situation, the chest pain is not a symptom of an MI but a result of ischemia caused by the excessive tachycardia. Slow the rate, and the chest pain should resolve by itself. Although antiarrhythmics are allowed during the unstable tachycardia sequence, they should not interfere with immediate synchronized cardioversion. It would be appropriate to rule out an MI after the tachycardia has been terminated.

41. (b) 1, 3, and 4. Like other ventricular antiarrhythmics in normal doses (1.0 to 1.5 mg/kg), lidocaine elevates the ventricular fibrillation threshold but has no significant effect on contractility. Doses over the maximum dose of 3 mg/kg cause toxic effects.

42. (c) 12 L/min of oxygen flow to a BVM with a reservoir. All cardiac arrests, regardless of preexisting lung pathology, should receive as close to 100% oxygen as possible. Even with 12 to 15 liters of supplemental oxygen, without a reservoir, a BVM cannot deliver more than 50% oxygen.

43. Ventricular fibrillation. This patient is in obvious ventricular fibrillation. The key here is to obtain a defibrillator as quickly as possible. Remember that if you do not deliver an initial shock quickly, the amount of high energy phosphates dwindles rapidly. If you are alone and

the defibrillator is close at hand (available within 1 to 2 minutes), you should leave the patient and bring it back and deliver the shock, rather than waiting for it to be brought to you. Timely defibrillation is the main strategy. A precordial thump might be considered since the arrest was in the CCU and therefore of short duration.

44. (d) Immediate defibrillation at 200 joules. The scenario describes a witnessed arrest that includes ventricular fibrillation, with a monitor-defibrillator immediately available. In this situation, CPR is inappropriate because immediate defibrillation takes precedence over basic life support in a witnessed situation. Ventricular fibrillation has no R wave to synchronize on, so (b) is incorrect. Finally, lidocaine, a class IIa treatment, should not take precedence over a class I treatment—immediate defibrillation.

45. Unstable atrial fibrillation. The rhythm's rate of 130 beats/minute and its gross R-R wave irregularity, combined with a narrow QRS complex, indicate a diagnosis of atrial fibrillation with a rapid ventricular response. Even though the rhythm's rate of 130 beats/minute is consistent with a *compensatory* rate, both atrial fibrillation and flutter are exceptions to the rate–volume–pump rule. These two arrhythmias have to be recognized as exceptions before treatment can commence. If the patient is deemed *stable*, these two arrhythmias are treated with a specific medication protocol. If the patient has been diagnosed as *unstable*, synchronized cardioversion is appropriate. The patient's compromised status, as noted by depressed level of consciousness and hypotension denotes, that the unstable tachycardia algorithm should be chosen. Although antiarrhythmics are allowed during the unstable tachycardia sequence, they should not interfere with immediate synchronized cardioversion.

46. (b) Ventricular tachycardia. Unlike the other rhythm selections that could present without a pulse, *pulseless* ventricular tachycardia is neither defined nor treated as a PEA rhythm.

47. Torsades de pointes: magnesium sulfate. The rhythm is torsades de pointes—twisting around a point. Torsades is a variation of ventricular tachycardia and may appear in several ways. In this rhythm strip, the QRS complexes appear positive for a while and then flip over to become negative—twisting around a point. This patient appears stable with no cardiovascular compromise, so a stable protocol (medication) is indicated. The problem with torsades is that if you follow the standard stable ventricular tachycardia protocol, procainamide may be employed. Procainamide increases Q-T intervals. *Torsades does not tolerate widening Q-T intervals well.* Therefore, do not use the standard ventricular antiarrhythmics such as procainamide; employ magnesium sulfate.

48. (b) False. When verifying a rhythm in a different lead with quick-look paddles, you cannot just reverse your hand placement. You must place the paddles in a configuration angle other than 180 degrees to your original paddle placement. The best paddle configuration is 90 degrees to an imaginary line from the right shoulder to just below the left armpit.

49. (c) Torsades de pointes. Procainamide is indicated in (a), (b), and (d). Torsades has difficulty with medications that cause widening Q-T intervals—a main side effect of procainamide.

50. The patient is in respiratory arrest, and there is no specific respiratory arrest algorithm for this situation other than the universal algorithm. Perform a primary survey. Start by making certain that the airway is open. A head-tilt and chin-lift maneuver is acceptable when there is no history of trauma. After the airway has been secured, check for any rudimentary breathing attempts. Because this patient is apneic, immediately perform positive-pressure ventilation by a BVM, mouth-to-mask, or barrier device or a demand valve. While the patient is being adequately ventilated, continue with the primary survey. From the scenario, the respiratory arrest appears to be the only problem. The patient should be put on a ventilator until she regains control of her own breathing.

51. (a) True. Although the bradycardia protocol appears linear, only progressing to the next treatment when the one before appears fruitless, it is not. If necessary, clinicians are encouraged to be as aggressive as required to increase the heart rate in order to raise the blood pressure. This means that atropine may be administered while simultaneously hooking up a TCP and a dopamine drip.

52. (a) 2 and 3. Although endotracheal intubation reduces the risk of aspiration, it should not be attempted by inexperienced clinicians. Although an open airway is a necessity, intubation is not always necessary for adequate lung ventilation. When performed in ventricular fibrillation, intubation should be initiated after the initial stack of defibrillations.

53. Acute coronary syndrome. The scenario is the picture of an acute MI. The patient's rhythm in lead II is evidencing an elevated ST segment (indicative of myocardial injury). Lead II views the inferior aspect of the heart, so the infarct is probably inferior. The patient should be treated for an MI and judged for thrombolytic criteria or angioplasty possibilities as soon as possible.

54. (b) Peripheral arterial vasoconstriction. At dosages above 20 mcg/kg/min, dopamine primarily stimulates α-adrenergic receptors (peripheral arterial vasoconstriction). Only at lower dosages does it affect dopaminergic receptors (mesenteric vasodilation and renal arterial vasodilation). Dopamine does not cause respiratory depression.

55. Unstable tachycardia. The patient's compromised status, as noted by pulmonary edema, denotes that the unstable tachycardia algorithm should be chosen. Even though the patient's vital signs make her appear stable, the difficulty breathing alters that status. In this situation, the pulmonary edema is not a symptom of chronic CHF that is now becoming acute; rather, it is the result of preload backing up into the lungs caused by the excessive tachycardia. If the clinician slows the rate with synchronized cardioversion, the pulmonary edema should resolve by itself. Although antiarrhythmics are allowed during the unstable tachycardia sequence, they should not interfere with immediate synchronized cardioversion.

56. (a) True. When treating what appears to be stable SVT, at any point at which the QRS complex becomes wide, it is inappropriate to continue with verapamil. Verapamil is known to exacerbate Wolff-Parkinson-White syndrome and ventricular rhythms in general. The clinician should change to the suspected ventricular tachycardia protocol and administer lidocaine. If the wide complex rhythm can be verified by a 12-lead ECG or a cardiologist as supraventricular—*without a doubt*—verapamil may be employed.

57. Ventricular fibrillation. This patient is in obvious ventricular fibrillation. The key here is to defibrillate as quickly as possible. Remember that if you do not deliver an initial shock quickly, the amount of high-energy phosphates dwindles rapidly. Defibrillation is the key strategy. You must deliver defibrillation within 10 minutes to have any chance of success. The quicker the defibrillation is delivered, the higher the rate of success.

58. (d) 4 mg/mL loading dose: 2 to 4 mg/min.

59. Unstable tachycardia. The pulse rate, 186 beats/minute, is faster than that of a routine *compensatory* tachycardia (usually less than 170 beats/minute). Because it is combined with a narrow QRS complex, the rhythm is identified as SVT. The excessively high rate is consistent with a rate problem causing chest pain, so the patient should be treated with the tachycardia protocol rather than the acute MI protocol. If the clinician only focuses on the chest pain symptoms, the underlying cause—the excessively fast rate—is not treated. In this situation, the chest pain is not a symptom of an MI; rather, it is the result of ischemia caused by the excessive tachycardia. Slow the rate by cardioverting the patient, and the chest pain should resolve by itself. Although antiarrhythmics are allowed during the unstable sequence, they should not interfere with immediate synchronized cardioversion. It would be appropriate to rule out an MI after terminating the tachycardia.

60. (c) Insertion of the tube into the right main-stem bronchus. Because the right main-stem bronchus is more parallel to the trachea than the left, pushing the ET tube past the level of the carina usually results in intubating the right main-stem bronchus. Both (a) and (d) do not have any validity if lung sounds are auscultated. Underinflation of the cuff would allow lung sounds but not necessarily only on the right.

61. (b) Lighter paddle pressure. Light paddle pressure *increases* transthoracic resistance. The other possible selections (successive countershocks, successively higher joule settings, and lower body weight) *decrease* the transthoracic resistance. Increasing the resistance makes the passage of defibrillating current through the chest more difficult; whereas decreasing the resistance makes the passage easier.

62. Significant bradycardia. The rhythm on the monitor is a sinus bradycardia with a second-degree, type II heart block. The scenario paints a picture of an unstable bradycardia. The patient's heart rate of 30 beats/minute, combined with hypotension, nausea, diaphoresis, and fainting, indicates that the heart rate is probably causing the instability. With the exception of a right ventricular infarction, which could benefit from a cautious fluid challenge, accelerating the rate should increase the blood pressure, discontinuing the compromising symptoms. The definitive treatment should include a permanent *transvenous* pacemaker because second-degree, type II blocks tend to progress to complete heart blocks.

63. (c) 1 and 4. Sodium bicarbonate is used in the treatment of acute hyperkalemia as well as other preexisting bicarbonate-responsive situations, such as aspirin overdose, DKA, and TCA overdoses. Sodium bicarbonate is not given either routinely in a cardiac arrest or prophylactically, even if blood gases are unavailable. In a routine cardiac arrest, the cause of the acidosis is carbon dioxide retention, which does not respond to bicarbonate administration.

64. Shock. The rate of this narrow complex tachycardia is 130 beats/minute—lower than any rate-driven tachycardia. This rate puts it in the realm of hypovolemia or CHF. The history noted that the patient was probably hypovolemic from the prolonged nausea and vomiting. There is a certain tendency in ACLS to treat all tachycardias with the tachycardia protocol. This would be disastrous in this case because the patient needs fluids, not medications. A word of caution: this patient has been compensating for his hypovolemic condition for a lengthy period. This situation, combined with his advanced age, should clue the clinician to be less aggressive in initially administering fluids. The above notwithstanding, the rate is the key: compensatory tachycardias usually do not go at SVT speeds (more than 170). In summary, with the exception of atrial fibrillation or flutter, if the QRS complex is narrow and the rate is less than 170 but above 60, investigate for other causes of the symptoms, such as hypovolemia or pump failure.

65. (a) 1 and 4. Atropine sulfate, a vagal blocker, indirectly causes rate increases in both ventricular and supraventricular bradycardias. It has no value in ventricular tachycardia. Atropine is only required in hemodynamically significant bradycardias because not all bradycardias are associated with cardiovascular compromise. The initial loading dose should be 0.5 mg to 1.0 mg.

66. The monitor recorded the patient going from atrial fibrillation into a wide complex tachycardia. Because the patient is both pulseless and apneic, the resulting rhythm is assumed to be ventricular tachycardia and treated with the ventricular fibrillation and pulseless ventricular tachycardia protocol.

67. (a) 1, 3, and 4. All may cause hypotension, with the exception of magnesium sulfate. Magnesium sulfate can usually be used with impunity when administered correctly; however, if injected too rapidly, it may lead to a pressure problem.

68. (a) True. Although most people think of atropine as only increasing heart rates, it is actually classified as a vagal blocker. If the vagus nerve is the cause of a significant bradycardia or asystole, atropine is administered to rule out any possibility of vagal involvement. If the vagus nerve was the cause, atropine works. If atropine does not have an effect, vagal domination is ruled out.

69. Stable wide complex tachycardia of uncertain type. Because the pulse is tachycardic with a wide QRS complex, the rhythm is identified as either ventricular tachycardia or SVT with

aberrant conduction. A 12-lead ECG was not present to differentiate between the two rhythms; thus, the wide complex tachycardia of uncertain type protocol should be selected. The patient is not suffering from acute cardiopulmonary distress, so treatment can begin with the *stable* protocol. If the presenting wide complex rhythm cannot be documented as ventricular tachycardia with a 12-lead ECG interpreted by a knowledgeable clinician, the stable *uncertain type* protocol should be selected. This protocol contains medications that will be helpful in treating either a ventricular or a supraventricular ectopic pacemaker.

70. (a) Yes. Although the protocols make it appear that an unstable patient should only receive immediate cardioversion, this is not specifically the case. The priority is in delivering an immediate synchronized shock; however, it is acceptable to administer a quick dose of whatever antiarrhythmic is appropriate between the shocks or while the machine is being charged.

71. (c) The presence of bruits. All of the selections are important to check before initiating vagal stimulation; however, the most critical is the presence or absence of bruits. Bruits, the sound of fluid turbulence, indicate build up of plaque within the carotid artery. Massaging these areas may precipitate emboli, resulting in a cerebrovascular accident.

72. The patient is in respiratory arrest. There is no specific algorithm for this situation other than the universal algorithm. Perform a primary survey. Start by making certain that the airway is open. A head-tilt and chin-lift maneuver is acceptable if there is no history of trauma. After the airway has been secured, check for any rudimentary breathing attempts. Because this patient is apneic, immediately perform positive-pressure ventilation using a BVM, mouth-to-mask, or barrier device or a demand valve. While the patient is being adequately ventilated, continue with the primary survey. From the scenario, respiratory arrest appears to be the only problem. The patient should be put on a ventilator until she regains control of her own breathing.

73. (b) 2 and 4. Procainamide should be administered at 20 to 30 mg/min until one of the following occurs: the arrhythmia is suppressed, hypotension develops, the QRS complex widens more than 50% of its pretreatment width, or a total of 17 mg/kg is administered.

74. Shock. The rate of this narrow complex tachycardia is 120 beats/minute—lower than any rate-driven tachycardia. This rate puts it in the realm of hypovolemia or CHF. The history noted that the patient was admitted for unknown abdominal pain; something may have ruptured to cause the bleeding. The signs and symptoms may support this supposition. There is a certain tendency in ACLS to treat all tachycardias with the tachycardia protocol. This would be disastrous in this case because the patient may need fluid, not medications. The rate is the key: compensatory tachycardias usually do not go at SVT speeds (more than 170). With the exception of atrial fibrillation or flutter, if the QRS complex is narrow and the rate is less than 170 but above 60, investigate for other causes of the symptoms, such as hypovolemia or pump failure.

75. (b) False. Placement of an NPA is contraindicated in deviated septa, but OPAs are not.

76. Stable SVT. The rate of this narrow complex tachycardia is 210—higher than any routine compensatory tachycardia (e.g., hypovolemia, CHF). This rhythm, combined with a narrow QRS complex and an excessively rapid pulse, indicate that this patient should be treated with the SVT protocol. The patient is alert and coherent, the vital signs appear stable, and the patient denies chest pain or breathing difficulty. Because there are no signs of cardiovascular compromise, the stable protocol should be chosen.

77. (c) 2 and 4. When a patient is unable to control his airway, the clinician must act. It the patient is unlikely to wake up in the near future (i.e., is deeply unconscious or is in cardiac arrest), you should select the best airway—an ET tube. Patients who do not have this problem (answers 1 and 3) only should be oxygenated and observed.

78. (b) False. The electronics of every AED are designed to detect the slightest motion or electrical activity. If any motor or electrical activity is detected, the machine will halt in the

middle of the *analyze* cycle. The machine can easily differentiate between ECG patterns caused by artifact, patient movement, and ventricular fibrillation. Therefore, do not touch the patient when the AED is in the "analyze" cycle.

79. PEA. Any cardiac arrest rhythm not identified as ventricular fibrillation, asystole, or ventricular tachycardia should be treated as PEA. The rhythm presenting is sinus tachycardia. The scenario hints that the patient's long-term alcoholism may have induced an upper gastrointestinal bleed. The most common cause of PEA is hypovolemia, so a fluid challenge would be in order while searching for other treatable causes.

80. (d) All of the above. Atropine may assist in accelerating sinus bradycardia by decreasing vagal tone. The correct maximum dosage is 0.04 mg/kg. Atropine may rarely cause hypotension in second-degree, type II or complete heart block. Nevertheless, because the amount of vagal innervation is minimal, atropine may not have any effect on bradycardic rhythms arising from ventricles.

81. Shock. The rate of this narrow complex tachycardia is 140—lower than any rate-driven tachycardia. This rate puts it in the realm of hypovolemia or CHF. The history noted that the patient was probably hypovolemic from a delayed rupture of his spleen. There is a certain tendency in ACLS to treat all tachycardias with the tachycardia protocol. This would be disastrous in this case because the patient needs fluids, not medications. The rate is the key—compensatory tachycardias usually do not go at SVT speeds (more than 170). In summary, with the exception of atrial fibrillation or flutter, if the QRS complex is narrow and the rate is less than 170 but above 60, investigate for other causes of the symptoms, such as hypovolemia or pump failure.

82. (b) False. A TCP should be *considered* in asystole. It has been determined, however, that asystoles in the prehospital sector almost never respond to pacing and therefore are not routinely performed. The time interval when successful pacing might be achieved is brief. The shorter the period of time from arrest to initiation of pacing, the more likely that pacing will be successful.

83. Stable ventricular tachycardia. The patient described in this scenario appears stable without any overt signs or symptoms of cardiovascular compromise. If present, these would include, but are not limited to, a depressed level of consciousness, hypotension, chest pain, or difficulty breathing. The rhythm displayed looks like ventricular tachycardia, but there is a 20% chance of it being SVT with aberrant conduction. The 12-lead ECG verifies the ventricular pacemaker. Ventricular antiarrhythmics would be appropriate.

84. (b) Coronary heart disease. Although causes of sudden death, the other options are not the *most* common.

85. (b) False. When treating a symptomatic bradycardia refractory to atropine, other interventions—pacemakers, dopamine, and epinephrine drips—should be contemplated before more potentially harmful isoproterenol is considered.

86. Unstable tachycardia. The underlying rhythm is atrial fibrillation. The rate of 180 beats/minute affirms that it is uncontrolled. Because many atrial fibrillations or flutters may cause cardiovascular difficulty at rates below this, it is necessary for clinicians to recognize these specific rhythms because their treatment differs from compensatory tachycardias. Because the excessively high rate is consistent with a rate problem causing a depressed level of consciousness and hypotension, the patient should be treated with the tachycardia protocol. If the clinician only focuses on the hypotensive symptoms and the depressed level of consciousness, the underlying cause—the excessively fast rate—is not treated. The patient's symptoms are not mirroring that of fluid loss or pump failure; they are the result of an excessive tachycardia of uncontrolled atrial fibrillation. If the tachycardic ectopic pacemakers are stopped, the depressed level of consciousness and hypotension should resolve by themselves. Although antiarrhythmics are allowed during the unstable tachycardia sequence, they should not interfere with immediate synchronized cardioversion.

87. (b) False. The difference between emergent and elective cardioversion is how quickly the patient requires cardioversion. If the patient is hypotensive, cardioversion should be performed immediately. If the patient is not unstable but the rhythm is refractory to standard drug interventions, however, time is not a crucial factor. The procedure could be scheduled at a surgery center or an outpatient clinic. Premedication is appropriate for both situations. In emergencies, sedate the patient with a hypnotic if he or she is alert enough to remember what happened. In elective situations, sedation may consist of general anesthesia.

88. Pulmonary edema. The patient's underlying rhythm is sinus tachycardia. The rate of 130 beats/minute is commensurate with that of a compensatory tachycardia. Because the rate is not faster than 170, the QRS complexes are narrow, and the rhythm is not atrial fibrillation or flutter, the clinician should consider the rate–volume–pump rule. If the heart rate is not fast enough to precipitate the pulmonary edema, the clinician should consider a possible volume problem. The patient has signs and symptoms of fluid overload, however, so the clinician should consider a possible pump problem. The patient's symptoms reflect CHF—a pump problem—not the result of an excessive tachycardia. Consider treatment modalities for this problem, such as furosemide, morphine, nitroglycerin, and oxygen.

89. (b) Adenosine overdose. Calcium competes with calcium-channel blockers, such as diltiazem and verapamil, for receptor sites and, as such, provides an antidote in an emergency. Calcium is also the antidote for hypocalcemic situations. Calcium has no effect on adenosine administration.

90. Significant bradycardia. The ECG on the monitor is identified as a sinus bradycardia with a 1° block. The scenario paints a picture of a significant bradycardia. The patient's heart rate of 45, combined with hypotension, diaphoresis, and a depressed level of consciousness, make the heart rate the main possibility. Accelerating the rate should increase the blood pressure, discontinuing the other symptoms. Clinicians are cautioned that right ventricular infarcts may cause hypotension associated with bradycardia. Rather than increasing the heart rate, an increased preload—a cautious fluid challenge—may serve to correct the presenting problem.

91. (c) Postural hypotension. Although nausea and vomiting are adverse reactions, they are not the *most* common. Bretylium causes a sympathomimetic effect initially by escalating the pulse rate. Diuresis is not a side effect of bretylium.

92. (b) False. If indicated, intubation is encouraged during the advanced airway portion of the secondary survey. The use of common sense, however, is also encouraged: intubation should never be rushed. Proper execution requires preparation. Only intubate when the equipment and the patient are ready. Remember, as long as you have an open airway and the patient is being ventilated appropriately, do not rush the intubation procedure. Only in airway-endangering circumstances, such as anaphylaxis or inhalation burns, should preparation time be minimized and intubation performed without delay.

93. Asystole. The rhythm is identified as a primary standstill. The ventricles have ceased depolarizing, although P waves are present. The cause of the arrest appears to be vagal, judging from the use of carotid massage to stop the SVT. Thus, atropine, along with concurrent CPR, should be administered immediately.

94. (b) 1, 3, and 4. Infectious complications can be minimized by careful aseptic technique, removal of a cannula on a timely basis, and capping a stopcock when not in use. The use of prophylactic systemic antibiotics in everyone, however, is excessive.

95. Pulmonary edema. The patient's underlying rhythm is sinus tachycardia. The rate of 125 beats/minute is commensurate with that of a compensatory tachycardia. Because the rate is not above 170, the QRS complexes are narrow, and the rhythm is not atrial fibrillation or flutter, the clinician should consider the rate–volume–pump rule. If the heart rate is not fast enough to cause the pulmonary edema, the clinician should consider a volume problem. The patient has signs and symptoms of fluid overload, however, so the clinician should consider a possible pump problem. The patient's symptoms reflect CHF—a pump problem—not the

result of an excessive tachycardia. Consider treatment modalities for this problem, such as furosemide, morphine, nitroglycerin and oxygen.

96. (c) Jaw thrust. If spinal trauma cannot be absolutely ruled out, the jaw thrust is the selection of choice. All other choices compromise the spine.

97. Stable wide complex tachycardia of uncertain type. Because the pulse is tachycardic with a wide QRS complex, the rhythm is identified as either ventricular tachycardia or SVT with aberrant conduction. A 12-lead ECG was available, but no one could read it to differentiate between the two rhythms. In this situation, the clinician should select the wide complex tachycardia of uncertain type protocol. The patient is not suffering from acute cardiopulmonary distress, so the rhythm is treated with the *stable* protocol. If ventricular tachycardia cannot be specifically documented with a 12-lead ECG, the stable *uncertain* protocol should be selected because it contains medications that will be helpful in either a ventricular or a supraventricular ectopic pacemaker.

98. (c) 22 to 45 shocks. At first glance, this appears to be an incredibly large number of shocks, but it is reasonable for an AED-equipped rescuer. With an AED, defibrillations are administered in stacks of three, about every 1 to 2 minutes. If you shocked every minute during a 15-minute time span, the number of shocks would be 45. If you shocked every 2 minutes, it would be about 22 shocks. Remember that the key strategy with an AED is immediate defibrillation in stacks of three separated by 1 minute of CPR.

99. (d) All of the above. Cardiac tamponade, which could be caused by an intracardiac needle, involves both decreased preload and afterload—blood cannot get into, or out of, the heart. Symptoms center around increased venous pressure (jugular distention) and low arterial pressure (hypotension). At least initially, tamponade might profit from a fluid challenge to increase preload while preparing for the definitive treatment—pericardiocentesis.

100. The patient is in respiratory arrest. There is no specific algorithm for this situation other than the universal algorithm. Perform a primary survey. Start by making certain that the airway is clear and patent. A head-tilt and chin-lift maneuver is acceptable if there is no history of trauma. After the airway has been secured, check for any rudimentary breathing attempts. Because this patient is apneic, immediately perform positive-pressure ventilation using a BVM, mouth-to-mask, or barrier device or a demand valve. While the patient is being adequately ventilated, continue with the primary survey. From the scenario, the respiratory arrest is the most critical symptom; however, there appears to be ST elevation in lead II. There may be an underlying infarction. Clinicians would be well advised to consider this line of thought. In the meantime, the patient should be put back on a ventilator until she regains control of her own breathing.

101. (d) History of aspirin overdose. Exposure, alcoholism, and diabetes all can cause hypothermia. A history of aspirin overdose would not lead clinicians to contemplate a hypothermia cause specifically.

102. (b) False. Large doses of morphine sulfate can result in *hypo*tension as well as respiratory depression. Morphine does not cause hypertension.

103. Stable SVT. The rate of this narrow complex tachycardia is 190—higher than a routine compensatory tachycardia (e.g., hypovolemia, CHF). The patient is alert and coherent, the vital signs appear stable, and the patient denies chest pain or breathing difficulty. The patient should be treated with the stable SVT protocol because there is no hint of cardiovascular compromise.

104. (c) Atropine. Although epinephrine, dopamine, and isoproterenol are all part of the bradycardia protocol, atropine is the first used because it is the most benign and readily available. With atropine administration, clinicians can effectively rule out vagal involvement.

105. Unstable tachycardia (atrial flutter). The underlying rhythm is atrial flutter. The rate of 150 affirms that it is uncontrolled. The rate is less than 170, and the QRS complex is narrow, so

this may be confused with a compensatory tachycardia and treated with the rate–volume–pump rule. Atrial flutter may cause cardiovascular difficulty at rates below 170. Therefore, it is necessary for clinicians to recognize this arrhythmia before proceeding with standardized protocols because its treatment differs from that of compensatory tachycardias. Atrial flutter is consistent with a rate problem causing a depressed level of consciousness and hypotension. The patient should be treated with the unstable tachycardia protocol. If the clinician only focuses on the hypotensive symptoms and the depressed level of consciousness, the underlying cause—the fast rate—is not treated. The patient's symptoms are *not* mirroring fluid loss or pump failure; they are the result of a tachycardia of uncontrolled atrial flutter. If the tachycardic ectopic pacemaker is stopped, the depressed level of consciousness and hypotension should resolve by themselves. Although antiarrhythmics are allowed during the unstable tachycardia sequence, they should not interfere with immediate synchronized cardioversion.

106. (a) True. Location of an R wave in polymorphic ventricular tachycardia can be extremely difficult. If the machine cannot locate an R wave, it cannot deliver a synchronized shock. Therefore, if a patient is quickly decompensating, it is foolish to take the time to tinker with the machine. You should immediately turn off the synchronizer and defibrillate the patient.

107. PEA. Any cardiac arrest rhythm not identified as ventricular fibrillation, asystole, or ventricular tachycardia should be treated as PEA. The rhythm presenting is a borderline sinus bradycardia. The scenario hints that the cause is probably an MI reinforced by the ST elevation. Because the most common cause of PEA is hypovolemia, however, a fluid challenge would be in order while searching for other treatable causes.

108. (b) False. Twenty percent of all wide tachydysrhythmias present as SVTs with aberrant conduction.

109. (c) 1, 3, and 4. When ventilating an intubated patient, positive-pressure ventilation devices are indicated (e.g., demand valves and BVM devices). An OPA can be used in conjunction with an ET tube in case the patient becomes conscious and bites down. Pressure-cycled ventilators are contraindicated because they are influenced by transthoracic pressure during CPR.

110. Stable ventricular tachycardia. The patient described in this scenario appears stable without any overt serious signs or symptoms of cardiovascular compromise. If present, these would include, but are not limited to, a depressed level of consciousness, hypotension, chest pain, or difficulty breathing. The rhythm displayed looks like ventricular tachycardia but has a 20% chance of being SVT with aberrant conduction; however, the 12-lead ECG verified the ventricular pacemaker. Ventricular antiarrhythmics would be appropriate.

111. (b) False. The secondary survey is not only a reverification of the primary survey, it also serves to remind the clinician to institute a more advanced form of the ABCDs: airway control—intubation; beware—mini-thorax examination and history; circulation—vital signs and intravenous line; and drugs—differential diagnosis and medications required.

112. (c) Fibrillation consumes high-energy phosphates much more rapidly than normal cardiac rhythms. Statistics have shown that if ventricular fibrillation is not corrected by defibrillation within the first 10 minutes, the chance of survival rapidly approaches zero. Therefore, the faster the defibrillation, the more likely that ATP is present in sufficient quantity to allow contraction. If the myocardium is devoid of ATP, the heart will not contract. The other answers are not medically valid.

113. Shock. The rate of this narrow complex tachycardia is 130—lower than any rate-driven tachycardia. This rate puts it in the realm of hypovolemia or CHF. The history noted that the patient was struck in the area of the spleen and became hypotensive 2 days later, probably indicating splenic rupture secondary to a subcapsular hematoma. There is a certain tendency in ACLS to treat all tachycardias with the tachycardia protocol. This would be disastrous in this case because the patient needs fluids, not medications. The rate is the key—compensatory tachycardias usually do not go at SVT speeds (more than 170). In summary, if

the QRS complex is narrow and the rate is less than 170 but above 60, investigate for other causes of the symptoms, such as hypovolemia or pump failure.

114. (d) 1 and 3. If trauma is the cause, assess for chest trauma pathologies. Hypocalcemia and pulmonary edema are not normally associated with trauma.

115. (d) The interval between when a patient comes into the emergency room and when he receives thrombolytic therapy. The other answers have no medical validity.

116. Asystole or PEA. This rhythm could be treated as PEA or with the asystole protocol. Because there are no P waves and the ventricular rate is less than 30, it is referred to as a *secondary ventricular standstill*—essentially asystole. On the other hand, any pulseless rhythm not identified as ventricular fibrillation, asystole, or ventricular tachycardia should be treated as PEA. A case could be made for treating the patient with either of these protocols. The two protocols differ only regarding whether an external pacemaker is employed because both use epinephrine and atropine. A TCP can be considered. If the cause of the arrest was drug related, introducing a TCP into the PEA protocol might be appropriate. Some drugs interfere with the electrical conduction system, so a TCP might serve to pace the heart until the drug could be eliminated and conduction restored (see ACLS text p. 1-23).

117. (d) Atropine, 0.5 to 1.0 mg given intravenously. The question described a hypotensive bradycardia exhibiting occasional ventricular escape beats. Although selections (b) and (c) are part of the bradycardia protocol, they are not considered first line. Lidocaine is inappropriate in treating ventricular escape beats. Escape beats represent symptoms of a struggling, as opposed to an irritable, myocardium.

118. Stable tachycardia (atrial flutter). The rhythm's rate of 145 beats/minute and its sawtoothed baseline, combined with a narrow QRS complex, indicate a diagnosis of atrial flutter with a rapid ventricular response. Even though the rhythm's rate of 145 is consistent with a *compensatory* rate, both atrial flutter and fibrillation are exceptions to the rate–volume–pump rule. They have to be recognized as specific rhythms before treatment can commence. If the patient is deemed *stable*, these two arrhythmias are treated with a specific medication protocol. If the patient has been diagnosed as *unstable*, synchronized cardioversion is appropriate. However, the patient's status appears stable because no chest pain, hypotension, or pulmonary edema is present. Therefore, the stable tachycardia algorithm should be chosen. The clinician is encouraged to consider any of the following medications for their value in treating this condition: diltiazem, β-blockers, verapamil, digoxin, procainamide, quinidine, and anticoagulants. Procainamide and quinidine are helpful after the rhythm has been converted. The clinician is cautioned to maintain a high index of suspicion that atrial flutter may be a symptom of an underlying myocardial infarction.

119. (a) Your machine may be switched over to the "only synchronize on the P wave" move. This selection is erroneous; no such switch exists. The other options usually cause a monitor-defibrillator to fail to synchronize.

120. Stable wide complex tachycardia of uncertain type. The rhythm started off as a sinus rhythm that changed into a wide complex tachycardia. Because the pulse is now tachycardic with a wide QRS complex, the rhythm is identified as either ventricular tachycardia or SVT with aberrant conduction. A 12-lead ECG was unavailable to differentiate between the two rhythms. In this situation, the clinician should select the wide complex tachycardia of uncertain type protocol. The patient is not suffering from acute cardiopulmonary distress, so the rhythm is treated with the *stable* protocol. If ventricular tachycardia cannot be specifically documented, the clinician should select the *uncertain type* protocol because it contains medications that can be helpful in treating either tissue type.

121. (c) 1, 4, and 5. Adenosine is an *endogenous* (naturally occurring) nucleoside (ATP) with a 5- to 10-second half-life. It works primarily by inhibiting reentry mechanism narrow complex tachycardias in the AV node. Its side effects are facial flushing, chest pain, and a brief period of asystole. It is preferred over verapamil owing to its comparatively benign potential side effects.

122. (c) Sodium bicarbonate. Lidocaine, atropine, and epinephrine may be administered down the ET tube at 2 to $2^1/_2$ times their normal intravenous dosage. Although occasionally administered by respiratory technicians in small doses, bicarbonate is usually too alkalotic for routine ET administration.

123. PEA. Any pulseless rhythm not identified as ventricular fibrillation, asystole, or ventricular tachycardia should be treated as PEA. The rhythm presenting is a sinus tachycardia. The scenario hints that the cause of this PEA is probably DKA. Because the most common cause of PEA is hypovolemia, fluids would also be part of the treatment. Consider both insulin and sodium bicarbonate for their specific indications in this patient.

124. (b) False. When intubated, the overall rate of compressions is increased for two-person CPR. The dead air space in the oral cavity, oropharynx, and laryngopharynx is decreased when employing an ET tube so the compressor does not need to stop every five compressions to allow extra time for the second rescuer to ventilate. The ventilator breathes the patient asynchronously at a rate of 12 to 15 ventilations per minute.

125. (b) False. During the lengthy years of research, development, and field trials, AEDs as a class had only a few errors. All of these errors were related to the failure to recognize VT or VF. None involved team members or lay public individuals being shocked by mistake.

126. Ventricular fibrillation. This patient is in obvious ventricular fibrillation. The key here is to defibrillate as quickly as possible. Remember that if you do not deliver an initial shock quickly, the amount of high-energy phosphates dwindles rapidly. Defibrillation is the key strategy. You must deliver the defibrillation within 10 minutes to have any chance of success; but the quicker it is delivered, the greater is the chance of success.

127. (b) Hyperapnea. All of the above are major complications with the exception of answer (b). Hyperapnea has nothing to do with intracardiac injection.

128. (b) 1, 2, and 3. Maximum benefit is seen within 90 minutes of the onset of symptoms. Limited benefits are seen within 6 hours; however, some limited benefits are still seen as late as 24 hours. Administration after 12 hours, however, may embrace risks that are greater than any *potential* benefits. Clinicians are encouraged to consider this fact closely.

129. Pulmonary edema. The rate of this narrow complex tachycardia is 150—lower than any rate-driven tachycardia. This rate puts it in the realm of hypovolemia and CHF. The history noted that the patient was probably in pulmonary edema, cause undetermined. There is a tendency in ACLS to treat all tachycardias with the tachycardia protocol. This would be disastrous in this case because the patient needs medications to treat the pulmonary edema, not to slow down the heart rate. The rate is the key—compensatory tachycardias usually do not go at SVT speeds (more than 170). In summary, if the QRS complex is narrow and the rate is less than 170 but above 60, investigate for other causes of the symptoms; first consider hypovolemia, then pump failure.

130. (d) 2 and 4. Additional atropine should be given while simultaneously hanging a dopamine drip (and calling for a TCP). Because the patient weighs 100 kg, the maximum total dose of atropine should be 4 mg. Additional atropine can be given because the patient responded initially; however, 10 minutes has already passed, and the patient is still severely hypotensive, so it would be inappropriate to wait another 10 minutes to see if the last dose of atropine will work before considering another intervention. Therefore, consider dopamine simultaneously with successive doses of atropine. Both epinephrine and isoproterenol should be considered, but not initially.

131. (a) 1, 3, and 4. Level of stability is not linked to the origin of the pacemaker. In some patients, SVTs may be just as cardiovascularly devastating as ventricular tachycardias. Usually, conscious patients are considered stable; however, if symptoms of chest pain or pulmonary edema become evident, an otherwise stable patient would be considered unstable. All tachycardic patients that become hypotensive are considered unstable.

Answers 327

132. Significant bradycardia. The rhythm on the monitor is a sinus bradycardia with a third-degree heart block. The scenario paints a picture of a significant bradycardia. The patient's heart rate of 38, combined with hypotension and a depressed level of consciousness, make the heart rate the problem. Accelerating the rate should increase the blood pressure, discontinuing the other symptoms. The definitive treatment should include a permanent *transvenous* pacemaker. Clinicians are cautioned that right ventricular infarcts may cause hypotension associated with bradycardia. Rather than increasing the heart rate, an increased preload—a cautious fluid challenge—may serve to correct the presenting problem.

133. (b) Make the ET tube firmer and conform better. An optional device, the stylet allows the clinician to bend the ET tube to any angle that makes intubation easier. It does not manipulate the cords, affect the tracheal walls, or secure the tube to the laryngoscope blade.

134. (d) All of the above. In an inside-the-needle catheter, the catheter is threaded through the needle, making the holes in the skin and the vein larger than the catheter. Thus, infection, hematomas, and extravasation of fluid are common problems. If the catheter is retracted through the needle, the catheter may shear off—not an exciting prospect.

135. Asystole or PEA. This rhythm could be treated as PEA or with the asystole protocol. Because there are no P waves and the ventricular rate is less than 20 or 30, it is referred to as a *secondary ventricular standstill*—essentially asystole. On the other hand, any pulseless rhythm that is not identified as ventricular fibrillation, asystole, or ventricular tachycardia should be treated as PEA. A case could be made for treating the patient with either of these protocols. The two protocols differ only regarding whether an external pacemaker is employed because both use epinephrine and atropine. A TCP can be considered If the cause of the arrest was drug related, introducing a TCP into the PEA protocol might be appropriate. Some drugs interfere with the electrical conduction system, so a TCP might serve to pace the heart until the drug could be eliminated and conduction restored (see ACLS text p. 1-23). The cause of this arrest is probably hypothermia, so consider core rewarming along with either of the protocols.

136. (d) High dosage regimen of 0.1 mg/kg every 3 to 5 minutes. The standard dosage is 1 mg/kg every 3 to 5 minutes, and the intermediate dosage is 2 to 5 mg/kg every 3 to 5 minutes.

137. (a) True. Most view ventricular fibrillation as a linear protocol—sodium bicarbonate only being considered near the end. This is incorrect. Sodium bicarbonate is a class I drug (definitely helpful) in situations such as hyperkalemia. This drug should be administered when you suspect a treatable cause, not waiting until the end. It should be administered promptly near the start of the protocol after at least one dose of epinephrine. It should be introduced *after* epinephrine so that epinephrine can improve the efficiency of CPR *before* bicarbonate administration. Take care to flush the line well, because epinephrine is inactivated in an alkalotic environment.

138. Stable SVT. The rate of this narrow complex tachycardia is 210—higher than any routine compensatory tachycardia (e.g., hypovolemia, CHF). The combination of a narrow QRS complex and an excessively rapid pulse indicates that this patient should be treated with the SVT protocol. The patient is alert and coherent, the vital signs appear stable, and the patient denies chest pain or breathing difficulty. The patient should be treated with the stable SVT protocol because there is no hint of cardiovascular compromise.

139. (a) Less than 90 minutes. Although the time intervals in the other options all have some benefit, the maximum benefit of thrombolytics is obtained if administered within 90 minutes from onset of symptoms. For this reason, the American Heart Association strives to keep the door-to-drug time interval to within 30 to 60 minutes, thereby keeping the overall symptom onset time to within 90 minutes total. Thrombolytics administered after 24 hours have no discernible benefit.

140. Unstable tachycardia (atrial flutter). The underlying rhythm is atrial flutter. The rate of 150 affirms that it is uncontrolled. Although the rate is greater than 170 and the QRS complex is

narrow, it is not treated with the rate–volume–pump rule. Many atrial flutters may cause cardiovascular difficulty at rates below this, and it is necessary for clinicians to recognize these two arrhythmias before standard protocol begins because the treatment differs from that for compensatory tachycardias. Because the high rate is consistent with a rate problem causing a depressed level of consciousness and hypotension, the patient should be treated with the tachycardia protocol. If the clinician only focuses on the hypotensive symptoms and the depressed level of consciousness, the underlying cause—the fast rate—is not treated. The patient's symptoms are *not* mirroring those of fluid loss or pump failure; they are the result of an excessive tachycardia of uncontrolled atrial flutter. If the tachycardic ectopic pacemaker is stopped, the depressed level of consciousness and hypotension should resolve by themselves. Although antiarrhythmics are allowed during the unstable tachycardia sequence, they should not interfere with immediate synchronized cardioversion.

141. (a) Mesenteric and renal vasodilation. At low dosages of 1 to 2 mcg/kg/min, only dopaminergic receptors are stimulated. The other answers require higher dosage levels: increased inotropic and chronotropic activity requires more than 2 mcg/kg/min, and vasoconstriction and renal shutdown require more than 10 mcg/kg/min.

142. (PEA). Any pulseless rhythm not identified as ventricular fibrillation, asystole, or ventricular tachycardia should be treated as PEA. The rhythm presenting is an accelerated junctional rhythm. The scenario hints that the cause of this PEA is cardiac tamponade. Although many professionals think that cardiac tamponade is just an *afterload* problem (getting blood out of the heart), it is actually also a *preload* problem (getting blood into the heart). Therefore, fluids would also be appropriate initially to increase the preload while correcting the problem with the definitive therapy—pericardiocentesis.

143. (d) 12 mg. Another dose of 12 mg may be given if the rhythm is still refractory after the first two doses.

144. (b) False. An oxygen face mask must be supplemented with at least 5 to 6 L/min of oxygen, or the flow is not sufficient to wash out the exhaled carbon dioxide.

145. Ventricular fibrillation. This patient is in obvious ventricular fibrillation. The key here is to defibrillate as quickly as possible. Remember that if you do not deliver an initial shock quickly, the amount of high-energy phosphates dwindles rapidly. Defibrillation is the key strategy. You must deliver the defibrillation within 10 minutes to have any chance of success; but the quicker it is delivered, the greater are the chances of success.

146. (b) 1 and 3. All patients should receive an antiarrhythmic infusion of the agent that was successful in terminating ventricular fibrillation. If an antiarrhythmic had not been given, give a loading dose of lidocaine, and hang a maintenance drip. In addition, these patients should receive supplemental oxygen. Atropine, a vagal blocker, is inappropriate for ventricular fibrillation. A low dose of dopamine is not given because it would cause both kidney diuresis and mesenteric vasodilation, exacerbating a potentially hypotensive situation.

147. (d) None of the above. β-Blockers have been shown to reduce infarct size by decreasing the myocardial oxygen requirement. They decrease myocardial contractility, heart rate, and blood pressure. Although selection 1 is true, the rest are false. Selection 2 is incorrect because β-blockers decrease heart rates. β-Blockers do not stimulate catecholamine production, they block it. Blocking of β-adrenergic receptors does not affect the vagus nerve.

148. (PEA). Any pulseless rhythm not identified as ventricular fibrillation, asystole, or ventricular tachycardia should be treated as PEA. The rhythm presenting is sinus tachycardia. The scenario hints that the cause of this PEA is hypovolemia with probable electrolyte imbalance caused by the diuretics. Treatment would consist of the standard PEA protocol plus fluids and attention to electrolyte balance.

149. (a) True. Stimulation of the adrenergic receptors in the heart and lungs (β), combined with increasing systemic vascular resistance (α), while continuing renal perfusion (dopaminergic) is a key strategy in the treatment of cardiogenic shock.

150. Asystole or PEA. This rhythm could be treated as PEA or with the asystole protocol. Because there are no P waves and the ventricular rate is less than 30, it is referred to as a *secondary ventricular standstill*—essentially asystole. On the other hand, any pulseless rhythm that is not identified as ventricular fibrillation, asystole, or ventricular tachycardia should be treated as PEA. A case could be made for treating the patient with either of these protocols. The two protocols differ only regarding whether an external pacemaker is employed because both use epinephrine and atropine. A TCP can be considered. If the cause of the arrest was drug related, introducing a TCP into the PEA protocol might be appropriate. Some drugs interfere with the electrical conduction system, so a TCP might serve to pace the heart until the drug could be eliminated and conduction restored.

151. Unstable tachycardia. The pulse rate of 210 is faster than that of a routine *compensatory* tachycardia, such as CHF or hypovolemia (less than 170). The excessive rate, combined with a narrow QRS complex, means that the rhythm is consistent with a rate problem causing pulmonary edema and that the patient should be treated with the unstable tachycardia protocol rather than the acute pulmonary edema protocol. If the clinician only focuses on the dyspnea, the underlying cause—the excessively fast rate—is not treated. The pulmonary edema is not a result of a failing heart; it is caused by the excessive tachycardia backing up the preload into the lungs. Treatment should be focused on stopping the ectopic pacemaker with cardioversion. This should slow the rate, and the pulmonary edema should resolve by itself. Although antiarrhythmics are allowed during the unstable tachycardia sequence, they should not interfere with immediate synchronized cardioversion.

152. (a) None. In the routine cardiac arrest, sodium bicarbonate is considered class III (harmful). If a preexisting bicarbonate-responsive situation (hyperkalemia, aspirin overdose, or DKA) is discovered during assessment, however, sodium bicarbonate is considered early in the protocol. The dose is then 1 mEq/kg until blood gases are obtained.

153. (a) True. In some studies, intravenous nitroglycerin has been shown to have as powerful an effect as some thrombolytics in reducing overall mortality rates and infarct size. Its primary mechanism—reducing both preload and afterload—decreases the myocardial oxygen requirement. A 25% reduction in mortality rates has been noted in the literature.

154. Significant bradycardia with a suspected acute MI. The rhythm on the monitor is a sinus bradycardia with no noted ST elevation. The clinician suspected this from the patient's history and physical examination because lead II does not view the lateral side of the heart—the site of the suspected MI. Although the scenario paints a picture of a significant bradycardia, ignoring the MI ramifications would be regrettable. The patient's heart rate of 45 beats/minute, combined with hypotension and an altered level of consciousness, indicate that the heart rate is the problem, evidencing signs of cardiogenic shock. Accelerating the rate should increase the blood pressure and elevate the level of consciousness. After correcting the immediate problem, attention to treating the MI would be appropriate (with nitroglycerin, aspirin, thrombolytics, angioplasty, etc.).

155. (b) False. Magnesium levels in an electrolyte panel reflect *serum*, not intracellular, levels. A person could be hypomagnesemic while still reflecting a normal panel level.

156. (c) After epinephrine. The progression of medications in the ventricular fibrillation protocol should *not* be thought of as specifically linear. Any hypomagnesemic condition should be treated as soon as it is suspected. If your assessment reveals that the patient was an alcoholic, was elderly, had a chronic disease, or kept poor nutritional habits, administer the magnesium sulfate promptly. Give the drug as early in the protocol as possible after the first dose of epinephrine. Epinephrine improves overall perfusion of administered drugs owing to its vasoconstrictive properties.

157. Unstable tachycardia. The pulse rate of 188 is faster than that of a routine *compensatory* tachycardia, such as CHF or hypovolemia (usually less than 170). This excessive rate, combined with a narrow QRS complex, is consistent with a rate-driven problem causing

chest pain. The patient should be treated with the unstable tachycardia protocol rather than the acute MI protocol. If the clinician only focuses on the chest pain symptoms, the underlying cause—the excessively fast rate—is not treated. The chest pain is not a symptom of an MI; it is the result of ischemia caused by the excessive tachycardia. Stop the ectopic pacemaker by cardioverting the patient. The resultant lowered rate will resolve the chest pain by itself. Although antiarrhythmics are allowed during the unstable tachycardia sequence, they should not interfere with immediate synchronized cardioversion.

158. (b) False. Intravenous nitroglycerin is one of the drugs of choice for unstable angina because it lowers both the preload and afterload, reducing the myocardial oxygen requirement.

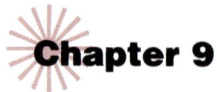

Chapter 9

Answers (p. 248)

1. 2.5 to 5 mg
2. 30 mg
3. He moved his left hand from directly overhead to pause one eighth of the way around, and then settled at the one-quarter mark, a spot perpendicular to his left side.

Answers (p. 249)

1. The warm sun
2. Teak
3. A rainbow

Answers (p. 250)

1. A piece of gray PVC pipe
2. Candy canes
3. They struck the door and laid down in front of it.

Answers (p. 251)

1. A candy cane and a cheerleader's baton
2. Tough one; better reread it if you didn't remember that you paused first, gazing at both
3. A total of three

Answers (p. 251)

1. Three candy canes: 3 mg/kg
2. Half of the initial dose (at whatever dosage you started with)
3. 1 to 1.5
4. No, the candy was struck poised over a cedar keg—a per-kilogram basis.

Answers (p. 252)

1. They are painted gray.
2. A keg
3. There are no windows.

Answers

Answers (p. 252)

1. The keg
2. The till
3. Flat black

Answers (p. 253)

1. The nest containing the pelican
2. The till
3. The pelican
4. The keg
5. The pelican
6. Live fish

Answers (p. 254)

1. A pack of cigarettes-not just cigarettes-a pack of cigarettes. You also threw in your watch.
2. A pack of cigarettes and a watch
3. It fell into the mouth of one of the fish.
4. The numbers from the face of the watch sparkled over the fish and the interior of the pelican's mouth.

Answers (p. 255)

1. Clockwise
2. That the pelican could ignore you by reading a magazine
3. *Seventeen*

Answers (p. 255)

1. The pelican is on top of the nest, and the nest is on top of the till: pro-nest-till (Pronestyl).
2. A pack of cigarettes and a watch. This reminds you of the dosage: 20 mg/min.
3. The maximum dose is *Seventeen*; 17 mg/kg.

Answers (p. 256)

1. You did.
2. On the head and body
3. Yes, the nest was precariously perched, so it fell easily once the pelican fell out.
4. A cash register till sitting on top of a keg

Answers (p. 256)

1. It was beaten with the rolled-up *Seventeen* magazine.
2. No, the nest disintegrated when the pelican rolled off.
3. Only one

4. Five

5. A second hand with 5 fingers sprouted from the till's opposite side, resulting in a total of 10 fingers.

6. Three times.

Answers (p. 257)

1. 1 g

2. 1 mg

3. 1 mg

4. Every 3 to 5 minutes

Answers (p. 258)

1. Brrr-till-ium (bretylium). The initial dose of bretylium is 5 mg/kg. Remember the frozen till. The hand with five gloved fingers coming out and waving at you. The till is sitting on top of the keg reminding you that this drug is given on a per-kilogram basis.

2. Every 3 to 5 minutes. Reverse the capital E in epinephrine, and it becomes a 3, reminding you to administer it every 3 minutes.

3. Wrap-a-meal (verapamil). Recall the aluminum-wrapped meal with the mouse on it. Watch his hands pass the initial dose of 2.5 to 5 mg. His hands stop, reminding you that there is an interval of waiting (15 to 30 minutes) between successive doses. Then visualize his hand returning to the 5 and progressing toward the floor, stopping at 10. Thus, the second dose is 5 to 10 mg.

4. If you don't recall the dose of any of the eight intravenous push drugs, say 1. The dose of atropine is 1 mg. In the bradycardia protocol, it is acceptable to administer 0.5 mg to 1 mg. But when in doubt, say 1.

5. Pro-nest-till (procainamide, Pronestyl). The pelican was sitting on the till. What did the pelican pick up on the floor and begin reading? Correct, *Seventeen* magazine. The maximum dose is 17 mg/kg (per keg). The entire structure is sitting on a keg, reminding you that the maximum dosage is in mg/kg.

6. If you don't recall the dose of any of the eight intravenous push drugs, say 1. The dose of magnesium sulfate is 1 g. It is administered by intravenous push, 1 to 2 g diluted in NS to 10 mL. However, when in doubt, say 1.

7. Li-dor-cane (lidocaine). Remember picking up a candy cane in front of the door where they were shot out of the mortar? Spying the keg and the baton leaning on it, you held the candy cane in one hand and the baton in the left. You paused as you contemplated that the first dose resembled the baton—the number 1. You then struck the candy cane, breaking it in half. The fracture of the candy cane reminded you that the larger initial dose is 1.5 mg/kg *and* that the second dose would be half of the first dose (0.5 to 0.75 mg/kg).

8. A-din-o-sin (adenosine). Sin begins at the witching hour—12 o'clock midnight. Thus, the second dose is 12 mg. The first dose was what time dinner began: 6 o'clock, or 6 mg.

Answers (p. 267)

1. Number 3: right rear leg

2. Number 5: left front leg

3. Number 1: head

4. Number 2: right front leg

5. Number 4: rear back leg

Answers (p. 268)

1. Number 2: right front leg
2. A trophy: atropine
3. Number 3: right rear leg
4. A trophy: atropine

Answers (p. 269)

1. Pacemaker
2. Atropine
3. Number 5: left front leg
4. Number 4: left rear leg

Answers (p. 269)

1. Dopamine
2. Pacemaker
3. Atropine
4. Pacemaker
5. Atropine
6. Dopamine

Answers (p. 270)

1. Adrenaline
2. Pacemaker
3. Atropine
4. Dopamine
5. Pacemaker
6. Adrenaline

Answers (p. 271)

1. Adrenaline or epinephrine
2. Pacemaker
3. Isuprel
4. Atropine
5. Pacemaker
6. Dopamine

Answers (p. 274)

1. The car

2. Glove box

3. Car radio; not radio—car *radio*

4. Speedometer needle

Answers (p. 275)

1. Purple

2. Bretylium

3. Violet

4. Adenosine

5. A glass antique syringe

6. No, only *stable* narrow complex tachycardias with hearts rates of more than 170 and wide complex tachycardias with rates over 100 are deemed rate driven. Atrial fibrillation and flutter are also treated in the speedometer, even though their heart rates are not fast enough to fall within the rate–volume–pump rule.

Answers (p. 277)

1. Question mark (wide complex tachycardia of uncertain type)

2. Documented V-tach

3. Question mark (w–c–t–of an un– ty–)

4. Obvious SVT

5. Documented V-tach

Answers (p. 278)

1. The mohawk was dyed lemon yellow, purple, blue, aqua, and violet (the drug colors).

2. Pink bunny slippers

3. An intravenous line

4. (a) "Kill them all and let God sort them out" or (b) "Mom," with skull and crossbones

5. The patient's rear

Answers (p. 278)

1. False. Only stable patients are treated in the speedometer.

2. False; it stands for stable.

3. False; unstable treatment takes place on the car radio. The patient loses consciousness or evidences other signs of instability (e.g., chest pain) and falls out over the car radio.

Answers (p. 279)

1. Question mark (wide complex tachycardia of uncertain type)

2. Documented V-tach

3. Vagal maneuvers

4. Obvious SVT

5. Vagal maneuvers

Answers (p. 280)

1. Vagal maneuvers

2. Documented V-tach

3. Adenosine

4. Obvious SVT

5. Vagal maneuvers

6. Adenosine

Answers (p. 281)

1. Obvious SVT

2. Vagal maneuvers

3. Adenosine

4. Verapamil

5. Vagal maneuvers

6. Verapamil

7. Adenosine

8. Adenosine

9. Vagal maneuvers

10. Verapamil

11. Adenosine

12. Verapamil

13. Vagal maneuvers

Answers (p. 282)

1. Head, eyes, eyelid

2. Lemons

3. Vagal maneuvers

Answers (p. 283)

1. Procainamide

2. Royal purple

3. Level with his pants

Answers (p. 283)

1. Procainamide

2. Lidocaine

3. Vagal maneuvers

4. Bretylium

5. Adenosine

6. Bretylium

7. Vagal maneuvers

8. Lidocaine

Answers (p. 285)

1. Lidocaine

2. Bretylium

3. Lidocaine

Answers (p. 286)

1. Procainamide

2. Vagal maneuvers

3. Lidocaine

4. Bretylium

5. Adenosine

6. Adenosine

7. Verapamil

8. Procainamide

Answers (p. 287)

1. The patient's head is pointed toward the steering wheel with his back toward the windshield.

2. No, he may be unconscious, going unconscious, or alert but showing signs of cardiovascular compromise.

Answers (p. 288)

1. False. Electrical therapy has a higher priority.

2. False. Both deliver electricity, but one is synchronized with the R wave, whereas the other is unsynchronized.

3. False. Medications can be employed during cardioversion, but they have a lower priority than electrical therapy.

Answers (p. 289)

1. The patient in the glove box is pulseless and therefore should be treated with the ventricular fibrillation protocol. On the other hand, the car radio has patients who are alive but need immediate synchronized electrical therapy to stop their rapid pulse and allow the normal pacemaker to resume.

2. Unstable patients are alive. Patients in the glove box are pulseless; hence, dead. Dead patients are not unstable, they are dead.

3. No. The ventricular fibrillation protocol is not in the car. Because the R waves of pulseless ventricular tachycardia vary so much in amplitude and width, they are difficult to synchronize upon. Therefore, this particular rhythm is treated with immediate defibrillation followed by the rest of the ventricular fibrillation protocol.

Answers (p. 292)

1. Pacemaker. Looking at the turtle from above, the head is number 1—atropine; number 2 is the right forearm, or the grandfather clock—pacemaker.

2. PEA helps to recall **p**ossibilities, **e**pinephrine, and **a**tropine.

3. Bretylium. The ventricular fibrillation mnemonic: shock, shock, shock, everybody, shock, little, shock, big—bretylium.

4. Pacemaker. The asystole protocol is exactly like the PEA—**p**ossibilities, **e**pinephrine, and **a**tropine—*with the addition of a pacemaker.*

5. Verapamil. Sit in the car and decide if the patient is stable (speedometer) or unstable (car radio). Because the question stated the stable protocol, look into the speedometer. See the patient point to the overhead monitor closest to the driver's car door; it states Obvious SVT. The first placard below the monitor states vagal maneuvers; the second placard is emblazoned with adenosine; and the third placard is painted in violet—verapamil.

6. Cardioversion. The correct sequence of therapy in treating noncompensatory tachycardias is to make a decision about the rhythm's stability before trying to interpret it. Only if the rhythm is stable would the rhythm be interpreted to decide on the appropriate drug. If the rhythm is unstable, interpretation is unnecessary because all noncompensatory tachycardias are put onto the car radio and cardioverted.

7. Epinephrine. Looking at the turtle from above, the head is number 1—atropine; number 2 is the right forearm, or the grandfather clock—pacemaker; number 3 is the dope-filled syringe—dopamine; and number 4 is the letter A drilling a hole in the leg—adrenaline.

8. Pronestyl (procainamide). Sit in the car and decide if the patient is stable (speedometer) or unstable (car radio). Because the question stated the stable protocol, look into the speedometer. See the patient point to the overhead monitor closest to the car radio; it states ventricular tachycardia. The first placard below the monitor states lidocaine; the second placard is emblazoned with procainamide.

9. Lidocaine. Sit in the car and decide if the patient is stable (speedometer) or unstable (car radio). Because the question stated the stable protocol, look into the speedometer. See the patient point to either the overhead monitor closest to the car radio (ventricular tachycardia) or the one directly overhead (question mark). The first placard below either of the monitors states lidocaine. Luckily, regardless of which protocol you decide on, the first drug is the same.

10. Adenosine. Sit in the car and decide if the patient is stable (speedometer) or unstable (car radio). Because the question stated the stable protocol, look into the speedometer. See the patient point to either the overhead monitor closest to the car radio (ventricular tachycardia) or the one directly overhead (question mark). The first placard below either of the monitors is lidocaine. Only under the question mark (wide complex tachycardia of uncertain type) monitor does the therapy differ after lidocaine administration because the protocol alters with the addition of adenosine before continuing under both sides with procainamide and bretylium.

GLOSSARY

Adrenergic receptor
- α_1: Postsynaptic; located on vascular smooth muscle; causes vasoconstriction.
- α_2: Presynaptic; inhibits the release of nonepinephrine.
- β_1: Causes increases in heart contractility and rate.
- β_2: Causes relaxation of smooth muscle in vascular compartment, mesentery, and bronchial tree.

Dopaminergic: In low levels, causes diuresis in kidneys and mesenteric vasodilation.

Afterload: (1) The amount of resistance that the heart must pump against. (2) Tension developed by the ventricle during systole. (3) Essentially, the arterial systolic pressure.

Chronotropic: This word means to affect the heart rate by increasing [+] or decreasing [−] the rate of contraction. Atropine, epinephrine, and isoproterenol are positive [+] chronotropes. Digitalis, verapamil, and adenosine are negative [−] chronotropes.

Inotropic: The word *inos* means strength. The suffix -tropic means to change. Thus, this word means to affect the force of contraction by increasing [+] or decreasing [−] contractility. Isoproterenol, digitalis, and dobutamine are positive [+] inotropes. Inderal and other β-blockers are negative [−] inotropes.

Preload: (1) The amount of blood returning to the heart, or the filling pressure of the right or left atrium. (2) The initial stretch of the myocardial fiber at end-diastole. (3) The ventricular end-diastolic pressure and the volume reflect this parameter. The central venous pressure (CVP) measures the preload of the right side of the heart, whereas the pulmonary wedge measures the left side.

Index

Page numbers followed by *f* indicate figures; those followed by *t* indicate tables.

A

ACE (angiotensin-converting enzyme) inhibitors, 83
ACLS course, 3–8
    changes in, 3
    discussion groups in, 4–5
    drug therapy in, 225–242
        memorization techniques for, 246–258
    enrollment requirements for, 3–4
    evaluation component of, 5–6
    megacode in, 217–223. *See also* Megacode
    memorization techniques for, 243–286
    organization of, 4–5
    posttest for, 175–213
    reverification program of, 5
ACLS team, monitoring of, in megacode, 220–223
Adenosine, 225*t*
    memorization techniques for, 247
    for tachycardia
        supraventricular, 135
        unstable, 119
        wide complex, 139
Adrenergic receptors, 333
    dopamine and, 105*f*
Advanced Cardiac Life Support. *See* ACLS course
Afterload, 333
Airway
    advanced
        in bradycardia, 102
        in coronary syndromes, 76
        in pulseless electrical activity, 53
        in respiratory arrest with pulse, 17–20, 18*f*, 20*f*
        in secondary survey of stroke, 151
        in stable tachycardias, 139
        in unstable tachycardias, 117
        in ventricular fibrillation, 39
    monitoring of, in megacode, 218
    primary assessment of
        in bradycardia, 102
        in coronary syndromes, 76
        in respiratory arrest with pulse, 13–15, 13*f*-15*f*
        in stable tachycardias, 133
        in stroke, 150
        in unstable tachycardias, 116
        in ventricular fibrillation, 34, 34*f*-35*f*
Altephase, for myocardial infarction, 81
Amaurosis fugax, 153
Amrinone lactate, 226*t*
Angioplasty, for myocardial infarction, 81–82
Angiotensin-converting enzyme (ACE) inhibitors, 83
Anticonvulsants, for stroke, 165
Arrhythmias. *See also under* specific types
    dopamine and, 96, 97*f*
    fluid volume in, 95, 95*f*
    heart rate in, 94–95, 94*f*
    hemodynamic compromise from, 93–94
    lethal, 29–69
    norepinephrine and, 96, 97*f*
Aspirin, for myocardial infarction, during prehospital phase, 78–79
Asystole, 61–67
    algorithm for, 62*f*
    assessment of, 64
    clinical features of, 63, 63*f*
    critical actions in, 61, 61*t*
    crossword puzzle for, 68*f*, 69
    defibrillation in, 64
    etiology of, 65
    interim evaluation questions for, 67
    memorization techniques for, 263–264
    termination of efforts in, 67
    treatment of, 66–67
    ventricular, 63, 63*f*
Atrial fibrillation, 94
    clinical features of, 114, 115*f*, 131–132, 131*f*
    stroke, assessment, 150, 150*f*
    treatment of, 119–120, 136–137
Atrial flutter, 94
    clinical features of, 115, 115*f*, 131, 131*f*
    treatment of, 119–120, 136–137
Atrial tachycardia, 130, 130*f*. *See* Supraventricular tachycardia
Atrioventricular (AV) block, clinical features of, 101, 101*f*
Atropine, 227*t*
    for asystole, 66
    for bradycardia, 103–104
    memorization techniques for, 257
    for pulseless electrical activity, 56–57
    reasoning behind usage, 103

B

Bag-valve-mask (BVM) ventilation
    in respiratory arrest with pulse, 16–17, 17*f*
    in ventricular fibrillation, 35*f*
Basic life support, certification in, as enrollment requirement for ACLS course, 4
Beta-blockers, 228*t*
    for myocardial infarction, 82
Blood gases, monitoring of, in megacode, 220
Blood pressure
    in bradycardia, 103
    hemodynamic significance, 93
    management of, in stroke, 163, 165, 166*t*
BLS, certification in, as enrollment requirement for ACLS course, 4
Bradycardia, 98–107
    algorithm for, 99*f*

Bradycardia (*Continued*)
    assessment of, 102
    clinical features of, 100–102, 100f-101f
    critical actions in, 98, 98t
    crossword puzzle for, 109–110
    and hemodynamic compromise, 103
    interim evaluation questions for, 107–108
    memorization techniques for, 265–270
    sinus, 12, 12f
    treatment of, 103–107
        atropine in, 103–104
        dopamine in, 105–106, 105f
        epinephrine in, 106
        isoproterenol in, 106
        pacemakers in
            transcutaneous, 104–105
            transvenous, 106–107
Breathing, primary assessment of
    in respiratory arrest with pulse, 15–17, 16f-17f
    in stroke, 150–151
    in ventricular fibrillation, 34, 35f
Bretylium, 229t
    memorization techniques for, 255–256
    for ventricular fibrillation, 42–43
    for wide complex tachycardia, 139–140
Bundle branch block, 128f
BVM (bag-valve-mask) ventilation. *See* Bag-valve-mask (BVM) ventilation

C

Calcium channel blockers, for myocardial infarction, 83
Calcium chloride, 229t
Cardiac arrhythmias. *See* Arrhythmias
Cardiac conduction system, and electrocardiogram, 128f
Cardiac tamponade, and pulseless electrical activity, 55
Cardiopulmonary resuscitation (CPR)
    ACLS team member's role in, 221
    in megacode, 219–220
    therapeutic interventions in, classification of, 8
Cardioversion
    elective, for atrial fibrillation or atrial flutter, 137
    synchronized
        for unstable tachycardia, 118–119
        for wide complex tachycardia, 140
Carotid circulation, and stroke, 154–155, 154f
Case studies, organization of, 6–7
Catheters, for suctioning, tonsil tip, 13f
Chest pain
    algorithm for, 72f
    in myocardial infarction, 74. *See also* Myocardial infarction (MI)
Chronotropic, definition of, 333
Cincinnati Prehospital Stroke Scale, 160t
Circulation
    in assessment of stroke, 151
    carotid, and stroke, 154–155, 154f
    primary assessment of
        in respiratory arrest with pulse, 17
        in ventricular fibrillation, 35
    secondary survey of
        in respiratory arrest with pulse, 21
        in ventricular fibrillation, 40
    vertebrobasilar, and stroke, 155, 155f
Compensatory tachycardia, clinical features of, 115–116, 116f, 132, 132f
Conduction system, and electrocardiogram, 128f
Consciousness, level of
    monitoring of, in megacode, 217–218
    in stroke, 162, 162t-163t
Coronary syndromes, 71–91. *See also* Myocardial infarction (MI)
CPR. *See* Cardiopulmonary resuscitation (CPR)

D

Defibrillation
    in asystole, 64
    role of ACLS team member in, 221–222
    in ventricular fibrillation, 36–39, 37f-38f, 42
Defibrillators
    automated, external, 38, 38f
    manual, 37, 37f
Digitalis, 230t
Diltiazem, 230t
Discussion groups, in ACLS course, 4–5
Dobutamine, 231t
Dopamine, 231t
    for bradycardia, 105–106, 105f
    for non-hypovolemic hypotension, 96, 97f
Dressler beat, 113–114
Drug overdose
    and asystole, 65
    and pulseless electrical activity, 56
Drug therapy, 225–242
    memorization techniques for, 246–258

E

Electrical activity, pulseless, 50–57. *See also* Pulseless electrical activity
Electrocardiogram, conduction system and, 128f
Electromechanical dissociation, true *vs.* false, 54
Embolism, pulmonary, and pulseless electrical activity, 56
Emergency department, interventions for stroke in, 161–163, 161f, 162t-163t
EMS dispatch, in stroke chain, 159, 159f
Endotracheal intubation, in respiratory arrest with pulse, 17–20, 18f, 20f
    in ventricular fibrillation, 39
Epinephrine, 232t
    for asystole, 66
    for bradycardia, 106
    for pulseless electrical activity, 56
    for ventricular fibrillation, 41
Evaluation, in ACLS course, 5–6

F

Face masks
    for mouth-to-mask ventilation, 16f
    for oxygen therapy, 20, 20f
Fibrillation, ventricular, 30–44. *See also* Ventricular fibrillation
Fluid therapy
    in pulseless electrical activity, 54
    in ventricular fibrillation, 40
Fluid volume, in arrhythmias, 95, 95f
Furosemide, 233t

G

Glasgow Coma Scale, 162t

H

Head-tilt/chin-lift
    in respiratory arrest with pulse, 14, 14f
    in ventricular fibrillation, 35f
Heart failure, memorization techniques for, 285–286
Heart rate, in arrhythmias, 94–95, 94f
Hemodynamic compromise
    arrhythmias and, 93–94
    bradycardia and, 103
    tachycardia and, 93–95
Hemorrhage
    intracerebral, 153–154, 156
    subarachnoid, 153, 156
Hemorrhagic stroke, 157

Hyperkalemia
    and asystole, 65
    and pulseless electrical activity, 55
Hypertension, in stroke, 163, 165, 166t
Hypotension, treatment of, in megacode, 218–219
Hypothermia
    and asystole, 65
    and pulseless electrical activity, 56
    and ventricular fibrillation, 40
Hypovolemia, in pulseless electrical activity, 54

I

Impedance, transthoracic, reduction of, 36
Inotropic, definition of, 333
Intracerebral hemorrhage, 153–154, 156
Intracranial pressure, in stroke, 165
Intravenous fluids. *See* Fluid therapy
Intravenous lines, monitoring of, role of ACLS team member in, 222–223
Intubation, endotracheal, in respiratory arrest with pulse, 17–20, 18f, 20f
Ischemic stroke, 157
Isoproterenol, 233t
    for bradycardia, 106

J

Jaw-thrust technique
    in respiratory arrest with pulse, 14f
    in ventricular fibrillation, 34f
Junctional rhythm, high, clinical features of, 100, 100f

L

Left-brain processing, 243–244
Lethal arrhythmias, 29–69. *See also* Asystole; Pulseless electrical activity; Ventricular fibrillation, Pulseless ventricular tachycardia
Level of consciousness
    monitoring of, in megacode, 217–218
    in stroke, 162, 162t-163t
Lidocaine, 234t
    memorization techniques for, 248–251
    for myocardial infarction, 84–85
    for supraventricular tachycardia, 136
    for unstable tachycardia, 119
    for ventricular fibrillation, 42
    for wide complex tachycardia, 138–139

M

Magnesium sulfate, 235t
    for myocardial infarction, 84
    for torsades de pointes, 43, 140
    for ventricular fibrillation, 41–42, 43
Masks
    for mouth-to-mask ventilation, 16f
    for oxygen therapy, 20, 20f
Megacode
    cardiopulmonary resuscitation in, 219–220
    monitoring airway in, 218
    monitoring blood gases in, 220
    monitoring medications in, 220
    monitoring of level of consciousness in, 217–218
    monitoring of pulse in, 218–219
    monitoring of ventilation in, 218
    objectives of, 217
    perfusion in, 218
    team monitoring in, 220–223
    treatment of hypertension in, 218–219
Memorization techniques, 243–286
MI. *See* Myocardial infarction (MI)

Mnemonics, 245
Morphine, 235t
    for myocardial infarction, during prehospital phase, 79
Mouth-to-mask ventilation, 15–16, 16f
Myocardial infarction (MI), 71–91
    algorithm for, 72f
    assessment of, 76–77
    clinical features of, 74, 75f, 76
    critical actions in, 71, 72t
    crossword puzzle for, 90–91
    interim evaluation questions for, 88–89
    memorization techniques for, 265
    and pulseless electrical activity, 56
    treatment of, 77–87
        algorithm for, 86f
        angiotensin-converting enzyme inhibitors in, 83
        beta-blockers in, 82
        calcium channel blockers in, 83
        lidocaine in, 84–85
        magnesium sulfate in, 84
        nitroglycerin in, 79–80
        prehospital, 77–79
        reperfusion in, 81–82
        thrombolytic agents in, 81
        warfarin in, 83–84

N

Narrow complex tachycardia, 130–132, 130f-132f
    narrow versus wide, explanation of, 127–130, 127f–129f
Nasal cannula, in respiratory arrest with pulse, 20
Nasopharyngeal airway, for respiratory arrest with pulse, 15, 15f
Neurologic assessment, in stroke, 162–163, 162t-163t
Nitroglycerin, 236t
    for myocardial infarction, 79–80
        during prehospital phase, 78
Norepinephrine, 237t
    and compensatory tachycardias, 96, 97f

O

Oropharyngeal airway, for respiratory arrest with pulse, 14, 15f
Oxygen, 237t
    for myocardial infarction, during prehospital phase, 78
Oxygen therapy, in respiratory arrest with pulse, 20

P

Pacemakers
    transcutaneous
        for asystole, 66
        for bradycardia, 104–105
    transvenous, for bradycardia, 106–107
Percutaneous transluminal coronary angioplasty (PTCA), 81–82
Perfusion, in megacode, 218
Pneumothorax, tension, and pulseless electrical activity, 55
Preload, 333
Procainamide, 238t
    memorization techniques for, 251–255
    for supraventricular tachycardia, 136
    for ventricular fibrillation, 43
    for wide complex tachycardia, 139
PTCA (percutaneous transluminal coronary angioplasty), 81–82
Pulmonary edema
    indications for instability, 117
    memorization techniques for, 285–286
Pulmonary embolism, and pulseless electrical activity, 56
Pulse, monitoring of, in megacode, 218–219

Pulseless electrical activity, 50–57
   algorithm for, 51*f*
   assessment of, 53–54
   clinical features of, 52, 52*f*-53*f*, 54
   critical actions in, 50, 50*t*
   crossword puzzle for, 60*f*
   electrochemical dissociation in, true *vs.* false, 54
   etiology of, 54–56
   interim evaluation questions for, 57–59
   memorization techniques for, 262–263
   treatment of, 56–57
Pulseless ventricular tachycardia, 30–44. *See also* Ventricular fibrillation

Q

QR complex, 128*f*
QRS complex, wide, in supraventricular tachycardia, 114
QRS complexes
   narrow, in stable tachycardia, 130, 130*f*
   narrow *vs.* wide, in stable tachycardia, 127–130, 127*f*-129*f*

R

Recertification. *See* Reverification program
Rehabilitation, after stroke, 169, 169*f*
Reperfusion, in myocardial infarction, 81–82
Respiratory arrest, with pulse, 9–22
   algorithm for, 11*f*
   critical actions in, 9, 10*t*
   crossword puzzle for, 26–27
   interim evaluation questions for, 22–25
   primary assessment in, 13–17, 13*f*-17*f*
     for airway, 13–15, 13*f*-15*f*
     for breathing, 15–17, 16*f*-17*f*
     for circulation, 17
   secondary survey in, 17–22, 18*f*, 20*f*
     for advanced airway, 17–20, 18*f*, 20*f*
     "beware blinders" in, 21
     for circulation, 21
     thoracic examination in, 21
   sinus bradycardia in, 12, 12*f*
   sinus tachycardia in, 11–12, 12*f*
Respiratory team member, role of, 221
Reverification program, of ACLS course, 5
Right-brain processing, 243–244
RS complex, 128*f*
RS waves, 129*f*
R waves, 129*f*

S

Secondary ventricular standstill, 52, 53*f*
Seizures, in stroke, 165
Sinus bradycardia, 12, 12*f*
   clinical features of, 100, 100*f*
Sinus rhythm, with atrioventricular block, 101, 101*f*
Sinus tachycardia
   clinical features of, 132, 132*f*
   in compensatory tachycardias, 93–95, 115–116, 116*f*
   in respiratory arrest with pulse, 11–12, 12*f*
Sodium bicarbonate, 239*t*
   for asystole, 67
   for pulseless electrical activity, 56
   for ventricular fibrillation, 41, 43–44
Sodium nitroprusside, 240*t*
Streptokinase, for myocardial infarction, 81
Stroke, 147–170
   acute ischemic, 157
   algorithm for, 149*f*
   anterior territory, 154, 154*f*
   assessment of, 150–151
   "beware blinders" in, 152
   carotid circulation and, 154–155, 154*f*
   classification of, 156–157
   clinical features of, 150, 150*f*
   critical actions in, 147, 148*t*
   crossword puzzle for, 173–174
   diagnosis of, 151
   differential diagnosis of, 152–153, 153*f*
   hemorrhagic, 157
   interim evaluation questions for, 170–172
   level of consciousness in, 162, 162*t*-163*t*
   neurologic assessment in, 162–163, 162*t*-163*t*
   physical examination in, 154
   posterior territory, 155, 155*f*
   rehabilitation after, 169, 169*f*
   risk factors for, 157, 158*t*
   treatment of. *See* Stroke chain
   vertebrobasilar circulation and, 155, 155*f*
Stroke chain, 158–169, 158*f*-169*f*
   blood pressure management in, 163, 165, 166*t*
   detection in, 158*f*, 159
   emergency department intervention in, 161–163, 161*f*, 162*t*-163*t*
   EMS dispatch in, 159, 159*f*
   intracranial pressure management in, 165
   rehabilitation in, 169, 169*f*
   seizure management in, 165
   steps in, 158, 158*f*
   thrombolytic therapy in, 165, 167*f*, 168, 168*t*
   transport in, 159–160, 159*f*-160*f*, 160*t*
   treatment planning in, 163, 164*f*, 165, 166*t*
   triage in, 160*f*, 161, 161*t*
ST depression, in stable tachycardia, 129*f*
ST segment, elevated
   in myocardial infarction, 74, 75*f*, 76, 129*f*
Subarachnoid hemorrhage, 153, 156
Suctioning, in respiratory arrest with pulse, 13–14, 13*f*-14*f*
Supraventricular tachycardia (SVT), 94
   clinical features of, 113, 113*f*, 130, 130*f*
   treatment of, 134–136
Synchronized cardioversion
   for unstable tachycardia, 118–119
   for wide complex tachycardia, 140

T

Tachycardia
   algorithm for, 97*f*
   atrial, 130, 130*f*
   compensatory, clinical features of, 115–116, 116*f*, 132, 132*f*
   narrow complex, treatment of, 134–137
   sinus
     clinical features of, 132, 132*f*
     compensatory, 96, 97*f*
     in respiratory arrest with pulse, 11–12, 12*f*
   stable, 125–140
     algorithm for, 126*f*
     assessment of, 133–134
     clinical features of, 127–133, 127*f*-133*f*
       QRS complexes in
         narrow, 130–132, 130*f*-132*f*
         narrow *vs.* wide, 127–130, 127*f*-129*f*
         wide, 132–133, 132*f*-133*f*
     critical actions in, 125, 125*t*
     crossword puzzle for, 144–145
     interim evaluation questions for, 141–143
     memorization techniques for, 270–282
   supraventricular. *See* Supraventricular tachycardia (SVT)
   unstable, 111–120
     algorithm for, 111*f*
     assessment of, 116–117
     clinical features of, 112–116, 113*f*-116*f*
     critical actions in, 111–112, 111*t*
     crossword puzzle for, 122–124

interim evaluation questions for, 120–121
memorization techniques for, 282–284
treatment of, 117–120
adenosine in, 119
lidocaine in, 119
synchronized cardioversion in, 118–119
ventricular, 132–133, 132f. See Ventricular tachycardia
pulseless, 30–44. See also Pulseless ventricular tachycardia
wide complex
differential diagnosis of, 137–138
of unknown origin, 114, 114f
Tamponade, and pulseless electrical activity, 55
Tension pneumothorax, and pulseless electrical activity, 55
Therapeutic interventions, in cardiopulmonary resuscitation, classification of, 8
Thorax, examination of, in secondary survey of respiratory arrest with pulse, 21
Thrombolytic therapy, 241t
for myocardial infarction, 79, 81
for stroke, 165, 167f, 168, 168t
TIAs (transient ischemic attacks), 152–153
Tonsil tip suction catheter, 13f
Torsades de pointes, treatment of, 43, 140, 140f
Transcutaneous pacemakers
for asystole, 66
for bradycardia, 104–105
Transient ischemic attacks (TIAs), 152–153
Transthoracic impedance, reduction of, 36
Transvenous pacemakers, for bradycardia, 106–107
Triage, in stroke chain, 160f, 161, 161t

V

Vagal maneuvers
for atrial fibrillation, 137
for supraventricular tachycardia, 135
Ventilation
monitoring of, in megacode, 218
mouth-to-mask, 15–16, 16f. See also Bag-valve-mask (BVM) ventilation
Ventricular asystole, 63, 63f

Ventricular defibrillation
procedure, 41–44
secondary survey in, drugs and diagnosis in, 40
Ventricular fibrillation, 30–44
algorithm for, 32f
critical actions in, 30, 31t
crossword puzzle for, 48–49
identifying features of, 33, 33f
interim evaluation questions for, 44–47
memorization techniques for, 260–261, 284–285
primary assessment in, 34–39, 34f-38f
for airway, 34, 34f-35f
for breathing, 34, 35f
for circulation, 35
for defibrillation, 36–39, 37f-38f
secondary survey in, 39–40
for advanced airway, 39
"beware blinders" in, 39–40
circulation in, 40
treatment of, 119
Ventricular standstill, 63, 63f
secondary, 52, 53f
Ventricular tachycardia
clinical features of, 113–114, 113f, 132–133, 132f
differential diagnosis of, 137–138
pulseless, 30–44. See also Ventricular fibrillation
Verapamil, 242t
danger of, in wide complex tachycardia, 136
memorization techniques for, 247–248
for supraventricular tachycardia, 135
Vertebrobasilar circulation, and stroke, 155, 155f
Visual images, as memorization techniques, 245–246

W

Warfarin, for myocardial infarction, 83–84
Wide complex tachycardia
clinical features of, 132–133, 132f-133f
of unknown origin, 114, 114f